Kinship and Cohort in an Aging Society

Kinship and Cohort in an Aging Society

From Generation to Generation

Edited by
Merril Silverstein
and
Roseann Giarrusso

The Johns Hopkins University Press
Baltimore

© 2013 The Johns Hopkins University Press
All rights reserved. Published 2013
Printed in the United States of America on acid-free paper
9 8 7 6 5 4 3 2 1

The Johns Hopkins University Press
2715 North Charles Street
Baltimore, Maryland 21218-4363
www.press.jhu.edu

Library of Congress Cataloging-in-Publication Data

Kinship and cohort in an aging society : from generation to generation /
edited by Merril Silverstein and Roseann Giarrusso.
   p. cm.
  Includes index.
   ISBN 978-1-4214-0893-4 (hardcover : alk. paper) — ISBN 978-1-4214-0894-1
(electronic) — ISBN 1-4214-0893-7 (hardcover : alk. paper) — ISBN 1-4214-0894-5
(electronic)
   1. Families.   2. Families—Cross-cultural studies.   3. Intergenerational relations.   4. Intergenerational relations—Cross-cultural studies.
5. Older people—Family relationships.   I. Silverstein, Merril.
II. Giarrusso, Roseann.
  HQ519.K56 2013
   306.85—dc23   2012037370

A catalog record for this book is available from the British Library.

Special discounts are available for bulk purchases of this book. For more informa-
tion, please contact Special Sales at 410-516-6936 or specialsales@press.jhu.edu.

The Johns Hopkins University Press uses environmentally friendly book materials, including recycled text paper that is composed of at least 30 percent
post-consumer waste, whenever possible.

Contents

Foreword, by Toni C. Antonucci   *ix*

Acknowledgments   *xiii*

Introduction. Solidarity as a Key Concept in Family
and Generational Research   1
Merril Silverstein and Roseann Giarrusso

PART I. FAMILY CONNECTIONS: SOLIDARITY WITHIN
AND ACROSS GENERATIONS   9

1   Differences in Mothers' and Fathers' Parental Favoritism in Later
    Life: A Within-Family Approach   11
    J. Jill Suitor and Karl Pillemer

2   Intergenerational Solidarity in Blended Families: The Inequality
    of Financial Transfers to Adult Children and Stepchildren   31
    R. Corey Remle and Angela M. O'Rand

3   Generational Contact and Support among Late Adult Siblings
    within a Verticalized Family   59
    Kees Knipscheer and Theo van Tilburg

PART II. GRANDPARENTS IN A CHANGING
DEMOGRAPHIC LANDSCAPE: MOTHERS AND MENTORS   77

4   Grandmothers' Differential Involvement with Grandchildren
in Rural Multiple Partner Fertility Family Structures   79
Linda M. Burton, Whitney Welsh, and Lane M. Destro

5   The Role of Grandparents in the Transition to Adulthood:
Grandparents as "Very Important" Adults in the Lives
of Adolescents   104
Miles G. Taylor, Peter Uhlenberg, Glen H. Elder, Jr., and Steve McDonald

PART III. OF GENERATIONS AND COHORTS:
MICRO-MACRO DIALECTICS   131

6   Who's Talking about My Generation?   133
Duane F. Alwin

7   Toward Generational Intelligence: Linking Cohorts, Families,
and Experience   159
Simon Biggs and Ariela Lowenstein

8   Biography and Generation: Spirituality and Biographical Pain
at the End of Life in Old Age   176
Malcolm Johnson

PART IV. RELIGION AND FAMILIES: CONTEXTS
OF CONTINUITY, CHANGE, AND CONFLICT   191

9   How Theory-Building Prompts Explanations about Generational
Connections in the Domains of Religion, Spirituality, and Aging   193
W. Andrew Achenbaum

10   The Transmission of Religion across Generations: How
Ethnicity Matters   209
*Norella M. Putney, Joy Y. Lam, Frances Nedjat-Haiem, Thien-Huong Ninh,
Petrice S. Oyama, and Susan C. Harris*

11 Church-Based Negative Interactions among Older African
    Americans, Caribbean Blacks, and Non-Hispanic Whites   237
    Karen D. Lincoln, Linda M. Chatters, and Robert Joseph Taylor

    PART V. GLOBAL, CROSS-NATIONAL, AND
    CROSS-ETHNIC ISSUES: WHO WILL CARE
    FOR THE YOUNG AND THE OLD?   263

12 Global Aging and Families: Some Policy Concerns about the
    Global Aging Perspective   265
    Victor W. Marshall

13 Social Change, Social Structure, and the Cycle of
    Induced Solidarity   284
    Dale Dannefer and Rebecca A. Siders

14 The Intergenerational Social Contract Revisited:
    Cross-National Perspectives   293
    Christopher Steven Marcum and Judith Treas

15 Aging, Health, and Families in the Hispanic Population:
    Evolution of a Paradigm   314
    Kyriakos S. Markides, Ronald J. Angel, and M. Kristen Peek

    Short Biography of Vern L. Bengtson   333
    List of Contributors   335
    Index   337

Foreword

In 1970 I had just completed my first year of graduate school and won a scholarship to the University of Southern California's Summer Institute of Gerontology. It was a fine time, with many new experiences for me. One I remember most clearly was meeting a new assistant professor who had just joined the faculty, Dr. Vern Bengtson. Everyone was very pleased that he had accepted USC's offer. They were especially excited about his special area of interest: generations. At the time few people thought about the life course, that is, anything past childhood or adolescence, never mind through adulthood and old age. Certainly most people studied each of these age periods as though they were static and occurred in isolation. USC had the Andrus Gerontology Center, but only four or five such gerontology centers existed around the country. People did recognize the importance of families, though most gerontological research focused on the family's role among clinical populations, and there was little talk about intergenerational family relations. Vern, because of his University of Chicago training, had the background to understand human development, including adulthood and aging. He understood quite early that generations might be important to understanding human development and behavior.

With the beginning of the Longitudinal Study of Generations (LSOG), Vern ventured into uncharted territory. It was a groundbreaking study in recognizing that generations within families are important sources of influence, change, and development. Vern knew it was important to study generations within families, but none of this early work was very sophisticated. We knew much less then about the importance of representative sampling and the perils and pitfalls of mailed questionnaires. Complex statistical modeling was basically nonexistent. But pioneers have to forge new paths regardless of the barriers they face. Despite limitations, LSOG brought us many fundamentals of intergenerational relations, including the initially counterintuitive finding that nonadjacent generation members tend to be closer than adjacent members and recognition that the perspective and developmental stake of the G1 family member (first/oldest generation member) differs from that of G2 or G3 (and later G4 and G5) members. Furthermore, the centrality of solidarity within families was developed from the study findings—later embellished upon with the important recognition of the role of conflict and, still later, of ambivalence.

Although grounded in sociology, Vern's home discipline, much of his work was interdisciplinary in nature and thus contributed to many different fields. I believe the study of adulthood and aging, in fact, gerontology in general, benefits most from an interdisciplinary perspective. Reflecting his early training at the Chicago School of Human Development, most of Vern's work on generations has this appeal. In addition, the early work on generations reflected some exciting times when we all began to think about the difference between intergenerational and intragenerational relations. We also came to understand that while there were unique characteristics of G1s as well as of G2s and G3s that were interesting and important, the same could be said of being within a single family, whether as a G1, G2, or G3. As times changed, generations changed as well, allowing us to begin to understand the place of individuals, families, and generations within society. The LSOG added G4s and G5s and collected data from generations as they lived through such diverse experiences as the Vietnam War, economic booms and busts, the dot.com world, and the environmental movement.

An important lesson learned from the seminal LSOG study is that families evolve just as societies do and that family members mutually influence one another. Vern's work demonstrated that families are dynamic, not static entities. It is certainly true that some families have more conflict, while others seem to have more positive emotional exchanges. The richness of the LSOG data taught us, however, that families are complex, they change, and they can be wonderfully supportive or heartbreakingly dysfunctional. The individual examples provided in the LSOG reports make clear the dynamism of families. There is always room for change and improvement, although sometimes breakdowns and conflict are all too predictable. Nevertheless, the LSOG gave us an initial understanding of how families and generations function. It helped lay the groundwork for an interdisciplinary field that seeks to understand people and families as they live and evolve.

The LSOG identified new issues to consider when seeking understanding of the family. Vern noted that the structure of the population and the form of the family were changing. Our population used to be pyramid shaped, with many young people and increasingly fewer people of older ages. People had many more children, but fewer people survived to old age. One might argue there was less of a need for a study of generations because there were fewer of them. Now the population is beanpole shaped, meaning more generations but fewer members in each. In addition, the very nature of families is changing. Although it is less recognized than it should be, early families often involved multiple marriages but these were usually the result of the early death by one partner, for example, of women in childbirth. Thankfully, this is much less likely now, but families do change form through divorce and remarriage, childbirth without marriage, and same-sex marriages. Families might easily include full siblings, half siblings, and stepsiblings as well as two sets of stepparents and multiple sets of grandparents and stepgrandparents.

In some ways the LSOG both prepared us for the changes and shed some early light on their influence. It was clear that families are important, that intergenerational relationships are crucially influential, and that formal ties or titles do not always tell the whole story. Thus, as we studied and learned more about the family, we came also to recognize that even the "synthetic" family—including all those "new" and "nontraditional" forms of the family—could also have an important influence on individuals and their ability to function productively.

While the LSOG was fundamentally a study of Californian families, the study has also had important implications for generations research internationally and cross-culturally. Although there are important cultural differences in the expression of family relations, constructs such as solidarity and conflict are nevertheless surprisingly universal. International scholars have found this work helpful as they attempt to understand families and intergenerational relations in their own societies.

Times have changed greatly since the early days of the LSOG. We have much more sophisticated ways to collect and analyze data. We now have national and international representative generational samples, and we can sample populations and subpopulations with surprising accuracy. We have impressive analytic techniques. Whereas early work used simple techniques such as *t*-tests and correlations, developments include the use of multiple-level modeling and impressive techniques for examining the individual within the family and the broader context. Similarly, in addition to mail-in questionnaires and face-to-face and telephone interviews, we now have web-based, daily dairy, and experience-based sampling technologies as well as nonintrusive methods for collecting biomarkers and other physiological measures. As the field moves forward in these many and impressive ways, it is clear that it builds on the important groundbreaking steps taken by Vern Bengtson and his colleagues.

TONI C. ANTONUCCI
Ann Arbor, Michigan

Acknowledgments

The editors are grateful to Retirement Living Television, the University of Southern California Davis School of Gerontology and College of Letters, Arts, and Sciences, and the John Templeton Foundation for their financial support of the conference from which most of the chapters in this volume were derived. In addition, great thanks go to Linda Hall, whose assistance in preparing manuscripts was invaluable to us, and to Norella Putney for her last-minute assistance. Finally, we acknowledge twenty years of research support from the National Institute of Aging, which brought Dr. Bengtson's ideas to fruition.

Kinship and Cohort in an Aging Society

Solidarity as a Key Concept in Family and Generational Research

Merril Silverstein and Roseann Giarrusso

The first line of Leo Tolstoy's epic novel *Anna Karenina* reads "all happy families are alike, each unhappy family is unhappy in its own way" (Tolstoy, 2004). Whether taken wryly or at face value, this dual view of family life rings true but is knowingly simplistic; almost all families manifest both positive and negative sentiments and indeed may shift from happiness to unhappiness and back again. Even families that are outwardly cordial and otherwise well-functioning belie a process of continual adjustment to internal and external stressors that threaten equilibrium. Dynamic tension between the centripetal forces that unite and the centrifugal forces that divide lies beneath the surface of virtually all contemporary families. Social science understandings of the family diverge from literary understandings in their emphasis on theoretical and conceptual development, use of systematically collected data, and reliance on rigorous methods to reach conclusions. Arguably no scholar of family science and social gerontology has added more to the scholarly toolbox of theory, data, and method than Vern Bengtson.

Bengtson, an American sociologist, social psychologist, and developmentalist, is best known for his contributions to family theory and his research on the topic of adult intergenerational relationships. Drawing in part from Durkheim's concept of social solidarity and Heider's (1958) and Homans's (1950) theories of small-group cohesion, Bengtson and colleagues developed a "periodic table" of the connective links between family generations—a model that became known as the intergenerational solidarity paradigm (Bengtson & Roberts, 1992; Roberts, Richards, & Bengtson, 1991). Both a conceptual scheme and a measurement model, the solidarity paradigm itemized the sentiments, behaviors, attitudes, values, and structural arrangements that bind generations, and it remains one of the most enduring and widely used schemes to represent adult family relationships. Later the paradigm evolved to include conflict as a seventh dimension, leading it to be renamed the intergenerational solidarity-conflict paradigm and allowing the incorporation of the concept of ambivalence (Bengtson et al., 2002). Among other topics Bengtson investigated over his career were generational equity, social breakdown, double jeopardy, grandparenting, and the beanpole family—all central to the social gerontology canon.

This volume brings together scholars whose common link is their intellectual intersection with Bengtson's body of work on families and aging. The fifteen chapters—most of which were presented in an earlier form at a conference following Bengtson's retirement—map major thematic areas to which Bengtson has contributed:

- Family connections: Solidarity within and across generations
- Grandparents in a changing demographic landscape: Mothers and mentors
- Generations and cohorts: Micro-macro dialectics
- Religion and families: Contexts of continuity, change, and conflict
- Global, cross-national, and cross-ethnic concerns: Who will take care of the young and the old?

Solidarity and Its Discontents

Insofar as solidarity represents the essential integrative features of interpersonal relations, it is an implicitly social psychological construct. Yet the power of the solidarity model lies in its parsimony and generalized utility—fulfilling the maxim that a good scientific theory ought to postulate little but explain a lot. On this count, the solidarity model holds up well, for it represents a comprehensive and systematic conceptual scheme that describes kinship relations along a circumscribed set of dimensions that can be applied under a variety of social conditions and family circumstances.

Popular paradigms that are in wide use in the social sciences are natural targets of critical appraisals, and the solidarity paradigm is no exception. These critiques include comments of the variety that solidarity as a concept and in its measurement gives short shrift to conflict, tends to focus on micro-social interactions, and does not well capture the subjective meanings of family life. Each of these concerns, while valid in its own right, is assuaged by the wide range of content areas informed by principles of solidarity, well beyond what Bengtson might have envisioned when he began to operationalize solidarity in his landmark Longitudinal Study of Generations (LSOG). The LSOG began in 1971 as a study of 2,044 individuals nested within 358 three-generation families. As the study progressed through the 1980s and 1990s, families changed in ways that were difficult to predict when the study started: the pro-test generation moved into careers and family life; women entered the labor force in large numbers so that two-earner families became the statistical norm; divorce and remarriage became more prevalent; families became smaller but more complex; and three- and four-generation families became increasingly common due to declines in mortality. If the legacy of a scholar's intellectual contribution is best judged by the echo it leaves in the work of new generations of scholars (rather than by whether it is replicated in an unaltered state), then solidarity, by virtue of its pliability, remains an enduring concept in family and aging studies even as it is reconsidered and adapted to new social realities. For instance, applications of the solidarity framework to vertical family relationships within traditional (see Suitor & Pillemer, Chapter 1) and nontraditional families (see Remle & O'Rand, Chapter 2) as well as to horizontal family relationships such as siblings (see Knipsheer & van Tilburg, Chapter 3) and spouses (see Markides et al., Chapter 15) have yielded promising results. The solidarity framework continues to help us to better understand the role of grandparents in a changing society (see Burton, Welsh, & Destro, Chapter 4; and Taylor, Uhlenberg, Elder, & McDonald, Chapter 5).

More recent intergenerational theories that formally recognize the simultaneous presence of countervailing forces in relationships—such as ambivalence theory—can be articulated within the solidarity-conflict paradigm and in fact are broadened by it (Bengtson et al., 2002; Silverstein et al., 2010). Several chapters in this volume acknowledge various dialectics in multigenerational families representing the tension between continuity and discontinuity, agreement and disagreement, affection and conflict, cohesion and entropy. That solidarity has its opposite or inverse in more negative attributes of family relationships should not be surprising; conflict has formally been part of the solidarity paradigm since the early 1990s and a formal part of classical sociological theory at least since Simmel (1955 [1918]).

With its functionalist roots, emphasis on social integration, and basis in formal model construction and codification, the solidarity paradigm represents (the best of) positivism in the social sciences; yet it has also provided insights into the negotiated nature of intergenerational family ties. Interpretative approaches have delved into various understandings of solidarity based on generation, such as whether social support (e.g., Pyke & Bengtson, 1996), religion (see Achenbaum, Chapter 9), religious instruction (see Putney et al., Chapter 10), and end-of-life care (see Johnson, Chapter 8) are ultimately viewed as divisive or bonding. Policy-relevant discussions may also emerge from these more qualitative accounts, such as whether middle-aged parents with "long-term lousy relationships" with their adult children can expect to receive social support from them when needed (Clarke et al., 1999).

The wider relevance of solidarity is brought to light by the idea that family relationships are embedded within larger social structures and contexts that give them shape and purpose. These structures range from ethnic-group membership (see Burton et al.; Lincoln, Chatters, & Taylor, Chapter 11; Markides et al.; and Putney et al. in this volume); voluntary organizations such as church groups (see Lincoln et al. and Markides et al. in this volume), nationality or citizenship/immigrant status (see Dannefer & Siders, Chapter 13; Marshall, Chapter 12; Marcum & Treas, Chapter 14; and Markides et al. in this volume), generational-historical location (see Alwin, Chapter 6; Biggs & Lowenstein, Chapter 7; and Johnson in this volume), and socio-political environment (see Marcum & Treas in this volume).

Origin and Organization of the Volume

In organizing the chapters for this volume, the editors asked prominent scholars in field of social gerontology—primarily but not exclusively those in family studies—to prepare original research or critical reviews in areas that directly or indirectly link to intellectual traditions pioneered by Vern Bengtson. What emerged is an eclectic collection of papers that reflect a rich diversity of applications and approaches to very different sociological questions that may on the surface seem dissimilar but ultimately build on a common intellectual foundation. Much like a river with branching tributaries, the chapters represented in this volume carve their own direction but maintain a discernible link to their scholarly source, the solidarity paradigm and subsequent paradigms inspired by it. Particularly noteworthy is that the chapters build on previous knowledge and paradigmatic structures while pushing in new directions.

Also noteworthy is the fact that each chapter in the volume focuses on a different population within the United States, or a different nation, and that the empirical chapters use very different data sets; only one uses the LSOG (Putney et al.). The other data bases include a Massachusetts-based sample of parents and their children (Suitor & Pillemer); the Health and Retirement Study (HRS) (Remle & O'Rand); a sample of older men and women in the Netherlands (Knipscheer & van Tillburg); a nationally representative sample of adolescents from the National Longitudinal Study of Adolescent Health (Add-Health) (Taylor et al.); data from the Family Life Project (Burton et al.); the National Survey of American Life (NSAL) (Lincoln et al.); the Hispanic subsample of the Established Population for the Epidemiological Study of the Elderly (EPESE) (Markides et al.); the Bennington longitudinal study (Alwin); the National Election Study (Alwin); and the International Social Survey Programme (ISSP) Social Network module (Marcum & Treas). These data were collected using qualitative as well as quantitative methods and longitudinal as well as cross-sectional designs. The quantitative data varied in terms of type and unit of analysis (social networks data; individual-, dyad-, and family-level survey). The studies included a broad range of cohorts, multiple nations, and an oversampling of particular racial and ethnic subgroups in the United States. This diversity of methodological approaches, sample characteristics, research designs, and types/units of analysis is significant because it demonstrates that the ideas generated by the LSOG can be tested on inner-city Blacks, older Dutch adults, Hispanic elders, and a nationally representative sample of adolescents. These chapters are a testament to the broad applicability of the theories and empirical findings of the LSOG—a study often criticized on the grounds of its non-representativeness (the sample is largely White and middle class).

The volume is divided into five sections. The first section, Family Connections, is devoted to the nature of personal relationships within families—how they are constructed enacted, and managed. The second section of the volume, Grandparents in a Changing Demographic Landscape, is devoted to the role grandparents play in families changed by demographic trends in fertility and family formation. The third section, Of Generations and Cohorts, examines the distinction between these two terms by showing how generational standing and cohort membership influence aging families. The fourth section, Religion and Families, focuses on the role of religion in family and institutional settings. The fifth section, Global, Cross-National, and Cross-Ethnic Concerns, examines globalization, cross-national, and cross-ethnic comparisons in who will care for the young and the old in aging families.

Concluding Thoughts

The social scientific literature and the chapters in this volume reveal that Tolstoy was not entirely correct about the unique characters of happy and unhappy families. Emotional closeness does not necessarily imply the absence of conflict; unpleasant circumstances may corrode even the happiest of families. Unhappy families may be anguished by interpersonal turmoil linked to economic downturns, political upheavals, cultural transformations, and the ineffable search for meaning in a society where social structures have softened if not withered or died. Happy families are not immune from stressors introduced by societal and family change, though they may be resilient to their effects even if exposed to their risks. Such coping may involve meaning-making activities such as those related to religious practice and spirituality or reliance on alternative social ties such as church members or siblings when children are not available.

Variegation of family structures due to divorce, remarriage, multiple parenting, low fertility, increased longevity, ethnic diversity, and immigration has altered the social terrain of family life, making it both more interesting and more challenging to study. Family sociologists and developmental scientists are less able to rely on a standard model of the family when considering this "new complexity"; but in compensation they are presented with new opportunities to examine change and variation in family styles and well-being as functions of these social transformations. The solidarity-conflict paradigm as an orienting schema continues to be a useful prism through which to view strengths and vulnerabilities in relationships between generations, cohorts, and age and peer groups, informing research on themes as disparate as intergenerational favoritism, blended families, grandparenting, spirituality, immigration, social movements, globalization, and public policies of the welfare state. By virtue of clarifying complex phenomena within a parsimonious framework, the solidarity-conflict paradigm fulfills the promise that a good theory postulates little but explains a lot.

REFERENCES

Bengtson, V. L., Giarrusso, R., Mabry, J. B., & Silverstein, M. (2002). Solidarity, conflict, and ambivalence: Complementary or competing perspectives on intergenerational relationships? *Journal of Marriage and Family, 64,* 568–576.

Bengtson, V. L., & Roberts, R. E. L. (1991). Intergenerational solidarity in aging families: An example of formal theory construction. *Journal of Marriage and the Family, 53,* 856–870.

Clarke, E. J., Preston, M., Raksin, J., & Bengtson, V. L. (1999). Types of conflicts and tensions between older parents and adult children. *The Gerontologist, 39(3),* 261–270.

Heider, F. (1958). *The psychology of interpersonal relations.* New York: John Wiley and Sons.

Homans, G. C. (1950). *The human group.* New York: Harcourt, Brace and World.

Pyke, K. D., & Bengtson, V. L. (1996). Caring more or less: Individualistic and collectivist systems of family eldercare. *Journal of Marriage and the Family, 58,* 1–14.

Roberts, R. E. L., Richards, L. N., & Bengtson, V. L. (1991). Intergenerational solidarity in families: Untangling the ties that bind. *Marriage and Family Review, 16(1/2).*

Silverstein, M., Gans, D., Lowenstein, A., Giarrusso R., & Bengtson, V. L. (2010). Older parent-child relationships in six nations: Comparisons at the intersection of affection and conflict. *Journal of Marriage and Family, 72,* 1006–1021.

Simmel, G. (1955 [1918]). *Conflict and the web of group affiliations.* Glencoe, IL: The Free Press.

Tolstoy, L. (2004). *Anna Karenina.* (Trans. R. Pevear & L. Volokhonsky.) New York: Penguin Books.

PART I / Family Connections

Solidarity within and across Generations

The solidarity-conflict theoretical perspective includes seven dimensions along which intergenerational relationships may differ including affectual solidarity (emotional closeness), consensual solidarity (attitude similarity), functional solidarity (the exchange of instrumental and emotional help and support), normative solidarity (feelings of family obligation), associational solidarity (frequency of contact), structural solidarity (geographic proximity, gender, and health), and conflict (disagreements). The chapters in this section use one or more of these dimensions to examine a variety of research questions about different types of family relationships.

Suitor and Pillemer raise the intriguing question of whether mothers and fathers show favoritism to the same adult child. To measure favoritism, they use functional as well as affectual solidarity. Although they found that mothers and fathers were equally likely to show favoritism (between 63% and 76% did, depending on the measure of favoritism used), mothers and fathers did not favor the same child. The contribution of this research is that it included the perspectives of fathers as well as mothers (most studies use only the mother as the informant) and it asked parents about each of their children rather than about their children as a whole—something few studies have done.

Remle and O'Rand examine economic transfers—a form of functional solidarity—from parents to adult biological children and stepchildren from the child's perspective. They found that relatively lower transfer rates to stepchildren are driven by restricted economic flows from remarried fathers. The significance of this chapter is that it shows that the solidarity-conflict paradigm can be adapted for use with changing family forms such as blended families and that biological children and stepchildren are treated differently by parents.

Although developed to examine the quality of relationships across generations (such as between parents and adult children), the dimensions of solidarity and conflict can also be used to examine the quality of relationships within generations (such as those among siblings and between husbands and wives). A further extension of the model would be the examination of how vertical family relationships influence horizontal family relationships—something done in the chapter by Knipscheer and van Tillburg. They use a social network approach to examine the interdependencies between sibling and parent-child ties in later life, finding that the presence of children is inversely related to the number and proportion of siblings in the support network of older adults.

CHAPTER ONE

Differences in Mothers' and Fathers' Parental Favoritism in Later Life

A Within-Family Approach

J. Jill Suitor and Karl Pillemer

In this chapter, we report on work that incorporates several dimensions of complexity in intergenerational relations. First, instead of comparing a single parent-child relationship between families, the research described here investigates how parents' relationships with individual children within the same family differ. Using a unique data set that includes parents' assessments of relationships toward all adult children, we focus on how individual relationships in the family may differ. Second, we extend an approach used extensively in the study of younger families to intergenerational relations in later life: parental favoritism.

Third, we move beyond the focus on mothers that is common in the study of intergenerational relations. Although the term "parent-adult child relations" implies an emphasis on adult children's relationships with both their mothers and fathers, the overwhelming majority of work on intergenerational ties in the middle and later years has been restricted to exploring mother-child relationships. Further, theoretical perspectives designed to frame research on parent-adult child relations have been developed with little question of whether children's relationships with their mothers and with their fathers can be explained by the same set of factors.

We attempt to extend understanding of the relationships between older fathers and their adult children, using a conceptual and analytic approach that allows us to explore within-family variations in father-child relations and compare these patterns to those found among older mother-child dyads. We focus on two specific research questions: (1) How do patterns of favoritism within the family differ by a parent's gender? and (2) Can mothers' and fathers' patterns of favoritism be explained by the same combination of social structural characteristics, attitudinal similarities, and contextual factors? To address these questions, we use data collected from 129 mothers and fathers 65 years of age and older as part of the Within-Family Differences Study (Pillemer & Suitor, 2006; Pillemer et al., 2007; Suitor & Pillemer, 2006a, 2007; Suitor, Pillemer, & Sechrist, 2006; Suitor, Sechrist, & Pillemer, 2007a,b; Suitor, Sechrist, Steinhour, & Pillemer, 2006).

Parental Favoritism in Later Life

Parents are commonly urged not to show favoritism (Cleese & Bates, 2001; Cohen & Cohen, 1997; Faber & Mazlish, 1987). However, research has shown that both mothers and fathers often differentiate among their young children and adolescents in terms of closeness and the provision of both emotional and instrumental support (Brody, Stoneman, & McCoy, 1992a,b; Kowal & Kramer, 1997; McHale, Crouter, McGuire, & Updegraff, 1995; Volling, 1997; Volling & Elins, 1998). Further, there is preliminary evidence that such patterns continue into adulthood. Studies by Bedford (1992) and Baker and Daniels (1990) showed that a substantial proportion of adult children believed that their parents favored some children in the family over others, whereas both Aldous et al. (1985) and Brackbill et al. (1988) found that most parents reported that they differentiated among their children in adulthood in terms of affection, pride, and disappointment. Although these studies were small and did not use representative samples, they suggest that within-family differences in parent-child relations occur in later life.

Despite this evidence regarding within-family differences, the designs of most studies of parent-adult child relations have not permitted further examination of these patterns. The majority of these studies have asked parents about their adult children in the aggregate, rather than about each child separately, or focused on only one child. Even the work on within-family differences in adulthood cited above did not collect data about both generations within the same family; thus, it is difficult to develop a picture of the extent of, explanations for, and consequences of within-family differences in parent-adult child relations.

Our previous work has demonstrated that mothers often differentiate among their adult children across a wide array of relational dimensions, including emotional closeness, confiding, preference for support, and the provision of support to children (Pillemer & Suitor, 2006; Pillemer et al., 2007; Suitor & Pillemer, 2006a,b, 2007; Suitor, Pillemer, & Sechrist, 2006; Suitor, Sechrist, & Pillemer, 2007a,b); further, children are aware of their parents' differentiation, although they are not always correct about which child is favored (Suitor, Sechrist, Steinhour, & Pillemer, 2006). The goal of this chapter is to shed new light on this critically important but under-researched topic by examining how older parent-adult child relationships vary within the family by parents' gender. We are responding to a call to increase scientific knowledge about how the relationship formed by each parent and child functions as an independent unit, different from other family dyads (Davey, Janke, & Salva, 2005; Lye, 1996; Troll & Fingerman, 1996).

Gender Differences in Whether Parents Express Favoritism

One question to be addressed in this chapter is, To what degree do mothers and fathers of adult children differ in whether they have favorite children? That is, are mothers or fathers more likely to declare a preference versus not choosing a specific child across relational domains? Studies of young children and adolescents have not found major differences between mothers and fathers in the degree to which they express favoritism (Kowal & Kramer, 1997; McHale, Updegraff, Jackson-Newsom, & Tucker, 2000; O'Connor, Dunn, Jenkins, & Rasbash, 2006; Tucker, McHale, & Crouter, 2003; Volling & Elins, 1998). Further, of the two studies that have examined gender differences in parental favoritism in adulthood, one showed no gender differences in whether a favorite was selected (Aldous, Klaus, & Klein, 1985) and one found greater favoritism on the part of mothers only in relation to birth order (Brackbill, Kitch, & Noffsinger, 1988).

These findings might lead to the hypothesis that no gender differences will exist between mothers and fathers in likelihood of favoritism. It is possible, however, that gender differences in parents' favoritism may emerge as children move into adulthood. In particular, mothers typically have closer relationships with their adult children than do fathers and interact with them more often (cf. Rossi & Rossi, 1990; Suitor & Pillemer, 2006a). For this reason, it is possible that mothers have greater opportunity to develop bases for favoritism than do than fathers. We believe that these gender differences in closeness and contact, as well as women's greater attention to the quality of interpersonal relationships in general, may lead to mothers being more likely than fathers to favor some children over others.

Gender Differences in Predictors of Parental Favoritism

Studies of within-family differences in early stages of the life course have documented the bases on which parents differentiate among their children (cf. Suitor et al., 2008). However, there has been little attention to systematic differences between predictors of mothers' and fathers' favoritism. We looked to theories of intergenerational relations in adulthood to guide our study of gender differences in mothers' versus fathers' favoritism. This line of scholarship, however, provided fewer guideposts than expected. For example, Bengtson's model of intergenerational solidarity, which has been the most influential theoretical development across the past three decades, does not detail different predictors of mothers' and fathers' relations with their adult children, despite the fact that Bengtson and colleagues have found substantial gender effects on affective relations (cf. Putney & Bengtson, 2001; Silverstein & Bengtson, 1997).

The empirical literature also provides few consistent bases upon which to develop hypotheses regarding gender differences in favoritism in later-life families. Although many data sets provide information on both mothers and fathers, surprisingly few studies of parent-adult child relations have explored the ways in which predictors of relationship quality vary by parents' gender. Further, studies that have explored this question provide few consistent patterns that can be used as a basis for developing hypotheses regarding either patterns or predictors of favoritism. For example, Rossi and Rossi (1990) and Aldous and colleagues (1985) found that adult children's becoming parents increased closeness between sons and fathers but not between mothers and sons, whereas Kaufman and Uhlenberg (1998) reported that parenthood decreased closeness for mothers and daughters but had no effect on the mother-son relationship. In contrast, Silverstein and Bengtson (1997) found that the presence of children in the household had little or no effect on either mothers' or fathers' relationships with their adult offspring. Inconsistent patterns have also been found regarding gender differences in the effects of adult children's other sociodemographic characteristics on parent-child relations.

In the absence of consistent findings regarding differences in predictors of mothers' and fathers' quality of relations with their adult children, we drew from the theoretical literature on gender to guide the development of our hypotheses. The classic arguments developed by Chodorow (1978), Gilligan (1982), and Williams (1993) posit that gender differences in socialization in childhood and adolescence lead women to emphasize expressive dimensions of their interpersonal relations, whereas men are socialized to emphasize instrumental dimensions. The empirical literature on gender differences in interpersonal relations provides support for this position. For example, Worthen (2000) found that adolescent girls place greater emphasis on empathy in the development and maintenance of friendships than do boys. Bank and Hansford (2000) found that differences in intimacy in men's and women's friendship were accounted for greatly by gender differences in emotional expressiveness.

In contrast, men emphasize instrumental issues in their interactions and relationships more than do women (Ali & Toner, 1996; Belansky & Boggiano, 1996; Pillemer, Landreneau, & Suitor, 1996; Reevy & Maslach, 2001). Thus, fathers are likely to tend to emphasize instrumental factors in their relationships with their adult children and with other associates. For example, fathers could be expected to differentiate on the basis of their children's status attainment, whereas mothers might differentiate among their adult children on the basis of values or expressive support. Further, men's more traditional gender-role attitudes (Powers et al., 2004; Rice & Coates, 1995) may lead them to value different dimensions of status attainment for their sons and daughters, with greater emphasis on daughters' traditional "women's statuses," such as marriage and parenthood, and on sons' education and employment.

Our previous work on favoritism provides support for these arguments in terms of mothers' differentiation among their adult children (Pillemer & Suitor, 2006; Suitor & Pillemer, 2000a,b, 2006a, 2007). In particular, children's gender, similarity of values, and religious participation played important roles in explaining mothers' favoritism among their adult children, whereas children's attainment of normative adult statuses had little or no predictive value. Because the analyses were restricted to women, Suitor and colleagues' study cannot shed light on gender differences in mothers' and fathers' favoritism.

Nevertheless, we suggest that our findings, in concert with the theoretical arguments regarding gender differences in men's and women's concern with expressive and instrumental dimensions of relationships, provide a basis for developing particular expectations. Specifically, we propose the following hypotheses: (1) expressive dimensions of the relationship, such as similarity of attitudes and attachment, will predict which children mothers favor; (2) children's attainment of normative adult statuses will predict which children fathers favor; and (3) fathers will emphasize traditional patterns of status attainment, focusing on marriage and parenting for daughters and focusing on employment and education for sons. Further, we also anticipate that mothers will be more likely than fathers to differentiate among their adult children.

Methods
Design Goals

The project was designed to provide data on within-family differences in parent-adult child relations in later life. The design involved selecting a sample of mothers 65–75 years of age with at least two living adult children and collecting data from them regarding each of their children. Only community-dwelling mothers were included in the sample to reduce the likelihood that the women would be in need of extensive caregiving, thus allowing us to study relationships outside of the context of caregiving.

Sample

Massachusetts city and town lists were the source of the sample. Massachusetts requires communities to keep city/town lists of all residents by address. Town lists also provide the age and gender of residents. The first step was to randomly select 20 communities from the total of 80 that were available. With the assistance of the University of Massachusetts, Boston, we drew a systematic sample of women ages 65–75 from the town lists from 20 communities in the greater Boston area. Once communities were selected and appropriate town lists obtained, equal numbers of women in the target age group were selected from each community.

We then sent a letter of introduction to each woman describing the study and explaining that an interviewer would contact her from the Center for Survey Research to determine her eligibility for participation and attempt to schedule a face-to-face interview if she met the study criteria. The interviewers began contacting potential respondents and continued until they had reached the target number of cases. Data were collected from 556 mothers, which represented 61% of those who were eligible for participation. The interviews were conducted between August of 2001 and January of 2003.

At the end of each interview, the mothers were told about the study component involving their husbands and were asked for their permission to contact them. Sixty-eight percent of the married mothers gave permission for the interviewers to contact their husbands; 78% of the husbands agreed to participate, resulting in a final sample of 130 husbands. In the present analyses, only 129 fathers were included because of missing data on the primary variables of interest. For this study, we included only those mothers whose husbands were interviewed; thus, only married couples are included. Each of the mothers was interviewed for between one and two hours; each of the fathers was interviewed for approximately one hour.

Sample Characteristics
Mothers' Characteristics

The mothers were between 65 and 75 years of age (mean = 69.6; SD = 3.3). Nine percent of the mothers had completed less than high school, 36% had completed high school, 18% had completed some college, and 36% had graduated from college. Seventy-one percent were not employed; 29% were employed. Twenty-six percent had a total family income of less than $30,000 in the previous year, 20% had an income of between $30,000 and $39,999, 11% had an income of between $40,000 and $49,999, 18% had an income of between $50,000 and $75,000, and 27% had an income of $75,000 or greater. Forty-five percent of the women were Catholic, 29% were Protestant, 15% were Jewish, and 11% reported another religion or said that they had no religious affiliation. Ninety-three percent of the mothers were Non-Hispanic White, 5% were Black, 1% were Hispanic, and 1% were Asian. The number of living children of women in the subsample for this analysis ranged from 2 to 13 (mean = 3.4; SD = 1.5). This married subsample is higher in socioeconomic status than would be expected for a random sample of individuals aged 65 and older. These differences reflect the cumulative advantage accrued by remaining married across the adult life course.

Fathers' Characteristics

The fathers were between 60 and 83 years of age (mean = 70.6; SD = 4.5). Only fathers who were married to the mothers participated; thus, all of the father participants were married. Twelve percent of the fathers had completed less than high school, 27% had completed high school, 12% had completed some college, and 49% had graduated from college. Sixty-two percent were not employed; 38% were employed. Forty-five percent of the men were Catholic, 32% were Protestant, 14% were Jewish, and 2% reported another religion or said that they had no religious affiliation. Ninety-three percent of the fathers were White, 4% were Black, and 3% described themselves as "mixed race."

Adult Children's Characteristics

Mothers provided demographic information for each of their adult children. This analysis included 441 adult children. The adult children ranged from 20 to 61 years of age (mean = 41.6; SD = 5.5). Forty-nine percent were daughters. Seventy-one percent of the adult children were currently married. Twenty-three percent of the adult children had completed high school, 11% had completed some college, 37% were college graduates, and 29% had completed some graduate work. Eighty-six percent of the children were employed. Seventy-one percent of the adult children were themselves parents.

Measures
Dependent Variables

To determine parental preference, we asked the mothers and fathers a series of questions that required them to select among their adult children, the method most commonly used in the literature on parental favoritism in childhood and adolescence. Specifically, each mother and father was asked to select which child (a) she or he would be most likely to talk to about a personal problem; (b) she or he would prefer help from if she (the mother) became ill or disabled; and (c) to whom she or he felt the most emotionally close. Each child was coded as 0 for each item for which he or she was not chosen and 1 for each item for which he or she was chosen. When respondents were initially unwilling to differentiate among their children, the interviewers were instructed to prompt the parent with a follow-up question (for example, "But is there one child to whom you are the most close?"). Analyses of the data revealed that less than 5% of the mothers were moved by the prompt to select a child, and there were no differences between mothers who did and did not respond to the prompt. Responses were similar for fathers.

Independent Variables

Each child was coded as first-born, middle-born, or last-born based on the mothers' reports of the children's ages. Child's gender was coded 0 = son, 1 = daughter. Marital status was measured by whether the adult child was currently married (0 = child not married; 1 = child married). Parental status was measured by whether the adult child had any children (0 = no children; 1 = had child). Mothers were asked to indicate the educational achievement category of each of their adult children: (a) less than high school; (b) some high school; (c) high school graduate; (d) post-high school vocational; (e) some college; (f) college graduate; or (g) completed graduate school.

Mothers were asked whether their children were employed but not the number of hours that they worked; thus, employment was coded 0 = not employed, 1 = employed. Proximity was measured in distance the child lived from the mother in terms of travel time by ground transportation. Categories were (a) same house; (b) same neighborhood; (c) less than 15 minutes away; (d) 15–30 minutes away; (e) 30–60 minutes away; (f) more than an hour but less than two hours; and (g) and two or more hours away.

Perceived value similarity was measured by the item: "Parents and children are sometimes similar to each other in their views and opinions and sometimes different from each other. Would you say that you and [child's name] share very similar views (4), similar views (3), different views (2), or very different views (1) in terms of general outlook on life?"

To measure attachment, we used a short version of the Cicirelli Adult Attachment Scale (Cicirelli, 1995), which focuses on parents' and children's current levels of attachment. The short version we used asks mothers whether they strongly agree (4), agree (3), disagree (2), or strongly disagree (1) with each of the following statements: (a) Being with [child's name] makes you feel very happy; (b) When you feel anxious or worried, [child's name] is one of the first people you want to be with; and (c) You feel lonely when you don't see [child's name] often. The scores on the three items were summed. The reliability coefficient (Cronbach's Alpha) on the present subsample was .65 for mothers and .66 for fathers.

Statistical Approach

Throughout, the adult child, rather than the parent, is the unit of analysis. In other words, the 441 adult children who constitute the units of analysis are nested within the 129 mothers and 129 fathers on whose reports the present analysis is based; thus, the observations are not independent. It is possible that characteristics we have not measured could have effects on parents' choices. To address this concern we used conditional logistic regression throughout the multivariate analysis. Conditional logistic regression is preferable to standard logistic regression in this case because the procedure controls on mothers' characteristics, much as would be the case if a dummy variable were created for each of the 129 parents and the set of dummy variables were included in the regression equations in which the mother-child pair was the unit of analysis

Table 1.1. Mothers' and fathers' differentiation among their children (*n* = 129)

	Percentage who named a preferred child	
Parent-child relationship contexts	Mothers	Fathers
Child that parent would most likely talk to about personal problem	75.8*	66.7
Child that parent prefers provide her/him with help if ill or disabled	69.5	70.5
Child that parent feels most emotionally close to	62.8*	68.0

* *p* < .05 (significance of difference between mothers and fathers)

(cf. Allison, 2005; Alwin, 1976; Suitor & Pillemer, 1996). Thus, conditional logistic regression allows us to focus on our primary question of interest—within each family, which child does the parent choose?—while controlling on parents' characteristics.

Results

Differences in Favoritism by Parents' Gender

Parents' reports revealed that mothers were not systematically more likely to express favoritism, contrary to expectations (table 1.1). Mothers were more likely to choose a particular child as confidant (76% vs. 67%; *p* < .05); however, they were *less* likely than fathers to name a child to whom they were most emotionally close (63% vs. 68%; *p* < .05), In the case of help during illness, mothers and fathers were equally likely to express a preference: 70% of both mothers and fathers chose a particular child as the one they would prefer to help them if they became ill or disabled.

Given the relatively high level of congruence in mothers' and fathers' likelihood of showing favoritism for a particular child, we might expect that they would have typically chosen the same child; however, this was not always the case. In families in which both parents differentiated among their children, mothers and fathers favored the same child only 52% of the time for confiding and for emotional closeness and only 64% of the time when naming a preferred source of care during illness. Thus, although mothers and fathers may be similarly likely to show parental favoritism, parents within the same family often choose different children.

In sum, there does not appear to be a consistent relationship between parents' gender and likelihood of favoritism toward adult children. Perhaps even more

Table 1.2. Conditional logistic regression analysis of parents' differentiation among children regarding emotional closeness

	Mothers			Fathers		
	B	(SE)	Odds ratio	B	(SE)	Odds ratio
Youngest child	.63[+]	(.37)	1.88	.47	(.34)	1.60
Oldest child	.80*	(.38)	2.23	.29	(.36)	1.33
Similarity of values	.91**	(.28)	2.48	.35	(.25)	1.41
Daughter	1.07**	(.32)	2.93	.31	(.30)	1.36
Child is married	−1.14*	(.53)	0.32	−.09	(.43)	0.91
Attachment to child	.17	(.15)	1.19	.37*	(.17)	1.45
Distance from child	−.05	(.10)	0.95	−.02	(.10)	1.02
Model χ^2			42.40**			21.82**
df			10			10
n^1			258			248

Note: Child's education, parental status, and employment status were not significantly associated with parents preferring one child over another with regard to emotional closeness, confiding, and receiving help when ill or disabled, and thus omitted from the tables.

[1] The n of cases differs across models because the only cases included in each analysis are those in which others were willing to choose among their children, which varied by the relational context.

$p < .10$, *$p < .05$, **$p < .01$

important, the findings indicate that the majority of both parents favored particular children across all three relational dimensions, and the differences between mothers and fathers were not large. In families in which both parents favor one child over others, mothers and fathers often favor different children.

Predictors of Parental Favoritism
Emotional Closeness

Table 1.2 presents the findings for favoritism regarding emotional closeness. Consistent with our hypotheses, mothers' favoritism appears to be influenced strongly by gender and perceived value similarity. Specifically, the odds of mothers choosing a daughter were approximately three times greater than the odds of choosing a son, and mothers were two and a half times more likely to choose a child who shared their outlook on life. Although being married increased children's similarity to their mothers, the odds of choosing a married child were only about one-third as great as those of choosing one who was single. Finally, the odds of mothers choosing first-borns or last-borns were, on average, about twice that of choosing middle-borns.

Table 1.3. Conditional logistic regression analysis of parents' differentiation among children regarding confiding

	Mothers			Fathers		
	B	(SE)	Odds ratio	B	(SE)	Odds ratio
Youngest child	.24	(.38)	1.27	.01	(.37)	1.01
Oldest child	.26	(.38)	1.30	1.03**	(.38)	2.81
Similarity of values	.54*	(.27)	1.71	.29	(.29)	1.34
Daughter	1.92**	(.40)	6.84	.03	(.31)	1.03
Child is married	.06	(.47)	1.07	-.40	(.47)	0.67
Attachment to child	.37*	(.18)	1.44	1.00**	(.24)	2.71
Distance from child	-.31**	(.10)	0.73	-.19	(.11)	0.83
Model χ^2		68.16**			38.84**	
df		10			10	
n[1]		288			256	

[1] The *n* of cases differs across models because the only cases included in each analysis are those in which others were willing to choose among their children, which varied by the relational context.

$p < .10$, *$p < .05$, **$p < .01$

The findings regarding fathers' favoritism regarding closeness were less consistent with our hypotheses. In particular, achievement of normative adult statuses did not influence fathers' likelihood of naming particular children as those to whom they were most close. In fact, attachment was the only factor that significantly predicted fathers' choices. Separate analyses not shown provided no support for our expectation that fathers would favor children who adhered to traditional family roles (i.e., daughters who were married homemakers and sons who were well-educated and employed).

The differences between the coefficients for mothers and fathers for several of these predictors were marginally statistically significant ($p < .10$), including the choice of first-borns, similarity of attitudes, and marital status.

Confiding

The predictors of mothers' and fathers' choices of confidants from among their adult children are presented in table 1.3. Consistent with our hypotheses, mothers chose daughters and children who shared their outlook on life; in fact, the odds of mothers choosing daughters were nearly seven times greater than the odds of their choosing sons. Mothers were also about 70% more likely to choose children who shared their values and to whom they reported high

Table 1.4. Conditional logistic regression analysis of parents' differentiation among children regarding help during an illness

	Mothers			Fathers		
	B	(SE)	Odds ratio	B	(SE)	Odds ratio
Youngest child	−.38	(.44)	0.69	.05	(.38)	1.05
Oldest child	−.70	(.49)	0.50	.36	(.37)	1.43
Similarity of values	.55+	(.30)	1.74	−.04	(.27)	0.97
Daughter	3.08**	(.41)	21.77	.60*	(.31)	1.83
Child is married	−.01	(.64)	0.99	−.25	(.47)	0.78
Attachment to child	1.21**	(.28)	3.34	1.18**	(.25)	3.26
Distance from child	−.46**	(.14)	0.63	−.17	(.10)	0.84
Model χ^2		83.25**			42.05**	
df		10			10	
n^1		284			264	

[1] The *n* of cases differs across models because the only cases included in each analysis are those in which others were willing to choose among their children, which varied by the relational context.

$p < .10$, *$p < .05$, **$p < .01$

attachment. Mothers were also less likely to confide in children who lived farther away.

In contrast, fathers' choices did not follow the patterns we hypothesized. The odds of fathers choosing first-borns and children to whom they reported high levels of attachment were nearly three times as great as that of choosing other children, whereas adult children's achievements of normative adult statuses did not predict fathers' choices. Two of the differences between the models for mothers and fathers were statistically significant—differences in the effect of child's gender ($p < .01$) and attachment ($p < .05$). Most interesting about the marked difference in the effect of attachment was that it was in the opposite direction from our expectations: attachment was a much stronger predictor for fathers than mothers.

Help during Illness

Table 1.4 shows the predictors of mothers' and fathers' choices of children to serve as sources of support when facing illness or disability. This was the only domain of favoritism in which predictors of mothers' and fathers' choices overlapped more than they diverged. Both mothers and fathers preferred that care be provided by daughters and by children to whom they reported high levels of attachment. The odds of mothers and fathers choosing children to whom they reported high levels of attachment were similar; this was not the case for child's gender. Although both mothers and fathers preferred daughters over sons as sources of support, the odds ratio for fathers choosing daughters was not quite twice that of choosing sons, whereas the odds of mothers choosing daughters was nearly *twenty-two* times the odds of choosing sons ($p < .01$), indicating that gender similarity was a very high priority in mothers' choices. Value similarity and proximity were also much stronger predictors of mothers' than fathers' choices, as expected ($p < .05$ for both factors). As was the case for emotional closeness and confiding, children's achievements had virtually no influence on fathers' choices of caregivers.

Discussion and Conclusions

Our goal in this chapter was to examine differences in patterns and predictors of fathers' and mothers' favoritism toward their adult children. Based on a combination of theory and empirical research we hypothesized that there would be consistent differences between mothers and fathers. First, we hypothesized that mothers would be more likely to express favoritism, as a result of women's tendency to emphasize details of their interpersonal relationships and the greater closeness and interaction between children and their mothers compared to their fathers. Second, we hypothesized that the same factors would lead mothers to favor children on the basis of expressive predictors, such as similarity and attachment, whereas the more traditional values typically held by men would lead fathers to favor on the basis of children's achievement of normative adult statuses.

Our findings revealed three important patterns. First, the majority of parents of both genders favored children across all three relational domains under investigation, demonstrating that fathers, as well as mothers, tend to differentiate among their adult children. Second, there were neither consistent nor large differences in mothers' and fathers' likelihood of favoritism among their adult children. Mothers were more likely than fathers to name a child as a confidant, whereas fathers were more likely to name a child to whom they were most emotionally close. Parents of both genders were equally likely to name a child as a preferred caregiver. Although there were not large differences in mothers' and fathers' likelihood of favoring, they chose the same child only about half of the time for emotional closeness and confiding. In families in which both parents named a preferred caregiver, about two-thirds of the time mothers' and fathers' choices agreed; the greater agreement can be attributed to the fact that both parents overwhelmingly chose daughters, thus reducing the range of children in the family likely to be chosen.

Third, the findings revealed gender differences in predictors of which children mothers and fathers favored. Consistent with expectations, both gender and value similarity were more important in shaping mothers' than fathers' choices of adult children, as we have previously found to be the case except under conditions of high levels of stress (Suitor & Pillemer, 2000b, 2002).

The unexpected findings regarding fathers are particularly interesting and call for future research on changes in the fathers' roles across the life course. Contrary to our hypothesis, attachment was a stronger predictor of child choice for fathers than mothers. Further, we had anticipated that fathers would particularly value gender-traditional achievements, such as education and employment for sons and marriage and parenthood for daughters. In almost no cases, however, did fathers explain their choices based on status attainment of children. Such findings are particularly surprising given that age is one of the best predictors of gender-role traditionalism among White men (Powers et al., 2004). However, studies of gender-role traditionalism usually focus on general attitudes regarding gender roles; perhaps older men relax those expectations regarding their own adult children. Such a reduced emphasis on traditional expectations for one's role partners and increasing attention to expressive aspects of roles would be consistent with Carstensen's (1992) theory of socioemotional selectivity.

In summary, the findings presented here suggest that despite strong norms regarding equal treatment of children, the majority of both mothers and fathers favor some of their adult children over others (for financial "favoritism," see Remle and O'Rand, Chapter 2). Neither the prevalence nor the predictors of mothers' and fathers' favoritism was entirely consistent with the conceptual framework we developed based upon theories of gender differences in interpersonal relationships. We hope that future research will expand the study of gender differences in parental favoritism in the later years, focusing particular attention on the meaning of fatherhood in the lives of older men. Further, we hope that future studies will examine these processes among other ethnic groups in the United States and cross-culturally. Our study has only begun to shed light on gender differences in favoritism in the later years; we expect that in the tradition set by Vern Bengtson, new studies will bring more sophisticated and innovative approaches to the study of this understudied and complex phenomenon.

Postscript on the Contributions of Vern L. Bengtson

The scholarly work of Vern Bengtson has been extraordinarily wide-ranging, covering a variety of subfields within social gerontology as well as broader issues relevant to sociology and social psychology at large. Across his distinguished career, Bengtson's theoretical and empirical work on intergenerational relations stands out as having particularly great impact. Indeed, it is fair to say that the intergenerational solidarity paradigm is the most influential framework for studying families in later life, having guided a generation of scholars internationally and in the United States.

We view our contribution to this volume as very "Bengtsonian" in its conceptualization and orientation. In particular, we see as a hallmark of the Bengtson approach a desire to recognize the complexity of later-life families. In contrast to much other research on later-life families, Bengtson's work from the 1970s to the present has developed conceptual approaches that correspond to the empirically demonstrated complexity of family life (Bengtson & Black, 1973; Bengtson & Kuypers, 1971; Bengtson, Giarrusso, Mabry, & Silverstein, 2002; Bengtson & Roberts, 1991). Thus, as the field has turned to the issues of conflict and contradiction within intergenerational relations, he has striven to expand the solidarity model to incorporate these factors. His and his colleagues' work on typologies of later-life families and on deconstructing the individual factors making up the phenomenon of solidarity, his pioneering inclusion of multiple generations in the same study, and his efforts to study changes in family processes and outcomes over time all have brought family complexity to center stage.

Indeed, this is how a scientific field should progress. In a classic article, the noted scientist and educator Warren Weaver described the key progression in the history of science as a movement from simpler models to more complex ones. In the early stages of a field, concern is with straightforward questions of categorization, description, and relatively simple hypotheses. As the discipline progresses, the "organized complexity" of systems is acknowledged and investigated (Weaver, 1948). It is clear that such a movement continues and is in fact growing in the scientific study of intergenerational relations among adults. Much of this work was anticipated by Bengtson and colleagues, and they continued to spearhead understanding of the complex world of families as they change over the course of history and individual lives.

ACKNOWLEDGMENTS

This project was supported by grants from the National Institute on Aging (RO1 AG18869-01; 2RO1 AG18869-04), J. Jill Suitor and Karl Pillemer, Co-Principal Investigators. Karl Pillemer acknowledges support from an Edward R. Roybal Center grant from the National Institute on Aging (1 P50 AG11711-01). Jill Suitor wishes to acknowledge support from the Center on Aging and the Life Course at Purdue University.

The authors would like to thank Jori Sechrist and Megan Gilligan for their helpful comments on earlier drafts of this chapter. They also wish to thank Michael Bisciglia, Rachel Brown, Ilana S. Feld, Alison Green, Kimberly Gusman, Jennifer Jones, Dorothy Mecom, Michael Patterson, and Monisa Shackelford for their assistance in preparing the data for analysis. Finally, they would like to thank Mary Ellen Colten and her colleagues at the University of Massachusetts, Boston, for collecting the data for the project.

REFERENCES

Aldous, J., Klaus, E., & Klein, D. M. (1985). The understanding heart: Aging parents and their favorite children. *Child Development, 56*(2), 303–316.

Ali, A., & Toner, B. B. (1996). Gender differences in depressive response: The role of social support. *Sex Roles, 35*(5–6), 281–293.

Allison, P. D. (2005). *Fixed effects regression models for longitudinal data using SAS.* Cary, NC: The SAS Institute.

Alwin, D. F. (1976). Assessing school effects: Some identities. *Sociology of Education, 49*, 294–303.

Baker, L.A., & Daniels, D. (1990). Nonshared environmental influences and personality differences in adult twins. *Journal of Personality and Social Psychology, 58*(1), 103–110.

Bank, B. J., & Hansford, S. L. (2000). Gender and friendship: Why are men's best same-sex friendships less intimate and supportive? *Personal Relationships, 7*(1), 63–78.

Bedford, V. H. (1992). Memories of parental favoritism and the quality of parent-child ties in adulthood. *Journal of Gerontology: Series A: Biological Sciences and Medical Sciences, 47*(4), S149–S155.

Belansky, E. S., & Boggiano, A. K. (1994). Predicting helping behaviors: The role of gender and instrumental/expressive self-schemata. *Sex Roles, 30*(9–10), 647–661.

Bengtson, V. L., & Black, K. D. (1973). Intergenerational relations and continuities in socialization. In P. B. Baltes & K.W. Schaie (Eds.), *Life-span developmental psychology: Personality and socialization* (pp. 207–234). New York: Academic Press.

Bengtson, V. L., Giarrusso, R., Mabry, J. B., & Silverstein, M. (2002). Solidarity, conflict, and ambivalence: Complementary or competing perspectives on intergenerational relationships? *Journal of Marriage and the Family, 64*, 568–576.

Bengtson, V. L., & Kuypers, J. A. (1971). Generational difference and the developmental stake. *Aging and Human Development, 2*, 249–260.

Bengtson, V. L., & Roberts, R. E. L. (1991). Intergenerational solidarity in aging families: An example of formal theory construction. *Journal of Marriage and the Family, 5*, 856–870.

Brackbill, Y., Kitch, D., & Noffsinger, W. B. (1988). The perfect child (from an elderly parent's point of view). *Journal of Aging Studies, 2*(3), 243–254.

Brody, G. H., Stoneman, Z., & McCoy, J. K. (1992a). Associations of maternal and paternal direct and differential behavior with sibling relationships: Contemporaneous and longitudinal analyses. *Child Development, 63*(1), 82–92.

Brody, G. H., Stoneman, Z., & McCoy, J. K. (1992b). Parental differential treatment of siblings and sibling differences in negative emotionality. *Journal of Marriage and the Family, 54*(3), 643–651.

Carstensen, L. L. (1992). Motivation for social contact across the life span. In J. E. Jacobs (Ed.), *Developmental perspectives on motivation* (pp. 209–254). Lincoln, NE: University of Nebraska.

Chodorow, N. J. (1978). *The reproduction of mothering.* Berkeley, CA: University of California Press.

Cicirelli, V. G. (1995). The measure of caregiving daughters' attachment to elderly mothers. *Journal of Family Psychology, 9*(1), 89–94.

Cleese, A. F., & Bates, B. (2001). *How to manage your mother: Understanding the most difficult, complicated, and fascinating relationship in your life.* New York: Gardeners Book.

Cohen, S., & Cohen, E. (1997). *Mothers who drive their daughters crazy.* New York, NY: Prima.

Davey, A., Janke, M., & Salva, J. (2005). Antecedents of intergenerational support: Families in context and families as context. In M. Silverstein, R. Giarrusso, & V. L. Bengtson (Eds.), *Annual review of gerontology and geriatrics* (Vol. 2): *Intergenerational relations across time and place* (pp. 29–54). New York: Springer.

Faber, A., & Mazlish, E. (1987). How to talk so students will listen and listen so students will talk. *American Educator: The Professional Journal of the American Federation of Teachers, 11*(2), 37–42.

Gilligan, C. (1982). *In a different voice: Psychological theory and women's development.* Cambridge, MA: Harvard University Press.

Kaufman, G., & Uhlenberg, P. (1998). Effects of life course transitions on the quality of relationships between adult children and their parents. *Journal of Marriage and the Family, 60*(4), 924–938.

Kowal, A., & Kramer, L. (1997). Children's understanding of parental differential treatment. *Child Development, 68*(1), 113–126.

Lye, D. N. (1996). Adult child-parent relationships. *Annual Review of Sociology, 22*, 79–102.

McHale, S. M., Crouter, A. C., McGuire, S. A., & Updegraff, K. A. (1995). Congruence between mothers' and fathers' differential treatment of siblings: Links with family relations and children's well-being. *Child Development, 66*(1), 116–128.

McHale, S. M., Updegraff, K. A., Jackson-Newsom, J., Tucker, C. J., & Crouter, A. (2000). When does differential treatment have negative implications for siblings? *Social Development, 9*, 149–170.

O'Connor, T. G., Dunn, J., Jenkins, J. M., & Rasbash, J. (2006). Predictors of between-family and within-family variation in parent-child relationships. *Journal of Child Psychology and Psychiatry, 47*(5), 498–510.

Pillemer, K., Landreneau, T., & Suitor, J. J. (1996). Volunteers in a peer support project for caregivers: What motivates them? *American Journal of Alzheimer's Disease, 11*, 13–19.

Pillemer, K., & Suitor, J. J. (2006). Making choices: A within-family study of caregiver selection. *The Gerontologist, 46*, 439–448.

Pillemer, K., Suitor, J. J., Mock, S., Sabir, M., & Sechrist, J. (2007). Capturing the complexity of intergenerational relations: Exploring ambivalence within later-life families. *Journal of Social Issues, 63*, 775–791.

Powers, R., Suitor, J. J., Guerra, S., Shackelford, M., Mecom, D., & Gusman, K. (2004). Regional differences in gender role attitudes: Variations by gender and race. *Gender Issues, 21*, 40–54.

Putney, N. M., & Bengtson, V. L. (2001). Families, intergenerational relationships and kinkeeping in midlife. In M. E. Lachman (Ed.), *Handbook of midlife development* (pp. 528–570). New York: John Wiley and Sons.

Reevy, G. M., & Maslach, C. (2001). Use of social support: Gender and personality differences. *Sex Roles, 44*(7–8), 437–459.

Rice, T. W., & Coates, D. L. (1995). Gender role attitudes in the southern United States. *Gender and Society, 9*(6), 744–756.

Rossi, A. S., & Rossi, P. H. (1990). *Of human bonding: Parent-child relations across the life course.* Hawthorne, NY: Aldine de Gruyter.

Silverstein, M., & Bengtson, V. L. (1994). Does intergenerational social support influence the psychological well-being of older parents? The contingencies of declining health and widowhood. *Social Science and Medicine, 38*, 943–957.

Silverstein, M., & Bengtson, V. L. (1997). Intergenerational solidarity and the structure of adult child-parent relationships in American families. *American Journal of Sociology 103*(2), 429–460.

Silverstein, M., Conroy, S. J., Wang, H. T., Giarrusso, R., & Bengtson, V. L. (2002). Reciprocity in parent-child relations over the adult life-course. *Journal of Gerontology: Social Sciences, 57*, S3–S13.

Silverstein, M., Parrott, T. M., & Bengtson, V. L. (1995). Factors that predispose middle-aged sons and daughters to provide social support to older parents. *Journal of Marriage and the Family, 57*, 465–475.

Suitor, J. J., Minyard, S.A., & Carter, R.C. (2001). Did you see what I saw? Gender differences in perceptions of avenues to prestige among adolescents. *Sociological Inquiry, 71*, 437–454.

Suitor, J. J., & Pillemer, K. (1996). Sources of support and interpersonal stress in the networks of married caregiving daughters: Findings from a 2-year longitudinal study. *Journal of Gerontology: Social Sciences, 52*, 297–306.

Suitor, J. J., & Pillemer, K. (2000a). Did mom really love you best? Exploring the role of within-family differences in developmental histories on parental favoritism. *Motivation and Emotion, 24*, 104–119.

Suitor, J. J., & Pillemer, K. (2000b). When experience counts most: Differential effects of structural and experiential similarity on men's and women's receipt of support during bereavement. *Social Networks, 22,* 299–312.

Suitor, J. J, & Pillemer, K. (2002). Gender, social support, and experiential similarity during chronic stress: The case of family caregivers. *Advances in Medical Sociology: Social Networks and Health, 8,* 247–266.

Suitor, J. J., & Pillemer, K. (2006a). Choosing daughters: Exploring why mothers favor adult daughters over sons. *Sociological Perspectives, 49,* 139–160.

Suitor, J. J., Pillemer, K., & Sechrist, J. (2006b). Within-family differences in mothers' support to adult children. *Journal of Gerontology: Social Sciences, 16B,* S10–S17.

Suitor, J. J., & Pillemer, K. (2007). Mothers' favoritism in later life: The role of children's birth order. *Research on Aging, 29*(1), 32–55.

Suitor, J. J., Sechrist, J., Pilkuhn, M., Pardo, T., & Pillemer, K. (2008). Within-family differences in parent-child relations across the life course. *Current Directions in Psychological Science, 17*(5), 334–338.

Suitor, J. J., Sechrist, J., & Pillemer, K. (2007a). When mothers have favorites: Conditions under which mothers differentiate among their adult children. *Canadian Journal on Aging, 26,* 85–99.

Suitor, J. J., Sechrist, J., & Pillemer, K. (2007b). Within-family differences in mothers' support to adult children in Black and White families. *Research on Aging, 29,* 410–435.

Suitor, J. J., Sechrist, J., Steinhour, M., & Pillemer, K. (2006). I'm sure she chose me! Consistency in intergenerational reports of mothers' favoritism in later-life families. *Family Relations, 55,* 526–538.

Troll, L. E., & Fingerman, K. L. (1996). Connections between parents and their adult children. In C. Magai & S. H. McFadden (Eds.), *Handbook of Emotion, Adult Development, and Aging.* San Diego, CA: Academic Press.

Tucker, C. J., McHale, S. M., & Crouter, A. C. (2003). Conflict resolution: Links with adolescent family relationships and individual well-being. *Journal of Family Issues, 24*(6), 715–736.

Vitulli, W. F., & Holland, B. E. (1993). College students' attitudes toward relationships with their parents as function of gender. *Psychological Reports, 72*(3), 744–746.

Volling, B. L. (1997). The family correlates of maternal and paternal perceptions of differential treatment in early childhood. *Family Relations, 46*(3), 227–236.

Volling, B.L., & Elins, J. L. (1998). Family relationships and children's emotional adjustment as correlates of maternal and paternal differential treatment: A replication with toddler and preschool siblings. *Child Development, 69*(6), 1640–1656.

Weaver, W. (1948). Probability, rarity, interest, and surprise. *The Scientific Monthly, 67*(6), 390–392.

Williams, C. L. (1993). Psychoanalytic theory and the sociology of gender. In P. England (Ed.), *Theory on Gender/Feminism on Theory.* New York: Aldine de Gruyter.

Worthen, M. F. (2000). The role of empathy in adolescent friendship. *Dissertation Abstracts International: Section B: The Sciences and Engineering, 61*(2–B), 1116.

CHAPTER TWO

Intergenerational Solidarity in Blended Families

The Inequality of Financial Transfers to Adult Children and Stepchildren

R. Corey Remle and Angela M. O'Rand

The dramatic increase of blended families over the past four decades has introduced new contexts for studying the dynamics of parent-child relationships in aging families. The growing diversity of family arrangements includes those who are related by marriage, birth, or adoption and those who join existing families voluntarily through remarriage (Ahrons, 1994; Marks, 1995) or as a result of intergenerational linkages (e.g., as children of a remarried partner). However this occurs, remarriages alter kinship statuses and probably affect family solidarity in ways we still do not understand. As such, a broader definition of family that includes blended families strengthens, but also complicates, our understanding of family solidarity (Amato & Booth, 1997).

In this chapter, we define blended families as kin networks that include biological kin and stepkin encompassing several generations and households (Cohler & Altergott, 1995; Riley & Riley, 1993). Riley (1983) conceptualized the kin network as a latent kin matrix of biologically and socially related individuals that transcends generations and households. Latency in the network reflects the underlying potential of members to share instrumental, emotional and other resources that is activated primarily when someone within the network is in need. Otherwise, family support systems are not always active or manifest. Silverstein, Bengtson, and Lawton (1997) stressed this aspect of the latent kin matrix: "If family relationships alternately shift between latency and activity, then it is important to consider the latent *potential* of kinship relations—insofar as it triggers or enables manifest functions" (p. 431, emphasis in the original).

The latent potential of stepkin relationships has received less attention than that of biologically related family members. Instead, theories of family solidarity have focused more on biological relationships (e.g., Bengtson, Biblarz, & Roberts, 2002; Bengtson & Harootyan, 1994). We argue that stepfamilies and the probable reconfiguration of family solidarity after remarriages deserve more attention and can extend our current understanding of latent and manifest patterns of family support.

We use several waves of the Health and Retirement Study (HRS) initiated in 1992 to examine patterns of financial transfer receipt by adult children from parents over time. We consider financial transfer as a form of solidarity and compare the prevalence of and conditions that precipitate transfers to biological children and stepchildren by biological parents and step-parents. Multi-level models permit us to examine these processes while controlling for non-independence of observations within families.

Stepfamilies

Bumpass, Sweet, and Castro-Martin (1990) reported that 42% of divorced parents in 1984 chose to remarry within five years—a decline from the 49% who reported having done so in 1970. They also estimated that over 70% of separated and divorced women would eventually remarry. A large majority of separated and divorced women at that time also had children under age 18. The high remarriage rate caused a sharp increase in the number of stepchildren in the United States (Bumpass, Raley, & Sweet, 1995). Depending on the timing of the remarriage, the structure of blended families could include children of either the father or the mother, children who were the biological progeny of both parents (i.e., those born after the remarriage), or a combination of both (Connidis, 2010; Rossi & Rossi, 1990). Thus, for this research, the term "blended families" refers to any remarriages that included children from previous relationships as well as to remarriages that included both children from previous relationships and children born after the remarriage (i.e., half siblings).

Estimates indicate that 30–35% of American children will live with a step-parent before turning 18 years old (Bumpass, Raley, & Sweet, 1995). However, little research has examined the impact of living with a parent and stepparent on intergenerational solidarity. While not all of the adult stepchildren of respondents in the HRS sample necessarily lived with a stepparent, it is reasonable to assume that many of them did and, further, that many lived with mothers and stepfathers. (The average length for HRS remarriages in the sample was 13.5 years. Many adult children in 1992 would likely have been minors at the time of remarriage. Physical custody was most often awarded to the mother after a divorce at the time.)

The Effects of Divorce and Remarriage on Family Solidarity

Previous work has demonstrated that divorce results in significant declines in intergenerational solidarity between parents and children and especially between noncustodial parents and their children (Lawton, Silverstein, & Bengtson, 1994; Silverstein, Bengtson, & Lawton, 1997; White, 1994). This pattern is more common between divorced fathers and adult children and probably reflects custody decisions that weaken ties (Amato & Booth, 1997; Aquilino, 1994). Other studies that do not employ the solidarity framework have examined aspects of solidarity between divorced fathers and their adult children. They have found that parental divorce results in less frequent contact, lower levels of affection, and reduced feelings of obligation (Cooney & Uhlenberg, 1990; Marks, 1995; Rossi & Rossi, 1990; Shapiro, 2004). Both physical and emotional distance can persist or increase between adult children and their divorced parents over time. Uhlenberg (1990) found this to be particularly true for divorced fathers, who have the lower likelihood of coresiding with adult children. Also, where children reside after parental divorce moderates the quality of their long-term relationships with their fathers (Cooney & Uhlenberg, 1990; Shapiro & Lambert, 1999).

Much of the research on family solidarity has defined solidarity as the strength of the ties either between mothers and adult children or between fathers and adult children. Analyses of affectual solidarity have shown that relations between adult children and parents are weakened by divorce and that this particularly differs in gender-based dyadic relations in late life (Connidis, 2010; Cooney, 1994; Cooney & Uhlenberg, 1990; Shapiro, 2003; Silverstein, Lawton, & Bengtson, 1994; White, 1994). Such studies make valuable contributions to the literature regarding family solidarity over the life course. However, the conceptual reduction of family solidarity to ties between adult children and each divorced parent disregards the complexity of intersecting adult lives when divorced parents remarry and introduce stepparents, potentially with their own ties to children from previous marriages, into the kin matrix.

The focus on specific parent-child ties deflects attention away from the family as a unit of analysis (Davey, Janke, & Savla, 2005; Hagestad, 2003). Consequently, the roles that stepparents play in altering intergenerational solidarity within families over time have been largely ignored. Most studies of stepfamilies have focused on the relationship challenges faced within stepfamilies that involve young or adolescent children. The addition of stepkin as part of the latent kin matrix provides a more detailed exploration of various family structures and intergenerational relationships. This expansion is essential to develop a fuller understanding of the individual life course, family dynamics, and the cobiographical influence they have on one another in relation to sharing valuable resources between generations.

Although the association between reduced contact and decreased affectual solidarity is well established, the effects of the construction of intergenerational linkages between stepparents and adult children—and reconstruction of family solidarity—have received limited attention. Regarding affectual solidarity, White (1992) reports that the quality of the ties between remarried parents and their children was not significantly different from the quality of the ties for parents and children from intact families. There were no significant differences for the quality of ties between adult children and remarried mothers compared to the ties between adult children and single mothers (White, 1994).

Further evidence indicates that custodial arrangements have mixed effects on relationship quality with biological parents who remarry (White, 1994). The quality of the father-adult child relationship for children who had lived with a remarried mother was not significantly different from the relationship quality with fathers for those children who lived in single-mother households. Conversely, if children lived with remarried fathers, the mother-adult child relationship quality was significantly lower. A negative correlation was reported between living with a custodial father and frequency of contact with the mother. Also, significantly more contacts and stronger relationships with stepfathers were identified, indicating that the addition of stepfathers to kin matrices improved family solidarity when stepfathers were accepted as family members (White, 1994). By comparison, the addition of a stepmother was not as well received by children who lived with remarried fathers.

However, in the case of functional solidarity (measured as financial assistance), multiple studies found that remarried parents were more likely to behave like divorced parents than to behave like continuously married parents, in spite of the typical increase in income and assets that accompanies remarriage (Clark & Kenney, 2010; Killian, 2004; White, 1992). Instead, researchers showed that the increase in the number of children of remarried couples was a primary reason for reduced financial assistance of adult children relative to children with continuously married parents (Killian, 2004; White, 1992). They speculated that the higher number of children and reductions in potentially transferable resources (in comparison to intact-marriage households) occurred because the parents were possibly supporting two families—the children/stepchildren from previous marriages and young children added to the family after the remarriage. The lack of social norms regarding how much responsibility midlife parents have toward adult children from previous marriages has led to ambivalence about financial obligations in exchanges within multigenerational kinship structures (Killian & Ferrell, 2005).

In another study, White (1994) compared single-mother families to remarried families and found that the likelihood of receiving instrumental support was significantly higher for adult children with remarried mothers. No effect was seen for adult children with remarried fathers. However, the summary measure of having received support did not include financial assistance. On the other hand, the summary measure of perceived support included whether children believed they could go to their parents for a loan of $200. For perceived support, there was no significant difference for those who had lived with a remarried mother, but those who had lived with a remarried father were much less likely to consider the father and stepmother as a source of emergency support. Though custodial arrangements are not legally binding after age 18, many parent-child ties remain altered by parental divorce and remarriage long after children have reached adulthood (Booth & Amato, 1994).

Stepfamilies and Normative Solidarity

Cherlin (1978) characterized stepfamilies as "incomplete institutions" primarily because social norms for them were not well established. The increase in cohabiting unions among divorced Americans since then has further complicated the development of social norms (Cherlin & Furstenberg, 1994). Nevertheless, research indicates that family structure mediates the willingness to honor kin obligations (Bengtson, 2001; Cherlin & Furstenberg, 1994; Killian, 2004). Obligations to assist biological children are felt more strongly than those to assist stepchildren—though not to the exclusion of stepchildren

(Aquilino, 2005; Ganong & Coleman, 2006; Killian & Ferrell, 2005). Rossi and Rossi (1990) attributed this to what they called "differentiated norms of family obligations."

Normative beliefs about responsibilities to other generations are generally weakened by remarriage, although a recent review of relevant literature identifies some shifts in stepparents' felt responsibility to children (Ganong & Coleman, 1999). Studies of biological fathers after divorce and stepfathers and biological fathers after a remarriage focus primarily on blended families with young children. However, some information drawn from these studies may be extrapolated to the normative financial obligations parents and stepparents have toward adult children. For example, Ganong, Coleman, and Mistina (1995) discovered the specific belief that coresident stepfathers should pay for tutoring services for a stepchild. However, remarriage moderated the obligations for biological fathers to pay for these services, either because remarried mothers had increased resources or because remarried fathers' resources would be limited by the higher number of children to be responsible for. In fact, many respondents explicitly stated that men should consider carefully their potential responsibilities in raising stepchildren before choosing to remarry (Ganong & Coleman, 1999). Some findings indicated that biological fathers' child support payments could be reduced if either parent remarried but especially if biological fathers remarried and assumed additional responsibilities for coresident stepchildren.

Later research demonstrated that financial matters cause conflict within stepfamilies. For example, some stepparents resent having to pay for stepchildren's college expenses, and some biological parents resent that stepparents do not contribute equally to expenses for young or adult stepchildren (Coleman et al., 2001). Aquilino (2005) found relationship quality to be an important determinant of stepparents' beliefs about financial obligations to adult stepchildren. Positive beliefs about providing financial support increased as relationship quality increased, but once baseline perceived obligations were included in the model, relationship quality stopped mediating the change in stepparents' beliefs when the child became a nonresident adult. These results are important for understanding normative solidarity or intergenerational obligations within stepfamilies and the latent potential support structure between generations, but closer attention should be paid to the elusive pattern of functional solidarity. This can be examined by researching the downward flow of financial transfers from older parents and stepparents to adult children.

Intergenerational Transfers

Since relationships are dynamic, there are observable fluctuations in the closeness, intensity, or frequency of contact within families over many years (Rossi & Rossi, 1990). However, the basic linkages between family members often remain lifelong influences on individual behavior in spite of changes in the nature or quality of relationships (Bengtson, Biblarz, & Roberts, 2002; Lawton, Silverstein, & Bengtson, 1994). Within an extended family, continuity and intergenerational bonds may be strengthened through the sharing of private economic resources between adult generations. The provision of monetary gifts is interpreted specifically as a behavioral indicator of functional solidarity (Bengtson & Harootyan, 1994; Kohli & Kunemund, 2003).

"Intergenerational transfer" is a broad term referring to the sharing of valuable resources across generations within a family. These resources can be redistributed in any of three instrumental currencies—space, time, and money—and can flow in two directions across generations (Soldo & Hill, 1993). Space transfers include shared housing or the coresidence of multiple adult generations. Time transfers are instrumental assistance between parents and adult children measured in the amount of time spent helping family members with various tasks. Money transfers come in two forms, *inter vivos* transfers and bequests. Financial assistance from midlife parents to adult children is a dynamic transaction affected by cobiographical trajectories for all involved.

Midlife adults who have living parents and progeny may engage in transfers with either generation in either currency, and the transfer may occur in one direction or, in the case of an exchange relationship, in both directions (Soldo & Hill, 1993). For life course researchers, transfer types and the flow of transfers are a valuable research area for understanding the importance of adult family relationships. For example, resource flows between generations tend to follow a life course pattern (Wong, Capoferro, & Soldo, 1999; Logan & Spitze, 1996; McGarry & Schoeni, 1995). Midlife adults with children are much more likely to be donors than recipients (Killian, 2004; Kronebusch & Schlesinger, 1994; Soldo & Hill, 1993). Parents tend to assist children through the transition-dense phase of young adulthood and often contribute to higher education costs (Hagestad, 2003). Financial transfers to adult children, regardless of the child's social status as student or worker, remain more common from midlife parents than transfers in the opposite direction (Berry, 2001; Kronebusch & Schlesinger, 1994; McGarry & Schoeni, 1995). As parents become incapacitated or need assistance in late life, adult children may begin providing support to parents.

In the Intergenerational Linkages Survey of 1990, nearly half of all parents had given large financial gifts to adult children (Harootyan & Vorek, 1994). Financial assistance occurred most among tight-knit families. Families weaker in affectual ties but with strong beliefs that parents and adult children should support each other were also more likely to make transfers than other family types, suggesting that perceived obligations were important to actual transfer behavior. This finding was later echoed by Silverstein, Bengtson, and Lawton (1997), who found that tight-knit and obligatory family types were more likely to give help than sociable and intimate but distant and detached family types.

Also using data from the Intergenerational Linkages Survey, Kronebusch and Schlesinger (1994) estimated that private transfers between age groups in 1990 in the United States equaled $1.1 trillion. However, this is an aggregate value that includes time transfers and coresidence that have been assigned monetary values (based on the purchase cost of comparable goods and services) as well as monetary transfers. Estimates based on these data indicate that approximately 30% of all transfers were in the form of monetary gifts. Thus, $330 million is the rough estimate of the total private financial transfers across the U.S. population in 1990. It may be more appropriate to examine transfer values at the individual or household level. Kronebusch and Schlesinger (1994) found that middle-aged adults gave between $1,500 and $2,000 to their college-aged adult children (18 to 24 years old) and that as children aged, the average amount of the transfer declined. Specifically, the groups who were most likely to give financial assistance to adult children were parents between ages 55–64 and ages 65–74. Cox and Raines (1985) found an average transfer to be $2,100 (in 1979 dollars).

Previous research has demonstrated that family structure affects the likelihood of financial transfers to adult children (Berry, 2001; Furstenberg, Hoffman, & Shrestha, 1995; Killian, 2004; Pezzin & Schone, 1999). Other research has found that the depletion of income and assets that often accompanies divorce is strongly correlated with a lower likelihood of providing financial assistance to adult children (Aquilino, 1994; Eggebeen, 1992; Cooney & Uhlenberg, 1992; White, 1992). Furstenberg, Hoffman, and Shrestha (1995) examined the influence of marital disruption on financial assistance to adult children. Divorced and widowed mothers were less likely than married parents to provide financial assistance, but there was no significant difference in the amount transferred when transfers were made. Divorced and widowed fathers were less likely than both married parents and single mothers to make transfers. The amounts transferred by divorced fathers were an average of 18% less than married parents' amounts. However, none of these studies differentiated continuously married parents from remarried parents, and only a few mentioned differences between biological children and stepchildren.

Studies of financial assistance from remarried households tend to show that remarried households make fewer transfers and transfer lower amounts than do intact-family households. Killian (2004) found that a lower percentage of households with at least one stepchild gave financial assistance to adult children than did households without stepchildren. The households of remarried parents who both had children from previous relationships made the lowest percentage of transfers and gave significantly lower average amounts compared to households without stepchildren. When the focus turned to stepchildren's receipt of transfers, Killian's (2004) results correspond with the findings of other studies that stepchildren were less likely to receive transfers than children from intact families (Berry, 2001; Eggebeen, 1992). The lone exception among such studies found that remarried parents provided lower financial amounts as well but found no significant differences between remarried and continuously married parents for the likelihood that such transfers were made (Pezzin & Schone, 1999).

Previous researchers have theorized that parents may feel less obligated to assist stepchildren but have only generalized this idea to cover all stepchildren without considering any differences between mothers' children or fathers' children (Ganong & Coleman, 1999; Killian & Ferrell, 2005; Rossi & Rossi, 1990; White, 1992). Killian (2004) used household-level data to differentiate between maternal children and paternal children as transfer recipients. He characterized HRS households from the 2000 wave as intact married households with biological children, households with maternal children only, households with paternal children only, and households with both maternal and paternal children. He found that while 32.5% of intact-marriage households had made financial transfers to children, the percentages were lower for households with stepchildren. Nearly 31% of households with only maternal children made transfers, 21.4% of households with only paternal children made transfers, and 11.7% of households with both maternal and paternal children provided financial assistance to nonresident adult children. In other words, all households with paternal children were much less likely to make intergenerational transfers than intact first-marriage households, while households with maternal children only made a slightly lower percentage of transfers.

The fraction of adult children identified across studies who receive transfers varies slightly (depending on sampling decisions) but tends to be less than one-fifth of adult children at any one time. Many studies limit their samples to adult children who do not reside with parents. Eggebeen and Hogan (1990) estimated that 17% of all nonresident adult children in the 1988 wave of the National Survey of Families and Households (NSFH) had received transfers of $200 or more from their parents over the previous five years. A similar percentage received transfers in the 1993–1994 wave of the NSFH. In the 1992 wave of the HRS, 16% received a financial transfer of $500 or more from their parents (Berry, 2001). In the 1994 wave of HRS, the gift threshold was lowered to $100, and the percentage of children who received transfers increased to 18.6% (Berry, 2001). These percentages included children of single parents as well. Among the children of HRS married and remarried parents, approximately 17.6% of adult children received financial assistance at each wave between 1992 and 1998. An examination of family transfers with a panel study across time should yield a higher percentage of adult children who received at least one transfer from parents as siblings or stepsiblings may receive financial support at different stages in the life course.

This chapter focuses on two intimately related issues regarding family-level transfer behaviors. First, we examine longitudinal data to reveal the effects of family structure on the likelihood of transfer receipt among adult children over time. Second, we examine the differential treatment of stepchildren based on whether the biological parent in the remarried household is the mother or the father.

Data

The HRS is a nationally representative survey of the 1931–1941 birth cohorts. Spouses of survey respondents were also interviewed, regardless of their age. The stratified, multi-stage area probability design included over-sampling of African Americans, Hispanics, and Floridians. The first wave, conducted in 1992, included face-to-face interviews with 12,652 individuals representing 7,607 households (Howell, 1995). This project uses four waves of HRS data: 1992, 1994, 1996, and 1998.

Data on family structure and intergenerational transfers were collected from one member of each household (the family respondent). Data on the financial status of the household were collected from one member of each household (the financial respondent). In married households, it was very rare for one person to be both the family and financial respondent. Instead, the wife was much more likely to answer the family structure and transfer questions, and the husband was more likely to answer the financial questions. Since information about transfers is child-specific, the family respondent answered transfer questions while discussing each child with the researcher rather than the financial respondent addressing the issue.

From 1992 to 1998, information about 16,263 adult children was provided by married family respondents who were mothers/stepmothers. In order to properly classify adult children of remarried parents as maternal children/paternal stepchildren or paternal children/maternal stepchildren for this research, HRS households where the father was the initial family respondent were excluded from the sample.

The biennial panel design of the HRS provides a unique opportunity to examine multiple opportunities for financial assistance and to reduce the limited information that derives from cross-sectional or two-wave studies. The HRS allows for a better estimation of routine assistance provided over a seven-year period since respondents were asked at four separate times whether a financial transfer of $500 or more had been given to an adult child since the previous wave (i.e., in the previous two years). (At baseline in 1992, the question specified "over the past year".)

Table 2.1 shows the descriptive statistics for the 15,689 adult children for whom information is available regarding kinship status, demographic characteristics, and transfer information in a minimum of two waves of data. Over 80% of the adult children remained in the sample for all four waves. For 1,540 individuals (9.8% of the sample), data are available for only two waves.

Comparisons of those lost to follow-up indicate that lost adult children were more likely to be older and of minority status and to have received a smaller percentage of financial transfers than those who remained in the sample. However, there were no evident differences by kinship status. In 1992, the median length of remarried parents' current marriages was 16.6 years, indicating that family structures were primarily stable once the parent remarried and that many of the adult children became stepchildren as youngsters or adolescents. Also, three-quarters of remarriages occurred after a divorce. Fewer stepfamily structures were the result of widowhood and remarriage. In this study, adult children were assigned kinship statuses as either biological children, maternal children/paternal stepchildren, or paternal children/maternal stepchildren based on the family respondents' first identification of each child's relation to her and to her spouse. Each household also counted the number of living parents (i.e., the eldest kin) at each wave of data collection.

Table 2.1. Descriptive statistics for adult children of married HRS parents

	All Children n = 15,689	Biological Children n = 10,225	All Stepchildren n = 5,470	Mothers' Children n = 2,718	Fathers' Children n = 2,752
Men[a]	51.2	51.5	50.7	49.7	51.7
Non-White	17.8	17.2	18.9	19.1	18.7
Hispanic	9.6	11.1	6.6***	7.1	6.2
30 and older at initial entry	49.4	46.3	55.9***	56.8	54.9
Average age (SE)					
in 1992[b]	29.6 (0.05)	29.1 (0.06)	30.7*** (0.08)	30.8 (0.12)	30.6 (0.13)
in 1994[c]	31.3 (0.05)	30.7 (0.06)	32.5*** (0.09)	32.5 (0.12)	32.4 (0.13)
in 1996[d]	33.1 (0.05)	32.4 (0.06)	34.3*** (0.09)	34.3 (0.12)	34.4 (0.12)
in 1998[e]	35.0 (0.05)	34.4 (0.06)	36.3*** (0.09)	36.2 (0.13)	36.4 (0.13)
Mean years of education	13.3 (0.02)	13.6 (0.02)	12.8*** (0.03)	12.8 (0.04)	12.9† (0.04)
Attended school between 1992 and 1998	18.2	20.9	13.1***	14.0	12.2†
Married before 1998	69.5	69.5	69.3	71.0	67.6†
Ever coresided 1992–1998	21.2	28.1	8.2***	12.1	4.3***
Returned to parents' home after living independently	7.5	9.1	4.3***	5.7	2.8**
Mean number of siblings	3.7 (0.02)	3.2 (0.02)	4.6*** (0.03)	4.6 (0.05)	4.6 (0.05)
Received 1 or more transfers during period	36.2	41.5	26.2***	30.2	22.3***
1 transfer	18.4	20.5	14.3***	16.2	12.8**
2 transfers	10.4	12.1	7.0***	8.7	5.6***
3 transfers	5.3	6.3	3.1***	4.0	2.7***
4 transfers	2.1	2.6	1.1***	1.2	1.1
Mean amount received overall (logged)	8.00 (0.02)	8.10 (0.02)	7.76*** (0.03)	7.79 (0.04)	7.71 (0.05)
Mean amount received overall (in 2005 $)	3,572	3,947	2,810***	2,906	2,684
Data available for sample:					
for 4 waves	81.0	81.6	79.9***	80.9	78.9
for 3 waves	9.2	8.6	10.3***	9.7	10.9
for 2 waves	9.8	9.8	9.8	9.4	10.2

Note: Various *t*-tests for between-group differences were significant as noted.

†p < .05, *p < .01, **p < .001, ***p < .0001

[a] All numbers are percentages unless otherwise noted

[b] n = 14,688

[c] n = 15,306

[d] n = 14,793

[e] n = 13,880

This variable was included to characterize the multigenerational relationships of the midlife adults' family structures.

Characteristics of Adult Children and Stepchildren in the HRS

The full sample of adult children ranged from 18 to 59 years in age. The average age for the sample was 29.6 years in 1992. For the analyses conducted in this chapter, adult children were divided into three age categories: college age (18–23), under 30 (24–29), and 30 and older. This category structure was assigned based on presumed normative, age-related life course transitions that are likely to occur for younger adults in particular. On the other hand, those who entered the sample at age 30 or older were more likely to have completed the major milestones associated with the transition-dense period of young adulthood (e.g., post-secondary education, establishing a separate residence, marriage). Education values ranged from 2 to 17 years, where 17 represented postgraduate education.

The majority (65.2%) of the adult child sample were the biological children of both parents (hereinafter referred to as "biological children"). The remaining individuals were biologically related to only one of the two parents and were stepchildren to the other parent. A nearly equivalent number were biologically related to only the mother or only the father: 2,718 were maternal children/paternal stepchildren, and 2,752 were paternal children/maternal stepchildren. Table 2.1 identifies key demographic and life course statuses of the adult children by kinship status. T-tests were completed for each characteristic to determine if there were any significant differences between kinship statuses. The table shows statistically significant results of the t-tests.

A substantial number of adult children in the sample—over 36%—received financial assistance, regardless of family structure. To explore this further, the subsample of all biological children was compared to the subsample of all adult stepchildren. This table provides the first indication that adult stepchildren were treated differently when it came to financial assistance from their parents/stepparents. From 1992 to 1998, stepchildren were significantly less likely to receive financial assistance than biological children. While over two-fifths of biological children received financial gifts of $500 or more, only 26.2% of stepchildren received similar assistance.

There were no significant differences between groups in relation to gender. Although stepchildren tended to be non-White, they were significantly less likely to be Hispanic. This was likely correlated with the fact that Hispanic marriages are significantly less likely to end in divorce and Hispanics are less likely to remarry than non-Hispanics (Bumpass, Sweet, & Castro-Martin, 1990; Sweet & Bumpass, 1987). The average age of stepchildren was nearly two years higher than the average age of biological children at each wave. However, as will be shown in the logistic regression analyses reported below, the adult child's kinship status as a stepchild did not moderate the significant effects of many other characteristics, including age, on the likelihood of receiving a financial transfer from parents. In other words, if remarriages accounted for the age differences between stepchildren and biological children, one would expect the effects of age to become insignificant or to be much less influential in predicting transfer receipt once kinship status is included in the model, but this did not occur.

On average, stepchildren had significantly less education than biological children (12.8 vs. 13.6 years). Even though stepchildren would have had more time to acquire more education, since a higher percentage of them had passed the normative ages for post-secondary education, their education levels were lower. This was also reflected in the significantly lower percentage of stepchildren who were reported to have attended school during the data collection period covered here. While 20.9% of biological children were still in or had returned to school at some point between 1992 and 1998, only 13.1% of stepchildren were in school during that time frame.

The percentage of biological children who coresided with parents at least once between 1992 and 1998 was nearly 350% greater than that of stepchildren. The mean number of siblings for stepchildren was 4.6 compared to 3.2 siblings for biological children. The construction of a second nuclear family typically brought together two parents with children from previous relationships. Depending on the life course timing of the remarriage for the parents, a binuclear family may have also included additional biological children (Ahrons, 1994). Marital histories and the growth of stepfamilies in recent decades may help explain some of the significant differences in ages between stepchildren and biological children if some of the younger adult children in the sample were products of second (or later) marriages.

As noted above, biological children and stepchildren differed significantly as recipients of any financial assistance from their parents (i.e., one or more transfers of $500 or more). Figure 2.1 shows that this was true for the number of each group who received multiple transfers as well. While 326 of all adult children received four reported transfers between 1992 and 1998, only 60 of those recipients were stepchildren. Nearly four times as many biological children as stepchildren received three transfers (644 individuals com-

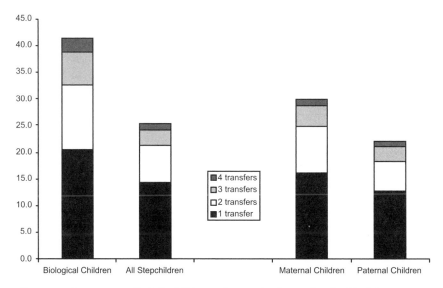

Figure 2.1. Percentage of adult children who received transfers by kinship status.

pared to 170). Of those who received two transfers, only 23.6% were step-children. In other words, relatively few stepchildren were transfer recipients, but comparatively, even fewer were recipients of multiple financial transfers from their parents. Only 23% of all multiple-transfer recipients were step-children. Transfer pattern differences between biological children and step-children as well as stepchildren by relation to one parent or the other are illustrated in figure 2.1.

Over all transfers, stepchildren also received over $1,000 less on average than biological children. (All monetary values are reported in 2005 U.S. dollars using the inflation calculator provided by the United States Bureau of Labor Statistics at http://www.bls.gov/cpi/.)

Comparisons of stepchildren based on their relationships to their respective mothers or fathers revealed interesting differences as well (columns 4 and 5 of table 2.1). Paternal children/maternal stepchildren were significantly less likely to receive financial transfers than maternal children/paternal step-children. Twenty-two percent of the paternal children/maternal stepchildren received at least one financial transfer over four waves of data collection while 30% of the maternal children/paternal stepchildren received financial transfers in that same time frame. This implies that remarried fathers were more likely to provide financial assistance to their stepchildren than to their adult biological children. (Another possible explanation for this finding is that if fathers provided financial gifts to their own children, they did not inform their wives, the family respondents who reported transfers during data collection. However, this potential explanation could not be explored because married fathers were not asked separately about financial transfers to children.) The significant differences regarding transfers received by stepchildren remained for multiple transfers over time with the exception of those few stepchildren on either side who received financial transfers consistently over time (i.e., transfers were repeated at each wave). The disparity for financial transfers existed despite the fact that there were no significant differences between paternal children/maternal stepchildren and maternal children/paternal stepchildren in terms of gender, race, ethnicity, or age.

Adult paternal children/maternal stepchildren were three times less likely to have coresided than adult maternal children/paternal stepchildren. This could be an echo of the custody arrangements regarding minors in which physical custody of young children was most often awarded to the mother (Cherlin & Furstenberg, 1994; Hoffman & Duncan, 1988). Coresiding adult stepchildren were very simply more likely to have stayed with the original custodial parent and family. Subsequently, 12.3% of the maternal children/paternal stepchildren coresided with the mother and stepfather, and 4.1% of the paternal children/maternal stepchildren coresided with the father and stepmother, within the four waves examined.

Multivariate Models Predicting Transfers from Kinship Status and Children's Characteristics

To investigate how kinship status was associated with financial transfers net of other individual and family characteristics, we used fixed-effects regression to predict (1) the likelihood that at least one financial transfer was received at any time between 1992 and 1998 and (2) the logged amount of money received during that time for the subsample of 5,535 adult children who received transfers. As noted above, 36.2% of the entire sample received one or more transfers during this time.

Model 2 of table 2A.1 provides clear evidence of the negative effect of being a stepchild on the likelihood of receiving a transfer: Stepchildren were 34% less likely to receive financial transfers than biological children based on a sample of 15,689 adult children drawn from 4,377 families. The inclusion of this variable had a strong effect on model fit (BIC difference = -29) when model 2 is compared to model 1. Parsing stepchildren into their kinship status as either maternal children/paternal stepchildren or paternal children/maternal step-children in model 3 shows that the former are not significantly different from biological children. However, the latter are 56% less likely than biological children to receive transfers of $500 or more. Not all stepfamilies are equal in terms of intergenerational transfers, with paternal children/maternal step-children at a significant disadvantage compared to children from other family structures.

Results in model 3 also showed the effects of adult child characteristics. Minorities were 25% less likely to receive transfers compared to Whites, and Hispanic children were 67% less likely to receive transfers than non-Hispanic children. Age was also an influential factor: College-aged adult children were nearly three times as likely as adult children over age 30 to receive a financial transfer from their midlife parents. If children had attended school at some point during the study period, they were nearly 2.2 times more likely to have received transfers as children who had completed school prior to 1992. Married adult children were 11% less likely to receive transfers than adult children who were not married when they entered the dataset and did not marry between 1992 and 1998. Those who coresided with their parents (or a parent and stepparent) were 2.2 times more likely to receive financial assistance than nonresident children. This included those adult children who coresided with the parents when they entered the dataset and those who returned to their parents' homes after living independently. As the number of siblings increased, the probability that any adult child received a transfer declined by 28%.

Factors that predict whether the amount of financial assistance from parents varied between biological children and stepchildren are shown in table 2A.2. Stepchildren received significantly less than biological children. However, when the stepchild variable was disaggregated according to parental relationships, there was no disadvantage experienced by maternal children/paternal stepchildren. However, an $820 disadvantage was experienced by paternal children/maternal stepchildren. (The equations to determine the logged value of money received in 2005 U.S. dollars are noted in table 2A.2.)

Other differences indicated a $1,134 disadvantage for African American children and a $912 disadvantage for Hispanic children. College-age adult children received $1,653 more than the "30-and-over" age group. Children who lived with parents/stepparents at some point between 1992 and 1998 received the equivalent of $771 more than nonresident children. With each additional sibling, transfers declined by $393.

Summary and Conclusions

We used data from the first four waves of the HRS (1992 to 1998) to demonstrate that kinship status was an important predictor of the likelihood that midlife parents provided financial assistance to their adult children or stepchildren. We observed several aspects of functional solidarity: how family and stepfamily members are linked via intergenerational transfers; what latent kinship matrix characteristics affect the activation of financial assistance; and how parent and adult child characteristics may influence the likelihood of instrumental support for adult children.

This research demonstrates that the likelihood of transfer receipt for adult children varies over time. Repeated measures of transfers over a short period of time (i.e., four measures over seven to eight years) reveal that more adult children receive financial transfers than previous research has indicated (Berry, 2001; Eggebeen & Hogan, 1990; McGarry & Schoeni, 1995). Over 36% of adult children received at least one transfer from parents, a higher percentage than cross-sectional studies have led us to believe. The majority of adult child recipients received only one transfer, which indicates that financial assistance is more likely to be episodic than routine (Eggebeen & Hogan, 1990). Yet a small percentage of the sample received multiple transfers over time, suggesting that some families develop a pattern of support over the life course.

This research also demonstrates that the likelihood of transfer receipt by adult children varied greatly based on family structure and kinship status across generations. Stepchildren were consistently less likely to receive transfers and to receive smaller amounts than biological children (for parental favoritism, see Suitor and Pillemer, Chapter 1). However, a closer examination uncovers the fact that this inequality in the likelihood of transfers given to adult children and stepchildren actually reflects the rarity of transfers from remarried fathers to their children from previous marriages. In contrast, the likelihood of transfers from remarried mothers and stepfathers to children from mothers' previous marriages is not significantly different from the likelihood of transfers to biological children of continuously married parents. Previous speculations suggested that all stepchildren would be less likely to receive transfers (Rossi & Rossi, 1990; White, 1994). Some previous study findings also appeared to support that assertion (Berry, 2001; Killian, 2004; Pezzin & Schone, 1999). However, there were no significant differences between biological children and maternal children/paternal stepchildren when kinship status was defined more carefully. Therefore, this study yields new information about the dynamics of intergenerational solidarity after parents' remarriages.

Primarily, our results identify the strong likelihood of weakened functional solidarity between biological fathers and children from previous marriages. This finding was not surprising in light of other research that has shown less frequent contact, less emotional closeness, greater geographic distance, and reduced feelings of obligation between divorced fathers and adult children (Cooney & Uhlenberg, 1990; Marks, 1995; Rossi & Rossi, 1990; Shapiro, 2004). Lower-quality relations between adult children and divorced fathers are clearly reflected in weakened solidarity across multiple dimensions. However, it is not clear if fathers' remarriages instigate further decline in solidarity beyond the effects of the initial parental divorce or if weaker functional solidarity is an aspect of the overall decline in the relationships between divorced fathers and adult children over the life course.

Secondly, the functional solidarity of relations between adult children, mothers, and stepfathers appears not to be different than the solidarity within intact families. Latent kin matrices that include stepfathers may be activated for financial assistance on par with the assistance provided to adult children by continuously married parents. This study shows that stepfathers' roles must be considered more carefully in future research about intergenerational solidarity. Ganong, Coleman, and Mistina (1995) determined that stepfathers are generally expected to assume at least some of the financial responsibilities for young coresident children. The results of this study indicate that stepfathers may maintain this commitment voluntarily, or from a sense of continued obligation, after the children reach adulthood.

There is insufficient information available to determine if stepfathers helped stepchildren but not their own children from previous marriages or if they were assisting more family members of the next generation equally regardless of kinship status. However, the results provide clues that family solidarity may be regenerated after parental remarriage and suggest that custody arrangements and coresidence probably play an important role in the linkages between adult children and stepparents later in life. Cherlin and Furstenberg (1994) asserted that given the tendency to award physical custody of young children to the mother after a divorce, it would seem logical that "kinship exchanges over the long-term are strongly tilted toward the (custodial) mother's side of the family" (p. 369). The findings of this study, which was designed to compare the effects of kinship status in remarriages for biological parents and stepparents, support that argument in the case of financial assistance.

Differences in coresidence patterns (i.e., structural solidarity) are likely related to weakened affectual, associational, and consensual solidarity within
families of divorce and remarriage (Aquilino, 1991; Shapiro & Lambert, 1999).
The significantly decreased likelihood of intergenerational coresidence with a
remarried parent (and stepparent) shown in table 2.1 reflects this change in
relationship quality and support, both in relation to any coresidence as well
as to returning to the parents' home to coreside after living independently.
Kronebusch & Schlesinger (1994) argue that coresidence is an intergenerational transfer with monetary value (i.e., the savings represented for the adult
child by not paying rent). In this respect, the study results show that paternal
children/maternal stepchildren were again at a disadvantage compared to maternal children/paternal stepchildren and biological children.

The inclusion of coresident adult children in the sample represented a
trade-off. When the data were collected, if an adult child was nonresident, the
parent was asked to estimate that child's household income. However, if the
adult child coresided, information was not requested about his or her income.
Previous studies that have examined financial transfers have limited the sample to nonresident children only (Eggebeen, 1992; Eggebeen & Hogan, 1990;
Killian, 2004; Pezzin & Schone, 1999). However, since coresidence has monetary value and may have been substituted for financial assistance, we included
coresident children. We found no evidence of a substitution effect. In fact,
since coresidence was associated with a higher likelihood for transfer receipt,
parents/stepparents apparently provided assistance in the forms of both living
space and money.

However, including coresident children meant that we were unable to determine whether transfers were motivated by financial need. Many have speculated that transfers are motivated by an adult child's financial need (Eggebeen, 1992; Furstenberg, Hoffman, & Shrestha, 1995; Rossi & Rossi, 1990).
Studies with samples limited to nonresident adult children have shown that
adult children with lower incomes are more likely to receive financial assistance from parents (Berry, 2001; Furstenberg, Hoffman, & Shrestha, 1995).
Even the results presented in this chapter showing that coresidence increased
the likelihood of transfer receipt suggest that adult stepchildren, in particular,
who lived with their parents/stepparents may have had greater financial need
for intergenerational assistance than their nonresident siblings. However, the
complexity and relativity of defining need for each child and the potential for
conflicting needs within families severely hamper our ability to determine

motives accurately. This requires information about parents' motives for giving (Silverstein, 2006).

By including coresident children in the sample, we also faced the risk that college students were counted as household members because they had not established a separate residence but, in actuality, only lived with the parents when school was not in session. An interaction effect was tested for coresidence and school attendance (analyses not shown). The interaction effect was significant but did not improve model fit. Concerns may be raised that parents may have counted college expenses as financial transfers, but various factors, such as the average and median amounts transferred as well as the high percentage of adult children not in school who received financial assistance, indicated that most respondents interpreted the survey question to not include college expenses.

Several researchers have demonstrated that as the number of siblings increased, the likelihood of transfer receipt decreased (Berry, 2001; Cooney & Uhlenberg, 1990; Killian, 2004). Some have argued that this supports the resource dilution hypothesis (e.g., Hogan, Eggebeen, & Clogg, 1993). If true, this would seem especially influential for remarriages where the average number of children per family was significantly higher than for intact families. However, while family size decreased the likelihood of transfer receipt generally, these analyses demonstrated that family size did not diminish the impacts of family structure or kinship status.

Some parents developed routines of downward transfers to the next generation by giving multiple transfers over time. The specific characteristics and life course statuses of biological children were collectively more predictive of multiple transfer receipt than those same factors were for stepchildren. It could not be determined if transfer behaviors reflected a blended family's degree of normative solidarity, but it was clear that biological children and maternal children/paternal stepchildren were favored for financial transfers.

The timing of remarriage may have been an important turning point that created greater unobserved heterogeneity within the stepchild categories. The greater variances in demographic characteristics, family structures, and life course patterns for blended families compared to intact two-parent families may make it more difficult to explain what factors are more influential for the likelihood of giving financial assistance to stepchildren. These issues should be explored further in future research.

Bengtson, Biblarz, and Roberts (2002) state, "The key is that family functioning is seen as an adaptive process, involving compensation by all of the family participants" (p. 33). Future studies must adopt a broader definition of families and acknowledge the complexity of maintaining—and in some cases, reconstructing—family solidarity across the life course. Theoretical development within the solidarity framework requires greater understanding of step-parents' roles in sharing household resources across the family life course.

Postscript

Since the conference presentation at the University of Southern California in 2007, Clark and Kenney (2010) reported similar findings using six waves of HRS data (1992–2002). They included adult children of married, remarried, and single parents in their sample to test hypotheses related to the "matrilineal tilt" of wealth flows between generations suggested by Cherlin and Furstenberg (1994). As in this chapter, their research demonstrated that the odds of financial transfer receipt were significantly lower for paternal children/maternal stepchildren than for children from any other family structure. However, their results showed a statistically significant difference for the odds of transfer receipt for maternal children/paternal stepchildren compared to biological children from continuously married families, whereas our results showed no significant differences between the two groups. The contrast may be the result of methodological differences between the two studies. Whereas Clark and Kenney (2010) generated a pooled cross-sectional sample from the six waves for a total of 80,007 single observations, we examined the likelihood of transfer receipt for each adult child *over time* with multiple opportunities to receive financial assistance (i.e., a repeated measures approach). This data construction method better matched our interest in examining intergenerational solidarity for blended families.

APPENDIX

Table 2A.1. Adult child characteristics predicting the likelihood of receiving one or more transfers between 1992 and 1998

Characteristics of the adult child	Model 1		Model 2		Model 3	
	Estimate	Odds ratio	Estimate	Odds ratio	Estimate	Odds ratio
Gender	-0.091†	0.91	-0.093†	0.91	-0.089	
(SE) *(ref = female)*	(0.05)		(0.05)		(0.05)	
Race	-0.294*	0.75	-0.298*	0.74	-0.301	0.74
(ref = white)	(0.09)		(0.09)		(0.09)	
Hispanic	-1.060***	0.35	-1.107***	0.33	-1.120***	0.33
	(0.12)		(0.12)		(0.12)	
Age 18–23 at entry	1.035***	2.82	1.020***	2.77	1.048***	2.85
	(0.08)		(0.08)		(0.08)	
Age 24–29 at entry	0.523***	1.69	0.511***	1.67	0.527***	1.69
(ref = 30 yrs and older)	(0.06)		(0.06)		(0.06)	
Attended school[a]	0.769***	2.16	0.764***	2.15	0.760***	2.14
	(0.07)		(0.07)		(0.07)	
Married[b]	-0.081		-0.099		-0.117†	0.89
	(0.06)		(0.06)		(0.06)	
Coresided with parents[c]	0.899***	2.46	0.832***	2.30	0.788***	2.20
	(0.07)		(0.07)		(0.07)	
Number of siblings	-0.346***	0.71	-0.320***	0.73	-0.324***	0.72
	(0.02)		(0.02)		(0.02)	
Stepchildren			-0.420***	0.66		
(ref = Biological children)			(0.07)			
Maternal children					-0.062	
					(0.08)	
Paternal children					-0.822***	0.44
(ref = Biological children)					(0.09)	
Intercept	-0.076		0.010		0.034	
	(0.08)		(0.08)		(0.09)	
Deviance statistic	1.459***		1.467***		1.499***	
	(0.04)		(0.07)		(0.05)	
BIC statistic		16,963.00		16,934.00		16,866.00
Difference from model 1				-29.00		-97.00
df		4376		4376		4376
n = 15,689						

[a] Adult child was in school during at least one wave.
[b] Reference group is adult children who were never married during the collection period.
[c] Adult child coresided with parents for at least one wave.
†*p* < .05, **p* < .01, ***p* < .001, ****p* < .0001

Table 2A.2. Adult child characteristics affecting the financial assistance received from parents 1992–1998

Characteristics of the adult child	Conditional amount[d]			Values of change for model 3[e]
	Model 1	Model 2	Model 3	
Gender	-0.046	-0.047	-0.046	
(SE)	(0.03)	(0.03)	(0.03)	
Non-White	-0.323***	-0.326***	-0.328***	-$1,134
(ref = White)	(0.05)	(0.05)	(0.05)	
Ethnicity	-0.247*	-0.257**	-0.255**	-$912
(ref = Hispanic)	(0.08)	(0.08)	(0.08)	
Age 18–23 at entry	0.340***	0.339***	0.342***	+$1,653
	(0.05)	(0.05)	(0.05)	
Age 24–29 at entry	0.098*	0.096†	0.099*	+$422
(ref = 30 yrs and older)	(0.04)	(0.04)	(0.04)	
Attended school[a]	0.304***	0.304***	0.304***	+1,441
	(0.04)	(0.04)	(0.04)	
Married[b]	-0.071†	-0.076†	-0.077†	-$300
	(0.03)	(0.03)	(0.03)	
Coresided with parents[c]	0.205***	0.182***	0.175***	+$771
	(0.04)	(0.04)	(0.04)	
Number of siblings	-0.111***	-0.100***	-0.102***	-$393
	(0.01)	(0.01)	(0.01)	
Stepchildren		-0.152**		
(ref = Biological children)		(0.04)		
Maternal children			-0.098	
			(0.05)	
Paternal children			-0.225**	-$820
(ref = Biological children)			(0.06)	
Intercept	8.100***	8.123***	8.126***	$4,053
	(0.05)	(0.05)	(0.05)	
BIC statistic	17,014.50	17,006.8	17,006.4	
Difference from model 1		-7.70	-8.10	
df	2576	2576	2576	
n = 5535				

Note: The last column converts each significant parameter by undoing the log transformation and then calculating the value of each variable's mean effect in 2005 U.S. dollars. Amounts were calculated by adding the parameter value to the intercept, re-exponentiating the log transformation of that total and then calculating the value of each variable's mean effect in 2005 U.S. dollars. The effect of each variable was calculated by the following steps:

Step 1: Calculate $e^{\beta_0 + \beta_1}$

Step 2: Subtract e^{β_0}

Step 3: Multiply the answer by the value of inflation between 1992 and 2005 to convert the value to 2005 U.S. dollars

Table 2A.2. (continued)

---

[a] Adult child was in school during at least one wave.
[b] Adult child was married at baseline or married during the data collection period.
[c] Adult child coresided with parents for at least one wave.
[d] Within-family regression model for amount received (logged) conditional upon receiving a financial transfer.
[e] Value reported in 2005 U.S. dollars.
[†]$p < .05$, [*]$p < .01$, [**]$p < .001$, [***]$p < .0001$

REFERENCES

Ahrons, C. R. (1994). *The good divorce*. New York: HarperCollins.
Amato, P., & Booth, A. (1997). *A generation at risk: Growing up in an era of family upheaval*. Cambridge, MA: Harvard.
Aquilino, W. S. (1991). Family structure and home-leaving: A further specification on the relationship. *Journal of Marriage and Family, 53*, 999–1010.
Aquilino, W. S. (1994). Impact of childhood family structure on young adults' relationships with parents. *Journal of Marriage and Family, 56*, 295–313.
Aquilino, W.S. (2005). Impact of family structure on parental attitudes toward the economic support of adult children over the transition to adulthood. *Journal of Family Issues, 26*, 143–167.
Bengtson, V. L. (2001). Beyond the nuclear family: The increasing importance of multigenerational bonds. *Journal of Marriage and the Family, 63*(1), 1–16.
Bengtson, V. L., Biblarz, T. J., & Roberts, R. E. L. (2002). *How families still matter: A longitudinal study of youth in two generations*. Cambridge, UK: Cambridge University Press.
Bengtson, V. L., & Harootyan, R. A. (1994). *Intergenerational linkages: Hidden connections in American society*. New York: Springer.
Berry, B. M. (2001). *Financial transfers from parents to adult children: Issues of who is helped and why*. Population Studies Center Research Report #01-485. Ann Arbor, MI: University of Michigan.
Booth, A., & Amato, P. (1994). Parental marital quality, divorce and relations with parents. *Journal of Marriage and the Family, 56*, 21–34.
Bumpass, L. L., Raley, R. K., & Sweet, J. A. (1995). The changing character of stepfamilies: Implications of cohabitation and nonmarital childbearing. *Demography, 32*(3), 425–436.
Bumpass, L. L., Sweet, J., & Castro-Martin, T. (1990). Changing patterns of remarriage. *Journal of Marriage and the Family, 52*, 747–756.
Cherlin, A. J. (1978). Remarriage as an incomplete institution. *American Journal of Sociology, 8*, 634–650.
Cherlin, A. J., & Furstenberg, F. F. Jr. (1994). Stepfamilies in the United States: A reconsideration. *Annual Review of Sociology, 20*, 359–381.
Clark, S., & Kenney, C. (2010). Is the United States experiencing a "matrilineal tilt?"

Gender, family structures and financial transfers to adult children. *Social Forces,* *88*(4), 1753–1776.

Cohler, B. J., & Altergott, J. (1995). The family of the second half of life: Connecting theories and findings. In M. Szinovacz & D. J. Ekerdt (Eds.), *Handbook of aging and the family* (pp. 59–94). Westport, CT: Greenwood Press.

Coleman, M., Fine, M. A., Ganong, L. H., Downs, K. J. M., & Pauk, N. (2001). When you're not the Brady Bunch: Identifying perceived conflicts and resolution strategies in stepfamilies. *Personal Relationships, 8,* 55–73.

Connidis, I. A. (2010). *Family ties and aging* (2nd ed.). Thousand Oaks, CA: Sage.

Cooney, T. M. (1994). Young adults' relations with parents: The influence of recent parent divorce. *Journal of Marriage and the Family, 56*(1), 45–56.

Cooney, T. M., & Uhlenberg, P. (1990). The role of divorce in men's relations with their adult children after midlife. *Journal of Marriage and the Family, 52,* 677–688.

Cooney, T. M., & Uhlenberg, P. (1992). Support from parents over the life course: The adult child's perspective. *Social Forces, 71*(1), 63–84.

Cox, D., & Raines, F. (1985). Interfamily transfers and income redistribution. In M. David & T. Smeeding (Eds.), *Horizontal equity, uncertainty, and measures of well-being.* Chicago, IL: University of Chicago Press.

Davey, A., Janke, M., and Savla, J. (2005). Antecedents of intergenerational support: Families in context and families as context. In M. Silverstein (Ed.), *Annual review of gerontology and geriatrics* (Vol. 24): *Intergenerational relations across time and place* (pp. 29–54). New York: Springer.

Eggebeen, D. J. (1992). Family structure and intergenerational exchanges. *Research on Aging, 14,* 427–447.

Eggebeen, D. J., & Hogan, D. P. (1990). Giving between generations in American families. *Human Nature, 1,* 211–232.

Furstenberg, F. F. Jr., Hoffman, S. D., & Shrestha, L. (1995). The effect of divorce on intergenerational transfers: New evidence. *Demography, 32*(3), 319–333.

Ganong, L. H., & Coleman, M. (1999). *Changing families, changing responsibilities: Family obligations following divorce and remarriage.* Mahwah, NJ: Lawrence Erlbaum Associates.

Ganong, L. H., & Coleman, M. (2006). Patterns of exchange and intergenerational responsibilities after divorce and remarriage. *Journal of Aging Studies, 20*(3): 265–278.

Ganong, L. H., Coleman, M., & Mistina, D. (1995). Normative beliefs about parents' and stepparents' financial obligations to children following divorce and remarriage. *Family Relations, 44,* 306–315.

Hagestad, G. O. (2003). Interdependent lives and relationships in changing times: A life-course view of families and aging. In R. A. Settersten Jr. (Ed.), *Invitation to the life course: Toward new understandings of later life* (pp. 135–159). Amityville, NY: Baywood Press.

Harootyan, R. A., & Vorek, R. (1994). Volunteering, helping and gift-giving in families and communities. In V. L. Bengtson & R. A. Harootyan (Eds.), *Intergenera-*

tional linkages: Hidden connections in American society (pp. 92–111). New York: Springer.

Hoffman, S. D., & Duncan, G. J. (1988). What are the economic consequences of divorce? *Demography, 25,* 641–645.

Hogan, D. P., Eggebeen, D. J., & Clogg, C. C. (1993). The structure of intergenerational exchanges in American families. *American Journal of Sociology, 98*(6), 1428–1458.

Howell, D. (1995). Health and retirement study wave 1 data: Data description and usage. Retrieved February 3, 2004 (http://hrsonline.isr.umich.edu/meta/1992/core/desc/hrs92dd.pdf).

Killian, T. S. (2004). Intergenerational money transfers to adult children and stepchildren: A household level analysis. *Journal of Divorce and Remarriage, 42,* 105–130.

Killian, T. S., & Ferrell, J. (2005). Perceived obligations of remarried households to provide assistance to younger family members. *Journal of Intergenerational Relationships, 3,* 23–43.

Kohli, M., & Kunemund, H. (2003). Intergenerational transfers in the family: What motivates giving? In V. L. Bengtson & A. Lowenstein (Eds.), *Global aging and challenges to families.* New York: Aldine de Gruyter.

Kronebusch, K., & Schlesinger, M. (1994). Intergenerational transfers. In V. L. Bengtson & R. A. Harootyan (Eds.), *Intergenerational linkages: Hidden connections in American society* (pp. 112–151). New York: Springer.

Lawton, L., Silverstein, M., & Bengtson, V. L. (1994). Solidarity between generations in families. In V. L. Bengtson & R. A. Harootyan (Eds.), *Intergenerational linkages: Hidden connections in American society* (pp. 19–42). New York: Springer.

Logan, J. R., & Spitze, G. D. (1996). *Family ties: Enduring relations between parents and their grown children.* Philadelphia, PA: Temple University Press.

Marks, N. (1995). Midlife marital status differences in social support relationships with adult children and psychological well-being. *Journal of Family Issues, 16,* 5–28.

McGarry, K., & Schoeni, R. F. (1995). Transfer behavior: Measurement and the redistribution of resources within the family. *The Journal of Human Resources, 30,* S184–S226.

Pezzin, L. E., & Schone, B. S. (1999). Parental marital disruption and intergenerational transfers: An analysis of lone elderly parents and their children. *Demography, 36*(3), 287–297.

Riley, M. W. (1983). The family in an aging society: A matrix of latent relationships. *Journal of Family Issues, 4,* 439–454.

Riley, M. W., & Riley, J. J. Jr. (1993). Connections: Kin and cohort. In V. L. Bengtson & W. A. Achenbaum (Eds.), *The changing contract across generations* (pp.169–189). New York: Aldine de Gruyter.

Rossi, A. S., & Rossi, P. H. (1990). *Of human bonding: Parent-child relations across the life course.* New York: Aldine de Gruyter.

Shapiro, A. (2003). Later-life divorce and parent-adult child contact and proximity: A longitudinal analysis. *Journal of Family Issues, 24*(2), 264–285.

Shapiro, A. (2004). *The hidden cost of being African-American: How wealth perpetuates inequality.* New York: Oxford University Press.

Shapiro, A., & Lambert, J. D. (1999). Longitudinal effects of divorce on the quality of the father-child relationship and on fathers' psychological well-being. *Journal of Marriage and the Family, 61,* 397–408.

Silverstein, M. (2006). Family structure and transfers. In R. H. Binstock & L. K. George (Eds.), *Handbook of aging and the social sciences* (6th ed., pp. 165–180). San Diego, CA: Academic Press.

Silverstein, M., Bengtson, V. L., & Lawton, L. (1997). Intergenerational solidarity and the structure of adult child-parent relationships in American families. *American Journal of Sociology, 103,* 429–460.

Silverstein, M., Lawton, L., & Bengtson, V. L. (1994). Types of relations between parents and adult children. In V. L. Bengtson & R. A. Harootyan (Eds.), *Intergenerational linkages: Hidden connections in American society* (pp. 43–76). New York: Springer.

Soldo, B. J., & Hill, M. S. (1993). Intergenerational transfers: Economic, demographic, and social perspectives. *Annual Review of Gerontology and Geriatrics, 13,* 187–216.

Sweet, J. A., & Bumpass, L. L. (1987). *American families and households.* New York: Russell Sage.

White, L. (1992). The effect of parental divorce and remarriage on parental support for adult children. *Journal of Family Issues, 13,* 234–250.

White, L. (1994). Growing up with single parents and stepparents: Long-term effects on solidarity. *Journal of Marriage and the Family, 56,* 935–948.

Wong, R., Capoferro, C., & Soldo, B. J. (1999). Financial assistance from middle-aged couples to parents and children: Racial-ethnic differences. *The Journals of Gerontology, 54B*(3), S145–S153.

CHAPTER THREE

Generational Contact and Support among Late Adult Siblings within a Verticalized Family

Kees Knipscheer and Theo van Tilburg

Since discussion of the isolated nuclear family and the modified extended family began in the 1960s, most empirical intergenerational family studies have focused on the structural and functional changes in the parent-child relationship. The verticalization of the family structure added an extra push to this direction in the discipline. The focus of the studies on sibling relationships has been quite different, however. These studies, very limited in number, are mainly on psychological and functional characteristics and only recently question the consequences of demographic changes in the structure of the multigenerational family. Focusing on the availability of siblings and on frequency of contact and exchange of support among older adults, we aim in this study to strengthen our understanding of the structural characteristics of the sibling relationship in late life by the end of the twentieth century.

In 1992, White and Riedmann made the point that they were not aware of any existing population studies on sibling relationships. Another publication by White (2001) appears to be the only publication on sibling relationships in the United States since 1992. This demonstrates that representative information about the sibling relationships on a national level is very limited. In the Netherlands, Voorpostel et al. (2007) published an article based on data from the Netherlands Kinship Panel Study. However, this article does not present much descriptive data on the composition and availability of siblings within the Dutch multigenerational family. This chapter, primarily focusing on availability, frequency of contact, and exchange of support among late adult and older siblings, will be based on data from a Dutch panel study that started in 1992.

In a review of the sibling literature, van Volkom (2006) opens by saying that the number of studies on siblings in general and siblings in late adulthood more specifically is very limited compared to the number of studies on romantic and parent-child relationships. She notes that this fact is not in harmony with her finding that "The majority of the work summarized here characterizes the sibling relationship as one of strong emotional ties, helping and importance for the adult's well-being" (van Volkom, 2006, p. 165). However, 44 of her 85 references were published between 1985 and 1995 and only 10 after the year 1999. This indicates no consistent tradition of sibling research and a recent decline in scientific interest in this type of relationship.

Scholars who have studied the role of siblings among older adults stress the importance of these relationships in late adulthood and old age because of their specific combination of characteristics. Siblings share the same biological parents (apart from half siblings and adopted siblings). This implies that the sibling relationship is in principle a given, not chosen, lifelong relationship and that siblings share a common educational history and may generally be considered age peers (van Volkom, 2006). Bedford (1996) describes the sibling relationship as an "elusive, emotionally charged, memory-laden tie" (p. 134). Adults feel close to their siblings because of their shared experiences, trust, concern for each other, and common enjoyment despite rivalries in a limited number of cases (Bedford, 1996). Cultural priority is placed on obligations to other family members (spouse, parents, and children), and the sibling relationship has been qualified as voluntary compared to the parent-child relationship, more expressive than instrumental, and based on equality (Avioli, 1989; van Volkom, 2006).

Important sources of variability within sibling relationships are evident. For example, differences in gender composition of the sibling relationship show up in most studies. The greatest levels of closeness are apparently between sisters, leaving cross-sex siblings somewhat behind (Cicirelli, 1985; White & Riedmann, 1992). Akiyama, Elliott, and Antonucci (1996) demonstrated that brothers' relationships appear to be the least close. Bedford (1996) and White (2001) demonstrated that sisters are more supportive than brothers. However, Bedford showed earlier that there can be a great deal of tension between sisters (Bedford, 1989). Sisters provide a great deal of emotional support and help to widows, although unmarried sisters do so more than married sisters (O'Bryant, 1988; White & Riedmann, 1992). In a later panel study over approximately five years among about 9,000 individuals aged 16–85, White (2001) confirms this increasing contact and exchange of support in case of marital dissolution.

Age effects appear to be stronger than family life course events. "Proximity and contact decrease modestly in early adulthood and then show long-term stability through old age. Giving and receiving help decline from age 16 until old age, however a substantial resurgence in sibling exchange is demonstrated after age 70 among those with nearby siblings" (White, 2001, p. 565). This demonstrates the importance of events related to family life course and fits with the original approach by Parsons (1943) arguing that siblings share in our "inner circle" of family of orientation but drop into the "outer circle" after marriage. This is supported by a convoy study by Antonucci and Akiyama (1987) showing that adult siblings are generally in the "second tier" (White & Riedmann, 1992). However, as White (2001) demonstrated and van Volkom (2006) stresses, family life course events, "such as widowhood and parental death, often lead to a sibling returning to the inner circle as a replacement for the person who was lost" (van Volkom, 2006, p. 153).

Just a few publications have examined the role of social class in sibling relationships. Avioli (1989) refers to some studies which show that working-class siblings exchange more instrumental support. These findings are supported by White and Riedmann (1992). Among middle-class siblings, expressive support was expected to be higher (Avioli, 1989). More specific findings became available in White's panel study (2001). Higher educated siblings move farther away, and their frequency of contact with siblings appears to be lower; however, exchange of support in both directions is higher among better-educated siblings. These somewhat paradoxical findings show that variability in sibling relationships according to social class is inconsistent.

The importance of sibling relationships is related to gender and age and is also linked to family life course events, including changes in partner status, having children, and parental loss as well as disruptive family life course events that became more common during the second half of the twentieth century, such as divorce and serial partner relationships. Riley (1983) referred to this "new family structure" as a matrix of latent relationships: a network potential that can be activated when appropriate. Van Tilburg and Thomése

(2010) stressed that these changed family structures did not provoke a decline in the importance of the family. In 2005, Connidis suggested considering siblings as part of a web of relationships that individuals have spun over time. This metaphor may be appropriate for conceptualizing the role of siblings in later life.

The limited number of sibling studies matches with the paucity of theoretical conceptualizations of this relationship. Among the earliest theoretical approaches are attachment theory (Cicirelli, 1996) and equity theory (George, 1986; Ingersoll-Dayton, Neal, Ha, & Hammer, 2003). Cicirelli argues that according to adult attachment theory (Bank & Kahn, 1982a,b), attachment is not restricted to the mother but can also develop to other individuals, including siblings who are responsive and supportive to their brothers or sisters. However, such an affective bond needs to fill several criteria to be considered as attachment. This chapter does not explore further the sibling relationship as an affectionate bond. Equity theory in sibling research originates from the distress experienced by siblings who assume the majority of caregiving responsibilities (Connidis, 2007; George, 1986; Ingersoll-Dayton, Neal, Ha, & Hammer, 2003). Several studies demonstrate the specific sensitivity of siblings to issues of inequity in caregiving, which extends both to those who deliver most care and to those who deliver less. Both attachment theory and equity theory focus on the individual relationships between siblings. Connidis (2005) argued in favor of a life course approach in combination with a consistent social structural perspective. "The compatibility of the life course perspective with feminist approaches . . . and the concept of ambivalence suggests a working perspective on sibling ties in which socially structured relations based on gender, class, race, age and sexual orientation shape the interdependent life course trajectories of siblings who engage in relationships characterized by ambivalence" (Connidis, 2005, p. 430). Her plea to use the life course perspective to conceptualize the sibling relationship seems to be in line with the importance of family life course events in shaping sibling relationships.

Still another structural factor supports the use of a life course perspective to study the sibling relationship. Most recent studies on sibling relationships stress the significance of demographic changes regarding both the increasing proportion of childless couples and the changing composition of the multi-generational family. A decreasing number of children per generation and the increase of life expectancy do not only cause a verticalization of the multigenerational family. They also increase the probability of sibling survival and in this way the availability of siblings in later life. As Connidis (2005) stresses,

"Living longer also increases the number of overlapping years and the number of significant transitions in their parents' and their own lives that siblings will share" (p. 431). These structural changes in the composition of the consecutive families of orientation may lead to an upswing of the role of siblings in later life, as White (2001) already demonstrated in her five-year panel study by showing a slight rise in exchange among siblings after the age of 70.

This chapter focuses on the availability of siblings to older adults and on the frequency of contact and exchange of support among them. We place siblings in the context of the social network of older adults. This offers two opportunities for insight into the role of siblings. First, we compare sibling relationships with two other relationship types within the social network, children and age peers, in terms of contact frequency and social support exchange. Second, we explore the main determinants of variability in sibling relationships and their place in social networks. The main questions we intend to answer are (1) To what extent are sibling relationships represented within the social network? Are there differences across generations, and what are main determinants of representation? and (2) What is the contact frequency and intensity of support exchanges among late adult siblings, and what can we learn from a comparison with older people's contact frequency and intensity of support exchanges with children and age peers?

Method
Respondents

Data were available for older people who participated in the Living Arrangements and Social Networks of Older Adults research program (Knipscheer, de Jong Gierveld, van Tilburg, & Dykstra, 1995). The program used a stratified random sample of men and women born between 1903 and 1937. The sample was taken from the population registers of eleven urban and rural municipalities in three regions that represent differences in religion and urbanization in the Netherlands. The oldest individuals in these areas, particularly the oldest men, were over-represented in the sample. In 1992, 4,494 respondents were interviewed in their homes. The cooperation rate was 62%. The interviews were carried out by interviewers who had received training for four days and who were intensively supervised, and the interviews were tape recorded to monitor and enhance the quality of data. Follow-ups were conducted in the context of the Longitudinal Aging Study Amsterdam, or LASA (Huisman et al., 2011). In 2002, LASA sampled a new cohort (birth years 1938–1947,

n = 1,002) from the same sampling frame as the earlier cohort, with a coopera-tion rate of 62%. There were various reasons not to have complete information for all respondents. Most frequently, respondents were too physically or cog-nitively frail to be interviewed with the full questionnaire, and an abridged version of the face-to-face interview was used (n = 361). Furthermore, data on the social network were not available for 61 respondents due to premature ter-mination of the interview or refusal for privacy reasons.

Measurements
Identification of Children and Siblings

At baseline, the identification of children followed a two-step procedure. First, the number of children was assessed by means of the following question: "How many children have you had? You should consider not only the children whose natural mother (father) you are but also stepchildren and adoptive chil-dren. Please do not forget to also count children who may have already passed away." In the second step, each child was identified by name. A similar proce-dure was followed for siblings of the respondent.

Child and Sibling Characteristics

After respondents identified their children, they were asked to give the children's gender; describe them as biological children, stepchildren, or adop-tive children; and state whether they were deceased. The frequency of contact was assessed by the question, "How often are you in touch with X?" The choice of answers and their numeric values were (1) never, (2) once a year or less, (3) few times a year, (4) once a month, (5) once a fortnight, (6) once a week, (7) few times a week, and (8) each day. Travel time to reach the child was asked in hours and minutes and scored in minutes. Data obtained within a side study showed that the traveling time reported by the older adults cor-related strongly (r > .80) with the time reported by the network members and with the figures given by public databases for traveling the distance by car. Among respondents born between 1903 and 1937, a similar procedure was fol-lowed for siblings; for later cohorts, these detailed data are not available for siblings.

Identification of Social Network Members

The main objective was to identify a network that reflected the socially ac-tive relationships of the older adult in the core as well as the outer layers of the larger network (van Tilburg, 1998). To ensure that all types of relationships had the same chance of being recorded, respondents' networks were identified with a domain-specific approach, using seven formal types of relationships: household members (including the spouse, if there was one), (other) children (including stepchildren) and their partners, other relatives, neighbors, colleagues (including from voluntary work or school), fellow members of organizations, and others (e.g., friends and acquaintances). To ensure that the socially active relationships were identified, but not individuals who were contacted frequently for non-personal reasons, such as shopkeepers, the importance of the relationship was added as a criterion in the stimulus question. After this inventory, we identified the top-12 network for all those respondents who listed thirteen or more relationships in the first step of the identification. In this case, the selection was based on frequency of contact. Support questions were limited to the relationships with members of the top-12 network.

In the domain of children, the following question was asked: "Earlier in the interview you provided the names of all your living children. You also told us whether they have a husband, wife or partner. We would like to know with which children and partners you have frequent contact and who are also important to you. Could you name them one at a time, by their first name and the initial letter of their surname?" These specific questions were repeated for other relatives, including siblings. Respondents were restricted to identifying only people above the age of 18 and a maximum of 80 people. No respondent reached this limit. Network members were identified by name. Contact frequency was assessed by means of the same question as above. The question was skipped for network members for whom the question had already been asked in the demographic section.

Supportive Exchanges

For the 12 relationships with the highest contact frequency, questions were asked about support. One question for each selected network member asked respondents about receiving instrumental support: "How often in the past year did X help you with daily chores in and around the house, such as preparing meals, cleaning the house, transportation, minor repairs, filling out forms?" One question asked respondents about receiving emotional support: "How often in the past year did you talk to X about your personal experiences and feelings?" For support given, the questions were reversed. The answer categories and their numeric values were never (0), seldom (1), sometimes (2), and often (3). To obtain an indicator of the intensity of support exchange, the four scores were summed.

Age Peers

Ninety percent of the respondents had siblings who were between 10 years younger and 15 years older. For respondents aged 55–64 years, nonkin network members in the age range of 10 years younger to 15 years older were considered to be age peers. For older respondents, we adopted a wider age range. For respondents aged 65–74 years, this age range was 15 years younger to 20 years older. For respondents aged 75 or older, the lower limit was 15 years younger and there was no upper limit. We differentiated the age ranges because we supposed that the older people are, the more broadly they understand their own age-peer groups.

Procedure

In answering the first research question, we made use of the complete inventory of children and siblings. We computed the average number of children and siblings born, the number still alive, and the number identified in the social network. We presented these data according to five-year birth cohorts characterized by 55–89-year-olds in 1992 and 55–64-year-olds in 2002. Next, we conducted by means of regression analysis a search for background variables to explain the variation in the number of siblings included in the network. Three dependent variables were distinguished. First, the absolute number of siblings identified as network members, ranging between none and 13. Second, the proportion of the network consisting of siblings. Third, the proportion of siblings represented in the network. Explanatory variables included in the regression equations were the number of siblings alive, the average traveling time to siblings, network size, having of children, average traveling time to children, partner availability, whether there is a parent alive, gender, level of urbanization, church membership, level of education, and geographical region. In a second step, we considered the importance of differentiation by cohort membership. Categorical variables were included as dummy variables.

In answering the second research question, frequency of contact and intensity of supportive exchanges within late-adult sibling relationships were assessed. To compare sibling relationships with child relationships, we selected respondents with living siblings and children. We decided further to select only one relationship with a sibling and one with a child for each respondent. We selected the one with whom there was the highest frequency of contact. Paired *t*-tests were conducted to evaluate whether the sample averages of both

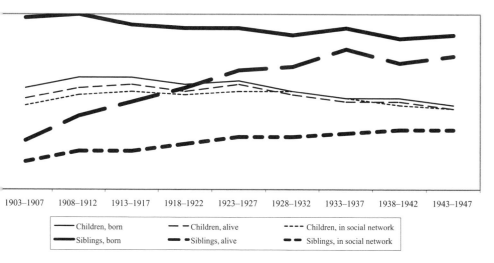

1903–1907   1908–1912   1913–1917   1918–1922   1923–1927   1928–1932   1933–1937   1938–1942   1943–1947

| —— Children, born | — — Children, alive | - - - - Children, in social network |
| ■■ Siblings, born | ■— ■ Siblings, alive | ■■ ■■ Siblings, in social network |

Figure 3.1. Average number of children and siblings born, alive, and in the social network. *Note:* Observations for cohorts 1903–1937 in 1992, for cohorts 1938–1947 in 2002. N = 5,199 and 5,135 for average number of children and siblings, respectively, born and alive. N = 4,365 and 4,345 for average number of children and siblings, respectively, in social network; respondents without children and siblings, respectively, are excluded.

categories differed. For the comparison with age peers, a similar procedure was adopted.

Results

Of the 5,135 respondents, 210 never had siblings and 519 no longer had living siblings. Figure 3.1 presents descriptive data about availability of children and siblings across 11 five-year cohorts born between 1903 and 1947. All cohorts consistently had about two more siblings than children. For siblings and children still alive, the figure shows that the youngest cohort had already lost on average almost one sibling; among the oldest cohort only about one sibling on average is left. This finding must be partly an outcome of early child death in the first half of the twentieth century and of the higher mortality rates over the age of 50 among these cohorts.

Respondents identified those children and siblings who were important to them and with whom they had frequent contact and as such who were members of their social networks. Figure 3.1 also displays the average number of liv-

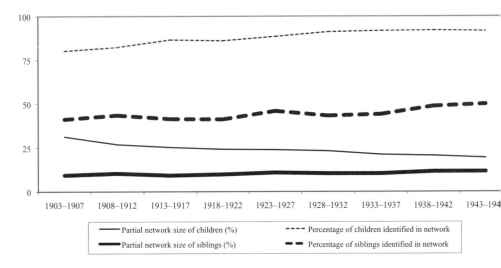

1903–1907	1908–1912	1913–1917	1918–1922	1923–1927	1928–1932	1933–1937	1938–1942	1943–194

———— Partial network size of children (%)   - - - - Percentage of children identified in network

■■■■ Partial network size of siblings (%)   ■ ■ Percentage of siblings identified in network

Figure 3.2. Partial network size of children and siblings (as percentage of total network size) and the percentage of children and siblings identified as social network members. *Note:* Observations for cohorts 1903–1937 in 1992, for cohorts 1938–1947 in 2002. *N* = 5,199.

ing children and siblings in the social network across birth cohorts. As is shown in figure 3.2, between 80% and 90% of living adult children were identified as social network members for all cohorts (i.e., the children are important to their parents and in relatively frequent contact with them). Between 40% and 50% of living siblings were in the respondents' social networks. Younger cohorts were more likely to identify children or siblings as network members.

The networks delineated in our study were large compared to those in other network studies (Broese van Groenou & van Tilburg, 2007). For the oldest cohort on average about eight network members are identified, and for recent cohorts the average size is about 14. On average, two-thirds of the network members are relatives (including in-laws), and children are proportionally a major part in the network. The proportion of children in the social network decreases over time (figure 3.2). For the oldest cohort, 31% of network members are children. This proportion decreases to 19% for the youngest cohort. The proportion of siblings within the social network is about 10% within all cohorts.

Table 3.1 presents the results of the regression of the number of siblings in the social network, the partial network of siblings as proportion of the social network, and the proportion of the siblings represented in the social network. Across the three regression equations the effects are remarkably similar, with

Table 3.1. Regression of the number of siblings in the social network, the partial network of siblings in the social network, and the proportion of siblings represented in the social network (n = 3,415)

	Number in social network	Partial network of siblings	Proportion of siblings in network
	Beta	Beta	Beta
Number of siblings alive	0.42 ***	0.30 ***	-0.14 ***
Average traveling time to siblings	-0.07 ***	-0.08 ***	-0.12 ***
Network size (siblings excluded)	0.29 ***	-0.15 ***	0.33 ***
Having children	-0.10 ***	-0.24 ***	-0.13 ***
Average traveling time to children	0.00	-0.01	-0.03
Having partner	-0.05 **	-0.07 ***	-0.03
Parents alive (versus both deceased)	0.01	0.00	-0.01
Female	0.07 ***	0.07 ***	0.09 ***
Level of urbanization	0.04 *	0.05 **	0.05 **
Religious denomination (*ref* = none)			
Roman Catholic	0.01	0.00	-0.01
Protestant	0.02	0.02	0.03
Educational level attained	-0.01	0.00	0.01
Region in the Netherlands (*ref* = South)			
Northeast	-0.01	-0.02	-0.02
West	-0.03	-0.03	-0.03

* p < .05, ** p < .01, *** p < .001

some exceptions. Respondents with more living siblings have more siblings in their network and their networks are more characterized by large numbers of siblings, but fewer of their siblings are identified as social network members. This suggests that siblings are an important category for older adults to have available in their network but that those with many siblings do not have frequent contact with all their siblings or do consider all of them important contacts. This is more true when siblings do not live nearby. For respondents with long traveling times from sibling to sibling, the network consists of fewer siblings. The positive effects for network size on the number of siblings and the likelihood of identifying a sibling as network member indicates that sociable older adults with many other relatives and nonkin contacts are more likely to include siblings in their networks than older adults with smaller networks. However, compared with childless older people, those with children have fewer siblings in their network. Similar effects are observed for respondents who have a partner available. Among those without a partner, siblings might compensate for relationship functions available within spousal and parent-child relationships.

A parent alive might be centrally positioned in a family and facilitate contact among siblings. However, whether a parent is alive does not matter for network membership of siblings. Female respondents have more siblings in their network, have a network composition characterized by a large partial network of siblings, and identify more of the siblings as social network members. Older people living in more urbanized areas, such as cities or large villages, have more siblings in their networks. Church membership, level of education, and geographic region do not help to explain variation in the respective sibling variables. The R^2 of these models were .28, .20, and .16, respectively. In a second model (results not shown), birth cohort membership was added to the equations. A significant increase in explanatory power was not observed in any model. Since birth cohort pertains to cohort differences as well as to age differences, an unambiguous conclusion cannot be drawn. It might indicate very little change over time among five-year cohorts born in the first half of the twentieth century. It also might indicate that the position of siblings in the personal network of older adult respondents does not change when they proceed from late adulthood to old age.

In answering the second research question, we assessed the contact frequency and the intensity of supportive exchanges within relationships with siblings. If there were numerous siblings, we selected the sibling most often contacted. By focusing on one sibling, we emphasize the specific meaning that a sibling relationship might characterize. To put the contact frequency and supportive exchanges in perspective, we compare the averages with those for a child and an age peer selected in a similar procedure. A comparison can only be conducted when a respondent has both categories available. On the scale for contact frequency, with a range from 1 to 8, the average for the selected sibling is 4.7 (SD = 1.8), which is close to once every two weeks. For the selected child this average is 7.0 (SD = 1.2), or several times a week, significantly more often than for selected siblings ($t(2976)$ = 63.5, p < .001). We observe that the average contact frequency with the selected child is much higher than with the sibling, showing the relative prominence of children in comparison to siblings. For the comparison with age peers, we have data available only from the top 12 of the network. There is more often contact with age peers: the average for the selected sibling is 5.3 (SD = 1.6), and for the age peer the average is 6.4 (SD = 1.5; $t(1672)$ = 21.3, p < .001). The intensity of support exchange was assessed on a scale from 0 to 12. The average for the selected sibling is 4.2 (SD = 2.7) and for the selected child 6.7 (SD = 2.9; $t(1171)$ = 29.6, p < .001). The average level of exchange of support with the child is considerably higher than with the sibling, showing again the prominence of children in comparison to siblings. For the comparison with an age peer, the average for the selected sibling is 4.5 (SD = 2.8) and for the selected age peer 4.2 (SD = 2.9; $t(1167)$ = 3.7, p < .001). Here we observe that support exchange is more intense among siblings than among nonkin age peers.

Discussion

We focused our analysis on the availability of siblings among older adults and on frequency of contact and exchange of support among them. Using the context of the social network of older adults for a comparative approach, we assessed how many siblings were identified as social network members with whom respondents had frequent and important contact. Sibling relationships were compared to those with children and nonkin age peers with respect to contact frequency and the intensity of social support exchanges.

Eighty-six percent of the older adults in our sample, aged 55 to 89 years, had at least one living sibling, a remarkable outcome of the increased life expectancy during the second half of the twentieth century. Additionally, about half of our respondents had at least one sibling in their social network.

The data presented in figure 3.1 show an interesting picture of family development in the Netherlands in the twentieth century. In contrast to discussions about the loss of the extended family, intergenerational conflicts, high divorce rates, and women's increased labor force participation, these figures demonstrate a remarkable stability in a number of family characteristics for those born in the first half of the twentieth century. Eleven five-year cohorts demonstrate hardly any change in the average number of siblings born for older adults among five-year cohorts from 1903 to 1947; due to mortality, the average number of siblings alive is much lower among the oldest cohort than the youngest one. During the same period, the average number of children among these cohorts is again quite stable; however, the average number of children is considerably lower than the average number of siblings. Both figures reflect the national birth rate during the twentieth century, which means that the average number of siblings will decrease among later cohorts after 1947. Given the fact that in the Netherlands the baby boom lasted up to 20 years after the Second World War, the average number of children among the cohorts of older adults born between 1947 and 1965 will be at about the same level as each other.

Having a complete inventory of children and siblings but also asking separately about those children and siblings who are considered members of the social network offers insight into the composition of the social network compared to the availability of children and siblings. For the oldest cohorts, the average numbers of children and siblings in the network are lower compared to the younger cohorts (see figure 3.1); however, these numbers are lower for quite different reasons. The smaller number of siblings in the social network among the older cohorts is mainly related to the death of siblings, whereas the smaller number of children seems to be related to deterioration of relationships with some children, as the lower proportion of children in the social network of the oldest cohorts indicates (figure 3.2). The decreasing average number of children in the social network for younger cohorts (figure 3.1) is related to the decreasing birth rate since 1965; however, it may also be related to a decreasing involvement of children in parents' social networks (figure 3.2), which may indicate a gradual shift in the significance of children in the social networks of older people. Apart from change in the availability of siblings, the partial network of siblings in the social network and the siblings as a proportion of the social network appear to remain remarkably stable among birth cohorts from the first half of the twentieth century. Undoubtedly, the role of the children is more prominent, but the role of siblings in the social network is also significant.

In addition to gender and age, family life course events have been identified as important determinants of the role of siblings in the lives of older adults. We explored these determinants by introducing several explanatory variables in the regression of the representation of siblings in the network. Women studied have more siblings in their social networks than men, a larger partial network of siblings, and a higher proportion of siblings in their social networks. Family life course events like childlessness and having no partner available result in an increased importance of sibling relationships. Number of living siblings relates significantly to two of the sibling variables of older adults social networks, but respondents with a high number of living siblings have a lower proportion of siblings in their social networks. However, the power of this regression needs a caveat: It is unreasonable to argue that number of siblings alive is conceptually completely independent of the three sibling variables. Network size appears to be positively related to the number of siblings alive and to the proportion of siblings in the social network but inversely related to the size of the partial network of siblings. This may be in some way related to our procedure for the network inventory, which tended to generate large networks (Broese van Groenou & van Tilburg, 2007). Within large social networks, a large proportion of siblings will be represented in the social network; however, the partial network of siblings will be relatively small. Travel distance seems to play an important role in interaction with siblings. Short distance offers easier access and may help maintain relationships. Living in the city also appears to promote contact with siblings.

Church membership, level of education, geographical region, and whether parents are alive did not contribute to the variables being studied. The fact that level of education had no effect was not surprising, and previous findings about variability in sibling relationships according to social class have been inconsistent. More surprising is that the death of both parents had no effects. White (2001) and van Volkom (2006) have suggested that siblings move back into the inner circle of a family of orientation after the death of the parents.

We observed cross-sectionally a great stability in the role of siblings among older adults over five-year birth cohorts between 1903 and 1947, as was clear from the descriptive results as well as from the regression analyses. The data show no evidence of historical variation of the three sibling variables in older adults' social networks. Important changes in family life during the second half of the twentieth century have not endangered the sibling constellation for generations from the first half of the twentieth century. Neither the verticalization of the multigenerational family nor the development of the family of orientation into a hazardous event shows a strong impact on sibling relationships in late life. Whether this will differ for future cohorts of older people is an open question.

The data demonstrated that siblings still play a significant role in terms of contact frequency and exchange of support, although children have a higher priority. Taking those respondents having both children and siblings and selecting the child and the sibling with the highest frequency of contact shows that the difference between the average frequency of contact with the child and the sibling is considerable, a few times a week for children and nearly once a fortnight for siblings. Nevertheless, that level of sibling contact is quite high. Relative to the level of contact, the role support exchange in sibling interactions is greater than in interactions with children. Those respondents with at least one sibling and one child in their top-12 social networks reported levels of support exchange with their siblings as being only slightly lower than levels of support exchange with their children. This again indicates that siblings are important in older adults' lives.

Comparing the roles of siblings and age peers in a similar way confirms the prominent role of siblings. Frequency of contact between respondents and their siblings and age peers (in networks including both siblings and age peers but not children) is higher than among siblings in networks that include children. This might be understood as siblings compensating for the lack of children. Nevertheless, age peers have a higher frequency of contact in these networks than siblings: siblings somewhat more than once in a fortnight and age peers more than once a week. Two observations can be made about networks with siblings and age peers: the contribution of siblings is on average higher than that of age peers, and it is also higher than siblings' contributions in networks that include both siblings and children.

In conclusion, our data illustrate the significant role of siblings in the social networks of many people in late adulthood and in old age. In coming decades it is expected that this picture of the late life family will change due to decreased birth rates, higher proportions of childless couples, and higher rates of divorce. More attention to the role of siblings in future studies on the family seems therefore to be required.

ACKNOWLEDGMENTS

The Living Arrangements and Social Networks of Older Adults research program was supported by the Netherlands Program for Research on Aging (NESTOR). The Longitudinal Aging Study Amsterdam is largely supported by a grant from the Netherlands Ministry of Health, Welfare and Sports, Directorate of Long-Term Care.

REFERENCES

Akiyama, H., Elliott, K., & Antonucci, T. C. (1996). Same-sex and cross-sex relationships. *Journal of Gerontology, 51B*, P374–P382.
Antonucci, T. C., & Akiyama, H. (1987). Social networks in adult life and a preliminary examination of the convoy model. *Journal of Gerontology, 42*, 519–527.
Avioli, P. S. (1989). The social support functions of siblings in later life. *American Behavioral Scientist, 33*(1), 45–57.
Bank, S., & Kahn, M. D. (1982a). Intense sibling loyalties. In M. Lamb & B. Sutton-Smith (Eds.), *Sibling relationships: Their nature and significance across the life span* (pp. 251–266). Hillsdale, NJ: Erlbaum.
Bank, S., & Kahn, M. D. (1982b). *The sibling bond*. New York: Basic Books.
Bedford, V. H. (1989). A comparison of thematic apperceptions of sibling affiliation,

conflict, and separation at two periods of adulthood. *International Journal of Aging and Human Development, 28,* 53–66.

Bedford, V. H. (1996). Relationships between adult siblings. In A. E. Auhagen & M. von Salisch (Eds.), *The diversity of human relationships* (pp. 120–139). Cambridge, UK: Cambridge University Press.

Broese van Groenou, M. I., & van Tilburg, T. G. (2007). Network analysis. In J. E. Birren (Ed.), *Encyclopedia of gerontology* (2nd ed., Vol. 2): *Age, aging, and the aged* (pp. 242–250). San Diego, CA: Elsevier.

Cicirelli, V. G. (1985). The role of siblings as family caregivers. In W. J. Sauer & R. T. Coward (Eds.), *Social support networks and the care of the elderly* (pp. 93–107). New York: Springer.

Cicirelli, V. G. (1996). Sibling relationships in middle and old age. In G. H. Brody (Ed.), *Sibling relationships: Their causes and consequences* (pp. 47–73). Norwood, NJ: Ablex.

Connidis, I. A. (2005). Sibling ties across time: The middle and later years. In M. L. Johnson (Ed.), *The Cambridge handbook of age and ageing* (pp. 429–436). Cambridge, UK: Cambridge University Press.

Connidis, I. A. (2007). Negotiating inequality among adult siblings: Two case studies. *Journal of Marriage and Family, 69*(2), 482–499.

George, L. K. (1986). Caregiver burden: Conflict between norms of reciprocity and solidarity. In K. A. Pillemer & R. S. Wolf (Eds.), *Elder abuse: Conflict in the family* (pp. 67–92). Dover, MA: Auburn House.

Huisman, M., Poppelaars, J., van der Horst, M., Beekman, A. T. F., Brug, J., van Tilburg, T. G., & Deeg, D. J. H. (2011). Cohort profile: The Longitudinal Aging Study Amsterdam (LASA). *International Journal of Epidemiology, 40,* 868–876.

Ingersoll-Dayton, B., Neal, M. B., Ha, J., & Hammer, L. B. (2003). Redressing inequity in parent care among siblings. *Journal of Marriage and Family, 65*(1), 201–212.

Knipscheer, C. P. M., de Jong Gierveld, J., van Tilburg, T. G., & Dykstra, P. A. (Eds.). (1995). *Living arrangements and social networks of older adults.* Amsterdam: VU University Press.

O'Bryant, S. L. (1988). Sibling support and older widows' well-being. *Journal of Marriage and the Family, 50,* 173–180.

Parsons, T. (1943). The kinship system of the contemporary United States. *American Anthropologist, 45,* 22–38.

Riley, M. W. (1983). The family in an aging society: A matrix of latent relationships. *Journal of Family Issues, 4,* 439–454.

van Tilburg, T. G. (1998). Losing and gaining in old age: Changes in personal network size and social support in a four-year longitudinal study. *Journal of Gerontology: Social Sciences, 53B,* S313–S323.

van Tilburg, T. G., & Thomése, G. C. F. (2010). Societal dynamics in personal networks. In C. Phillipson & D. Dannefer (Eds.), *The Sage handbook of social gerontology* (pp. 215–225). London: Sage.

van Volkom, M. (2006). Sibling relationships in middle and older adulthood: A review of the literature. *Marriage and Family Review, 40*(2/3), 151–170

Voorpostel, M., van der Lippe, T., Dykstra, P. A., & Flap, H. (2007). Similar or different? The importance of similarities and differences for support between siblings. *Journal of Family Issues, 28*(8), 1026–1053.

White, L. K. (2001). Sibling relationships over the life course: A panel analysis. *Journal of Marriage and Family, 63*(3), 555–568.

White, L. K., & Riedmann, A. (1992). Ties among adult siblings. *Social Forces, 71*(1), 85–102.

PART II / Grandparents in a Changing Demographic Landscape

Mothers and Mentors

R ecent demographic changes in longevity, fertility, and family formation have influenced the status and role of grandparents. In 1900 only about 50% of young adults had a living grandparent compared to about 90% in 2000. In addition to a decline in fertility over this same time, patterns of fertility, marriage, and cohabitation have grown increasingly complex. Multiple partner fertility, when men and women have biological children with more than one partner, has become common. The question addressed in this section is how the changing demographic landscape has influenced the involvement of grandparents in the lives of adolescent and young adult grandchildren.

Burton, Welsh, and Destro examine how maternal grandmothers differentiate among their grandchildren in rural families characterized by multiple partner fertility. They identify three main factors prompting greater involvement of grandparents and, in some cases, even taking on the role of mother to grandchildren: biological relatedness of grandchildren, marriage of the parent, and abusive behavior by the father. Taylor, Uhlenberg, Elder, and McDonald investigate the conditions under which grandparents enact a mentoring role toward their adolescent grandchildren and with what effect. The authors find that grandparents are particularly active in nontraditional families and exert a positive influence by lowering rates of depression and delinquent behavior among grandchildren in those families.

CHAPTER FOUR

Grandmothers' Differential Involvement with Grandchildren in Rural Multiple Partner Fertility Family Structures

Linda M. Burton, Whitney Welsh, and Lane M. Destro

Multiple partner fertility (herein referred to as MPF) involves men and women having biological children with more than one partner, frequently in the context of nonmarital romantic relationships (Carlson & Furstenberg, 2006). This fertility pattern creates diverse, complex, and transient multigenerational kinship networks that have quickly become one of the most prevalent extended family forms in America (Guzzo & Furstenberg, 2007; Manlove, Logan, Ikramullah, & Holcombe, 2008). In this chapter, we use longitudinal ethnographic data to identify and describe how MPF shapes the structure, roles, and relations of grandmothers and their grandchildren within a population that has been sorely neglected by aging and family researchers— low-income rural Americans. We address two research questions: (1) What types of family structures are emerging in rural populations as a result of MPF? and (2) How do these family structures differentially impact grandmothers' involvement in their grandchildren's lives?

We begin this investigation with a brief overview of the extant literature on MPF and grandparent-grandchild relations. Next, we describe the Family Life Project (herein referred to as FLP) ethnography, which is the dataset we used to examine MPF patterns and grandmothering in rural families. We present exemplar case studies from these data to illustrate representative forms of MPF family structures and patterns of grandparents' differential involvement in their grandchildren's lives. The implications of considering the structural and relational dimensions of MPF in future studies of grandparent-grandchild relations are also discussed.

Background
The Prevalence of MPF

Within the last decade, the extent to which unmarried romantic couples are embedded in MPF relationships is a topic that has appeared with increasing regularity in the family demography literature (Bronte-Tinkew, Horowitz, & Scott, 2009; Meyer & Cancian, 2011). Early in the decade, Carlson, McLanahan, and England (2004), alerted family scientists to the growing prevalence of MPF in the lives of couples involved in the Fragile Families and Child Well-Being Study. This study followed a cohort of nearly 5,000 children born in large U.S. cities between 1998 and 2000 (roughly three-quarters of whom were born to unmarried parents) to closely examine the nature and condition of relationships between unmarried and married parents of children. Analyses of these data by Carlson and Furstenberg (2006, p. 723) revealed that among the couples in the study who were unmarried at the time of their child's birth, in a majority of these cases (59%) "one or both parents already had at least one child by another partner; in 22% of the cases, only the father had another child, in 17% only the mother had a previous child, and in the remaining 20% of the cases, both the mother and the father had children by a previous partner." For both mothers and fathers, MPF occurred most often in "visiting relationships," or relationships in which partners were romantically involved but were living in different households. Although slightly less so, MPF was also prevalent among parents who were married at the time of their child's birth. "Overall, in 21% of the married couples, either one or both partners had children by another partner (8% the father only, 8% the mother only, and 5% both)" (Carlson & Furstenberg, 2006, p. 723).

Further, Meyer, Cancian, and Cook (2005) compiled data from Wisconsin's Client Assistance for Re-Employment and Economic Support program (CARES), the Unemployment Insurance System (UI), and the Kids Information Data System (KIDS) to study the impact of MPF on paternal child support. Of the mothers in this sample, 30% experienced MPF and 36% had children by only one partner. (Due to the incomplete establishment of paternity, MPF status could not be determined for the remaining 34% of mothers.) For 20% of all mothers in the study, the father of their children had additional children with another partner, which indicated that at least half of the mothers in this sample experienced MPF through their own partnerships or through their partners'. From the perspective of fathers with established paternities, 26% had simple partner fertility (e.g., only had children by one woman) and 28% had children with mothers who had children with another partner. Nine percent of fathers had children with multiple mothers but were the only fathers of those mothers' children. For 37% of fathers, both they and the mothers of their children had children with other partners. In an expanded and updated analysis of these data, Cancian, Meyer, and Cook (2011) found that the incidence of MPF in the sample increased over time. They reported that "60% of a 1997 birth cohort of 8,019 firstborn children of unmarried mothers in Wisconsin had at least one half-sibling by age 10" due to either the children's mothers having subsequent children with other men, their biological fathers having children with other women, or both biological parents having children with other partners (p. 957).

Other research also has observed notable rates of MPF. Data from the National Survey of Family Growth (NSFG) indicated that nearly 8% of all male respondents aged 15–44 had children with at least two women (Klerman, 2007). Looking at fathers exclusively, 17% of men in the NSFG reported MPF, as did 14% of mothers in the National Longitudinal Study of Adolescent Health (Add Health) who were unmarried at first birth (Klerman, 2007).

Overall, very complex and often transient multigenerational kinship networks are created as a function of MPF among couples. These networks comprise various structural configurations of biological and nonbiological grandparental figures; biological parents; stepparents; adult boyfriends, girlfriends, and fiancées as "temporary parents;" blood-related and "fictive" aunts and uncles; and children who are full siblings, half siblings, step siblings, and "siblings" who were unrelated biologically or through marriage or adoption (Burton & Hardaway, 2012; Cancian, Meyer, & Cook, 2011). The complicated and frequently transient structure of these networks inherently sets the stage for explicit and implicit power battles between current and former romantic partners and their children and for ambiguity within these networks about family membership, role expectations, and obligations (McLanahan & Beck, 2010; Roy & Dyson, 2005). For example, Burton, Cherlin, Skinner, and Destro (2006), reporting findings about MPF and sibling inequality from the Three-City Study ethnography, indicated that grandparents in these networks were often uncertain about whether they should provide resources for the biologically unrelated "siblings" (e.g., a mother's boyfriend's child by another woman) of their biological grandchildren. That uncertainty often led to emotional battles between biological parents and grandparents around grandparents' decisions concerning whether to claim the unrelated siblings as their grandchildren as well as about how involved they should be in these children's lives (e.g., by giving birthday presents).

MPF as a Context for Grandparent-Grandchild Relations

As interesting and pronounced as the MPF prevalence statistics are, they only scratch the surface of the complexity that MPF brings to family structures and relations. Unfortunately, detailed knowledge about that complexity is limited by the available empirical research. Most studies focus primarily on the relationships between past and current MPF partners and their perceptions of equity in familial support within and across the extended networks they share. For example, Harknett and Knabb's (2007) study of MPF and social support, using longitudinal data from the Fragile Families Study, suggested that both mothers' and fathers' MPF statuses were significantly related to lower perceptions of familial support toward them. How that extended family support translates into what children who are "siblings" in these structures receive, or how they are treated equitably by kin within these networks, is not clear from these types of analyses. Indeed, research focusing on siblings' equitable access to intergenerational support or children's differential involvement with kin in nonmarital MPF family structures, in particular, is virtually nonexistent.

Likewise, the intergenerational literature on grandparent-grandchildren relationships does not inform our understanding of how MPF might influence the ways in which grandparents may be differentially involved with their grandchildren as a function of the structural complexity of these family forms. To be sure, there is a small but influential body of literature that points to the distinct emotional relationships grandparents have with different grandchildren. Fingerman's (1998) study of emotional ties between grandparents and their grandchildren, for instance, demonstrated that grandchildren who were full biological siblings within the same nuclear family units were viewed differently by their grandparents: some were viewed as special, while others were seen as worrisome and irritating. The bases of grandparents' emotional differentiation of their grandchildren included their frequency of contact with particular grandchildren and grandchildren's personal attributes. However, Fingerman did not discuss whether the differentiation process of these grandparents might vary as a function of grandchildren's parents' fertility behaviors or the family structures these grandchildren were embedded within.

Perhaps the most relevant literature available for consultation about the differential involvement and treatment of grandchildren by their grandparents comprises studies of inequality among children in stepfamilies (Cherlin & Furstenberg, 1994; Cogswell & Henry, 1995; Ehrenberg & Smith, 2003). Overall, this literature indicates that stepfamilies, resulting from parents' divorce and remarriage to others, produce sibling inequalities at least at the level of relationships among parents, biological children, and stepchildren (O'Connor, Dunn, Jenkins, & Rasbash, 2006). The work of Manning and Smock (2000), for example, suggested that while divorced and remarried parents typically do not transfer resources from their nonresidential biological children to their residential stepchildren, new coresidential biological children reduced the support of parents to their other children (see also Furstenberg, 1995). One might hypothesize that the logic of parents' unequal treatment of their biological children and stepchildren in these cases may also extend to the potential for grandparents' differential involvement with their old and new biological grandchildren as well as their new step-grandchildren.

Taken together, the limited insights that these literatures provide intimate that MPF creates complex family structures that are likely mired in ambiguity and some conflict about family ties and norms (Brown & Manning, 2009; Meyer & Cancian, 2011). Our goal in this chapter is to explore the nature of that involvement relative to the roles and relations that rural maternal grandmothers have with their grandchildren in the context of MPF family structures.

Why a Focus on Rural MPF Families?

To date, urban families have been the primary focus in research on MPF. Although urban families are an important part of the story, we argue that MPF patterns in low-income rural families are equally important in light of current economic declines in those communities which have reshaped family structures and relations in fairly dramatic ways (King & Elder, 1995; Lichter & Graefe, 2011; Maggard, 1984). Specifically, in the context of community poverty and broader social changes, our preliminary observations of marriage and romantic couple relations in the FLP ethnographic sample suggested that, regardless of race, rural families often had highly complex MPF systems that were (1) surprisingly similar to, but in some instances more complex than, those in urban low-income families and (2) a source of within- and across-household patterns of differential treatment and economic and social inequality among children who were full, half, and biologically unrelated siblings in these networks. Indeed, the MPF families in FLP ethnography, in most cases, did not mirror the image of the simple, bucolic, direct-lineage extended family systems of rural yesteryear (Davidson, 1996). In ways that mimic family configurations in urban centers, MPF families appear to be growing in numbers and to have become a permanent fixture in the contemporary rural landscape (Snyder & McLaughlin, 2004).

Data and Methods

To investigate grandmothers' involvement with their grandchildren in MPF family structures, we used longitudinal ethnographic data on families who participated in the FLP ethnography. The FLP was designed to study young children and their families who lived in two of the four major geographical areas of the United States with high poverty rates (Dill, 1999). Specifically, three counties in eastern North Carolina and three counties in central Pennsylvania were selected to be indicative of the Black South and Appalachia, respectively. The FLP's primary goal was to develop a better understanding of how community, employment, family economic resources, family contexts, parent-child relationships, and individual differences among children influence development and competencies in children during their first five years. To this end, the FLP consists of two longitudinal components: a study of children's lives and development via a series of home visits, childcare visits, and phone interviews with a representative birth cohort sample of 1,292 children (and their families) whose mothers resided in one of the six counties at the time of the child's birth; and a longitudinal ethnographic component involving 101 families with young children residing in locales that range from small cities to remote rural areas within the six counties.

Sample Description

Families were recruited into the FLP ethnography from December 2002 to June 2003. Participants in the ethnography matched participants in the larger FLP component on some, but not all, demographic characteristics, and participation in one portion of the study permanently prohibited participation in the other. Respondents for the larger component were recruited exclusively in North Carolina and Pennsylvania county hospitals shortly after giving birth, whereas respondents in the ethnography were recruited when mothers were five to eight months pregnant. In this way, the families and children in the ethnographic component were developmentally ahead of those in the other component, which enabled the principal investigators of the study to gather ethnographic data to inform measurement and data collection strategies for the birth cohort sample.

Ethnographers recruited respondents in person at churches, grocery stores, WIC offices, social services offices, parks, and shopping centers, and by posting flyers and handouts in the same locations. Snowball sampling was also used to recruit respondents in selected instances to add racially diverse respondents to the study sample. Unlike the larger FLP component's sample, all of the ethnographic respondents were low income, with reported earnings and income at 200% of the poverty level or below.

Table 4.1 displays the demographic characteristics of the maternal grandmothers (G1), mothers (G2), and children (G3) in the ethnographic sample by state. The majority of families were Non-Hispanic Whites, followed by African Americans and Latinos/Hispanics (principally of Mexican and Central American origin). Well over half of the grandmothers were aged 45 or younger at the time families were recruited into the study, and the majority of their daughters (G2s) were age 29 or younger. Most of the G2s had a high school diploma or GED or attended trade school or college, and the majority were not receiving welfare (Temporary Assistance for Needy Families, or TANF) when they entered the study. Two-thirds of G2s were working. The sample of 101 G2s identified a total of 194 children (G3) in their households, with most children under 4 years of age. Most G2s indicated that they were neither married nor cohabiting with a partner at the start of the study. However, longitudinal interviews and observations of the sample revealed over time that more respondents were in marital or cohabiting relationships than they had initially reported.

Data about the education, income, and working and marital statuses of the G1s were not gathered systematically, as G1s were not the primary focus of this study. Also, our analysis concentrates on maternal grandmothers (G2s' mothers) because they were the grandparents we had the most detailed information about. Data on the G1s were gathered primarily through participant observations at family events, casual interviews, and their daughters' and grandchildren's accounts of them.

Likewise, while we describe the MPF behaviors of G2s' romantic partners in the results section of this chapter, we do not report demographic data about them. G2s typically had multiple partners during the course of the ethnography, and those relationships were frequently transient, making it difficult to

Table 4.1. Characteristics of Family Life Project ethnography sample (*n* = 101 families)

Characteristic	North Carolina (*n* = 42 families)		Pennsylvania (*n* = 59 families)	
	n	%[1]	*n*	%[1]
Ethnicity/race (family)				
African American	19	45	15	25
Latino/Hispanic	6	14	6	10
Non-Hispanic White	17	40	38	64
G1 ages				
32–35	2	5	3	5
36–40	8	19	12	20
41–45	19	45	2	37
46–50	6	14	5	9
51–55	1	2	2	3
56+	1	2	3	5
Unknown	0	0	6	10
Deceased	5	12	6	10
G2 ages				
15–19	8	19	6	10
20–24	10	24	24	41
25–29	17	40	12	20
30–34	5	12	9	15
35–39	2	5	2	3
40+	0	0	6	10
G2 education level				
Less than high school	11	26	18	31
Completed high school or GED	12	29	26	44
College or trade school	19	45	15	25

determine and thus report G2s' multiple partners' demographic characteristics (e.g., work status, completed education).

Ethnographic Methodology

To gather and analyze ethnographic data on the grandmothers, mothers, children, and other family members, a method of "structured discovery" was used to systematize and to coordinate the efforts of the FLP ethnography team. Structured discovery comprises an integrated and transparent process for collecting, handling, and analyzing ethnographic data (see Burton et al., 2009; Winston et al., 1999). In this process, there was consistent input about data collection and analysis from over 25 ethnographers, qualitative data analysts, and research scientists who worked on the project over the course of five

Characteristic	North Carolina (n = 42 families)		Pennsylvania (n = 59 families)	
	n	%[1]	n	%[1]
G2 TANF/work status				
TANF/working	0	0	7	12
TANF/not working	1	2	12	20
Non-TANF/working	28	67	32	54
Non-TANF/not working	13	31	8	14
G2 marital status/living arrangements [2]				
Not married, not cohabiting	19	45	24	41
Married, spouse in home	11	26	10	17
Married, spouse not in home/separated	3	7	4	7
Cohabiting (any marital status)	9	21	21	35
Number of G2s' children (G3s) [2]				
1	18	43	20	35
2	8	19	15	26
3	8	19	18	32
≥4	8	19	4	7
G3 ages [2]				
<2	52	53	65	68
2–4	16	16	12	13
5–9	17	17	10	10
10–14	10	10	7	7
15–18	3	3	2	2
Total	98		96	

[1] Percentages may not sum to 100 due to rounding.
[2] There are missing data for five cases in the marital status and living arrangements category, two cases in the number of children category, and four cases in the children's age category.

years. Interviews with and observations of the respondents focused on specific topics but allowed flexibility to capture unexpected findings and relationships among variables. The interviews covered a wide variety of topics that included intergenerational family relationships, intimate partner relationships, child development, health and health care access, family economics, formal and informal support networks, and neighborhood environments. Ethnographers also engaged in participant observation with respondents, attending family functions and outings, being party to extended conversations, and witnessing relationship milestones such as a couple's decision to cohabit, marry, or have a child. They accompanied mothers and their children to the welfare office, hospital, day care, or workplace and noted both context and interactions in each situation. Ethnographers met with each family once or twice per month for 12 to 18 months and then every six months thereafter through 2006. Respondents were compensated with grocery or department store vouchers for each interview or participant observation.

Data Sources, Coding, and Analysis

The ethnography generated multiple sources of data that were used to discern MPF patterns in these families and to identify and describe grandmothers' involvement with their grandchildren. Ethnographers in each site wrote detailed field notes about their interviews and participant observations with families, and all interviews were recorded and transcribed. In addition, transcripts of principal investigators' group and individual discussions with ethnographers and qualitative data analysts about the families were consulted in this analysis. During the data collection process, the principal investigators held monthly cross-site conference calls or in-person meetings to raise Thought Provoking Questions (TPQ) with ethnographers and qualitative data analysts. The purpose of these conference calls and in-person meetings was to discuss emergent themes in ethnographers' ongoing field observations and in the data analysts' synthesis of the ethnographers' field notes and transcribed interviews. The data were coded collaboratively by ethnographers and qualitative data analysts according to a general thematic coding scheme developed by the principal investigators. The coded data were then entered into a qualitative data management (QDM) software application and were summarized into detailed case profiles about each family. The QDM program and case profiles enabled counts across the entire sample as well as detailed analysis of individual cases. Overall, in this study, we enhanced data credibility and dependability (Lincoln & Guba, 1985) through prolonged engagement in the field, repeat coding techniques, member checks with participants, and triangulation through multiple data sources and multiple methods of data collection.

Three waves of coding were conducted for each family's data. First, field notes and family profiles were open coded with common codes and sensitizing concepts. Next, coding patterns were examined within and across all families using axial coding techniques adapted from constant comparison methods of analytic induction (Charmaz, 2006; LaRossa, 2005; Strauss & Corbin, 1998). In these analyses, we identified four types of MPF family structures and four themes that characterize grandmothers' involvement with their grandchildren. Below, we present the results of these analyses first by reporting the prevalence of types of MPF family structures in the sample and second by describing grandmothers' involvement with their grandchildren in the context of these structures. We use exemplars to illustrate the parameters of grandmothers' involvement. Exemplars, or representative illustrative cases, are an established form of presenting ethnographic data that give readers a sense of the reality of respondents' experiences—that is, the *verstehen* or viewpoint of the actors (Strauss, 1987). In the specific case examples used below, mothers and their family members have been assigned pseudonyms to protect their confidentiality.

Results
Types and Prevalence of MPF Family Structures

Within the sample a considerable number of the mothers (G2s) and their current and former romantic partners demonstrated patterns of MPF characterized (on the parts of both men and women) by early and compressed fertility. Stated another way, most of the G2s and their partners had their first child during their teen and early adult years and had other children shortly thereafter (83%) and often with other partners (58%). In some instances, mothers' partners had contemporaneously impregnated several women who bore children within weeks or months of each other. After several months of ethnographic data analysis, we identified four forms of family structures linked to specific fertility patterns. The four forms that emerged in the data are as follows:

Simple

G2 has

- Children with one partner and that partner does not have children with anyone else; partner may or may not be coresiding
- Children with one previous partner and new coresiding partner does not have any children
- Children with one previous partner and new coresiding partner has children with only one previous partner

Complex Mother

G2 has

- Children with multiple previous partners and no coresiding partner
- Children with multiple previous partners and a child/children with coresiding partner
- Children with multiple previous partners and no child with coresiding partner; co-residing partner does not have any children

Complex Partner

G2's coresiding partner has

- Children with multiple previous partners; no child with respondent (respondent has children, but only with one previous partner)
- Children with multiple previous partners; child with respondent (respondent only has child with coresiding partner)

Complex Both

G2 and coresiding partner both have

- Children with multiple previous partners and no child with each other
- Children with multiple previous partners and child/children with each other

The distribution of family structures is indicated in table 4.2. Forty-three percent of the G2s were in simple family structures; however, the majority (58%) were in complex MPF networks, with 23% representing the complex both category, 19% complex partner, and 16% complex mother. The MPF structures and prevalence distribution that emerged in our data analysis were consistent with those represented in the work of Carlson and Furstenberg (2006). Reporting MPF structure distributions using the unweighted sample of the Fragile Family Study, Carlson and Furstenberg (2006) indicated that 46% of the respondents were in simple family structures, 19% in both-parents-MPF structures, 17% in father-MPF-only structures, and 16% in mother-MPF-only structures. The Fragile Family Study's sample comprised urban couples, many of who were ethnic/racial minorities. Carlson and Furstenberg (2006) found that MPF was more prevalent among African American women in the sample than in the other racial/ethnic groups. In comparison, race/ethnicity and whether respondents lived in North Carolina or Pennsylvania did not differentiate the type or prevalence of MPF structures within the FLP ethnographic sample: African Americans, Non-Hispanic Whites, and Latinos/Hispanics in both Pennsylvania and North Carolina were equally likely to be members of any category.

The historical and current patterns of MPF in the FLP families created complicated family structures that were frequently characterized by ambiguous and transient relational ties involving variable configurations of biological and nonbiological grandparental figures; biological parents; stepparents; adult

Table 4.2. Distribution of family structures in the
Family Life Project ethnography sample (n = 101)

Family structure type	n	%[1]
Simple	43	43
Complex mother	16	16
Complex partner	19	19
Complex both	23	23
Total complex[2]	58	57

[1] Percentages may not sum to 100 due to rounding.
[2] Total complex category is equal to the sum of
complex mother, complex partner, and complex both
categories.

boyfriends, girlfriends, and fiancées as "temporary parents;" blood-related and "fictive" aunts and uncles; and children who are full siblings, half siblings, stepsiblings, and "unrelated" siblings. Within these structures, parents and parental figures frequently manifested a number of challenges in assuming parental responsibility for their children, particularly their eldest children. Maternal grandmothers (G1s) often took responsibility for raising the eldest children (G3s) in these families because those children had typically been born to teen parents (G2s). In contrast, the elder children's younger siblings were born when their parents were much older and, in some cases, more mature and responsible. As such, parents in these MPF structures typically took responsibility for rearing their children who were later in the birth order (e.g., fourth-born).

Other features that characterized the MPF family structures included (1) power struggles and physical and emotional fights between current and former partners about intimate relations and the equitable distribution of resources to children; (2) the disavowing of children by relatives depending on how well members of these family networks were getting along at any point in time; (3) the absorption of non-biologically related children from previous partners into current unions because ex-partners "were not good parents and the children would suffer if someone didn't step up to the plate and take care of them;" (4) the biological grandparents of G2s' children competing with and being "thrown off balance by" new grandparents and new grandchildren being introduced into the family system via a "temporary romantic relationship" of G2; and (5) a tenuous clarity among adults and children about family obligations and legal rights concerning the "ownership" of children. This is not to say that similar issues were not experienced in some of the simple family structures. Ethnographers, however, clearly noted that the issues mentioned above were more pronounced in the MPF families in the sample and that these issues likely set the stage for maternal grandmothers' differential involvement with their grandchildren within these structures.

Grandmothers' Involvement with Grandchildren

How does MPF shape the roles and relations of grandmothers and their grandchildren? Does MPF promote grandmothers' differential involvement in their grandchildren's lives? Our data analysis indicated that MPF was indeed associated with grandmother-grandchild relations and that it shaped grandmothers' differential involvement with their grandchildren in profound ways. For instance, one ethnographer characterized G2 respondent Denise's family as follows:

> After seeing this very complicated family with so many children with different fathers, I knew from jump street that the children were going to have "unequal childhoods." The grandparents clearly had preferences for their own biological grandchildren although one of the grandmothers did extend herself to the children who were not her son's. And Denise [G2 respondent] does not appear to get along with most of the grandparents of her children, as several of them do not like her. In fact they despise her. I suspect that Christmas is a difficult time in this family with Denise and the grandparents feuding and the children receiving different amounts of presents from their respective grandparents.

As this ethnographer's assessment suggested, the sheer complexity in the number of actors in this MPF family structure, coupled with the conflictual tenor of the relationships between Denise and her children's grandparents, would likely lead to grandmothers' assuming different roles with each of their grandchildren.

In general, our analysis identified three broad themes that distinguished grandmothers' involvement with their grandchildren in the context of MPF structures: (1) the relationships between children's fathers' behaviors and grandmothers roles; (2) how family health shaped grandmothers' responsibilities for their grandchildren; and (3) whether grandmothers co-opted their firstborn grandchildren from their daughters' (G2s) MPF relationships as their own children. Owing to limitations in the depth of data gathered about the children's paternal grandparents and the grandparents of children who were not G2s biological children, our findings focus specifically on the involvement of maternal grandmothers (G2s' mothers) with the children in G2s' lives (e.g., G2s' biological children, G2s' romantic partners' children with other women). The data on G1s are also not as comprehensive as we would have liked, but they provide some general insights on the issues that clearly raise questions to be addressed in future research.

Fathers and Grandmothers

The first theme we identified concerned how the children's (G3s) fathers' behaviors created the contexts for grandmothers (G1s) to differentially inter-vene in some, but not all, of their grandchildren's lives in fairly demonstrative ways. Let us consider the case of Cassie's MPF family. Cassie is a 26-year-old Non-Hispanic White mother of four children, David, Andrea, James, and Mary, each by a different father. As Cassie's MPF diagram (figure 4.1) illus-trates, David's father has children with other partners, and only two of her children, James and Mary, have paternal grandparents who are involved in their grandchildren's lives. Cassie's mother, Clara, also has an MPF structure of her own creation, having borne children by two different men and having married another man, her granddaughter Mary's father's father, with a child from a previous relationship (Cassie's stepbrother).

The data indicated that Clara assumed different levels of involvement with her four grandchildren in large part because of the unique circumstances Da-vid's and Andrea's fathers' violent behaviors toward Cassie created, and because of James' and Mary's fathers' expectations about Clara's role as a caregiver. The ethnographer's field notes stated:

> David's father raped Cassie and Andrea's father was violent, abusive, and often incarcerated. James' father was also abusive, but Cassie has a positive relation-ship with his parents. Mary's father is Cassie's stepbrother and she has a good relationship with him. Consequently, Cassie's mother is raising David and An-drea, and Cassie is raising her two younger children. Cassie's current boyfriend won't buy things for Andrea because he believes that her grandmother, Clara, will just take care of it.

Although Cassie's family's case is extreme in terms of her particular expe-riences with sexual abuse and domestic violence, it demonstrates a clear pat-tern that we observed in the data. Essentially, the individual characteristics of children's (G3s) fathers' and mothers' (G2s) mental health and developmen-tal maturity at the time the children were born played a major role in shap-ing grandmothers' (G1s) involvement with their grandchildren. Troubled

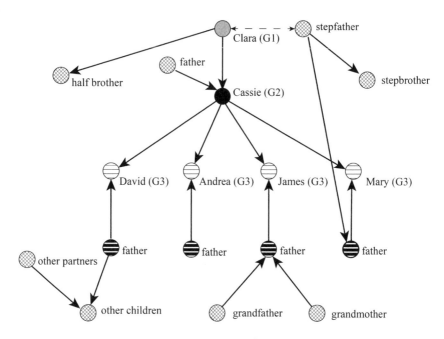

Figure 4.1. Cassie's multiple partner fertility family structure.

fathers engaged in the abusive treatment of mothers (G2s) that ultimately resulted in maternal grandmothers' assuming responsibility for the care of some, but not all, of their grandchildren. In Cassie's case, she did not want her two oldest children because one child, David, was a product of rape, and the other, Andrea, had a father who violently abused Cassie. As Cassie went on to have other children, one with a man she loved and another with a man whose parents loved their grandson, Clara was "not expected to raise her two youngest grandchildren" as their fathers had qualities that facilitated their assuming responsibility in parenting their children. In this context, Clara declared that she had different feelings about and commitments toward her grandchildren. She definitively stated, "The first two are mine, the last two belong to their mother and their fathers. They know Andrea and David are my responsibility and that James and Mary are not. I will never give up David and Andrea."

In line with Clara's engagement in different levels of caregiving with her grandchildren based on their fathers' attributes, some grandmothers defined their involvement with their grandchildren according to whether their daugh-

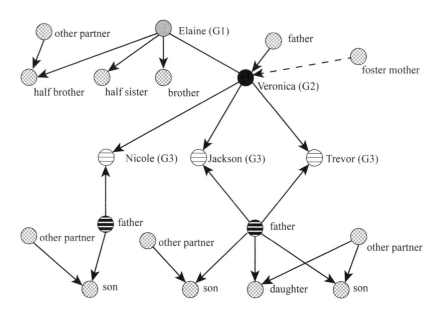

Figure 4.2. Veronica's multiple partner fertility family structure.

ters (G2s) were legally married to their grandchildren's fathers. For example, Veronica, a 25-year-old mother of three children, was married to the father of her two youngest children, Jackson and Trevor (see figure 4.2), but not to the father of her first child, Nicole.

Moreover, Veronica acquired stepchildren in marrying Jackson and Trevor's father. The ethnographer described the views of Veronica's mother, Elaine (G1), about how the marital status of her biological grandchildren's fathers and her daughter's stepchildren affected her involvement with them as follows:

> Elaine has established rules of engagement with her daughters' children and stepchildren. She explicitly indicates that she will give Trevor and Jackson the world because at least Veronica is married to their father, even though she isn't crazy about him. She says that she tries to get close to Nicole, but she just can't. Her father is in jail and she is so grown that she will probably be just like him. As for her daughter's husband's other children, she doesn't claim them as her grandchildren at all. She said, "Let their grandparents deal with them. Even though my daughter claims them, they are not my blood. I will protect what I give Trevor and Jackson, and make sure that none of those kids get what rightly belongs to them."

Grandmothering and Family Health

A second theme that emerged in the data involved the differential involvement of grandmothers in their grandchildren's lives as a function of MPF and
the health of grandmothers (G1s) and their daughters (G2s). Barbara's MPF
family network is the exemplar we use to illustrate this theme. As figure 4.3
shows, 25-year-old Barbara (G2) was the mother of six children: a set of twin
girls, one additional girl, and three boys. Her children Gregory, Vivian, Roger,
and Jerome each have different fathers, and the twins, Sharice and Denise,
share the same father. Similar to Cassie's situation, at least one of the fathers
of Barbara's children had a child with another partner, and only one paternal
grandmother was involved in this MPF network. Barbara's mother, Hilda,
also contributed to the MPF complexity of this network by having had a son,
Barbara's half brother, with another man and also by having married a third
partner who "occasionally" claims to have several children with other women.

Both Barbara and Hilda suffered from severe health problems including
morbid obesity, hypertension, and cardiovascular disease. Poor health across
two generations of caregivers in the context of MPF had serious implications
for Hilda's involvement in the lives of her grandchildren. After a year of participating in the study, Barbara, at age 26, unexpectedly dropped dead from
a heart attack while attending church with her children and Hilda. Upon
Barbara's death, Hilda, at nearly 50 years of age, was left to negotiate the care
of her six grandchildren with their respective fathers, none of whom Barbara
had legally married. The ethnographer reported that

> When Barbara died, three of the children's fathers came to claim them, and the
> other three children's fathers disavowed them. Hilda, who was in very poor
> health, had to assume total responsibility for three of her grandchildren and
> say goodbye to the three younger ones. Even though she won't see them often,
> it may be OK because she can't take care of them anyway.

Barbara's death due to her extremely poor health, coupled with MPF, created a situation in which Hilda became the primary caregiver of her three eldest grandchildren and also was relegated to having a distant relationship with
her three younger grandchildren as their fathers removed them from her care.
Hilda remained concerned that her younger grandchildren would grow up
thinking that she did not want them and that her older grandchildren would
likewise believe that their fathers, who did not come for them, did not want
them. Hilda believed that her life, as a function of Barbara's MPF behaviors,

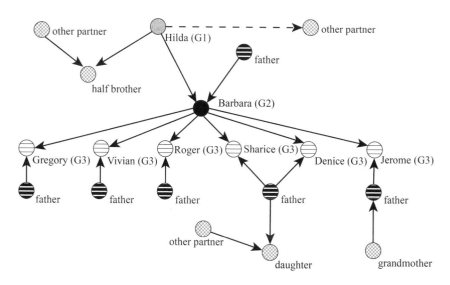

Figure 4.3. Barbara's multiple partner fertility family structure.

would forever be difficult. She said, "These babies will always be asking why they were picked over, even if it wasn't my fault. Even though I'm sick, I have to make it better for at least the three that I have. Don't know when I'll ever get to have a relationship with the other three."

Grandmothers Who Co-Opt Their Grandchildren as Their Own

The third theme that emerged in the data involved grandmothers (G1s) claiming their daughters' (G2s) firstborn child as their own and leaving their daughters' subsequent children for them to raise. In these instances, the G2 had typically been a teen mother. Grandmothers in these cases, who essentially co-opted their daughters' first children, also had been teen mothers and saw the opportunity for rearing their grandchildren as a second chance at parenting. As the family of Mandy, our exemplar for this theme, shows (see figure 4.4), G2s often went on to have children by other men who they claimed as "their own and not their mothers'." Renee, Mandy's mother, said of her grandchildren:

Abby belongs to me and her sister Amelia to her mother, Mandy. No one else can have her. She *is* my child . . . my second chance.

The ethnographer went on to note:

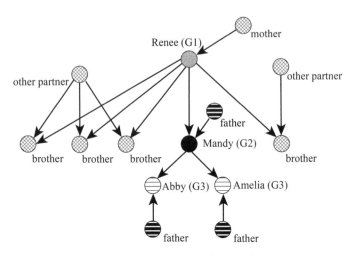

Figure 4.4. Mandy's multiple partner fertility family structure.

The difference in how Renee treats Abby over Amelia is scary. Renee acts as if the only child in the world is Abby. She totally ignores Amelia and dares Mandy to exert her parental role with Abby. This is a mess. And it doesn't help that the two girls have different fathers which further exacerbates the paramount inequalities that exist between these two siblings.

Discussion and Conclusion

The purpose of this chapter was to give honor to the mentoring and scholarly contributions of Vern Bengtson by exploring a topic that occupies center stage in his program of research, grandparenthood, and doing so with an ethos that Bengtson inspires in his students, an emergent science perspective. Using longitudinal ethnographic data from the FLP, we examined grandparenthood in the context of an emergent demographic phenomenon that has yet to be considered systematically in aging and intergenerational family research—multiple partner fertility. We addressed two research questions: (1) What types of family structures are emerging in rural populations as a result of MPF? and (2) How do these family structures differentially impact grandmothers' involvement in their grandchildren's lives?

Overall, the results of our study indicated that the prevalence of MPF in rural communities was similar to patterns observed in urban centers. Essentially, women and men were having children with other partners with increasing frequency in rural places. That being said, MPF in the FLP sample created complex family structures that had a major impact on grandmothers' differential involvement with their grandchildren. As the exemplar cases in our study show, grandmothers had distinct levels of involvement with their grandchildren based on the assorted qualities of their grandchildren's fathers, their grandchildren's parents' marital status, their grandchildren's birth orders, intergenerational health (for other health effects, see Markides, Angel, & Peck, Chapter 15), and the grandmothers' perceptions of raising their grandchildren as a second chance at parenting.

The work we presented here is very preliminary, in large part because of data limitations. As we noted earlier, this study was not designed to gather comprehensive data about grandparenting and MPF, although through the ethnographic data collection process we were able to garner information that allowed us to address the research questions at a very basic level. Rather than view our chapter as a defining discussion of this topic, we saw it as an opportunity to pursue a line of inquiry that Vern Bengtson, as an advocate of exploring emergent topics in intergenerational relationship science, would surely support. What we found, despite its preliminary nature, has piqued our interest such that we are likely to pursue further investigation of these issues in a study designed specifically to explore them.

Postscript

Vern Bengtson has successfully cultivated several generations of social scientists who have the conceptual and methodological talent, skills, and rigor to move the fields of gerontology and family science forward in very significant ways. His efforts will stand the test of time, forever prodding scholars to "make the fields better." And, his heart will always be a source of inspiration for those who seek to be the best scholars they can be (Burton, 2005, p. 92).

In 2005, Linda Burton had the distinct honor of writing a tribute about Vern Bengtson's numerous mentoring and scholarly contributions to the fields of gerontology and family science (see Burton, 2005). As the above-cited excerpt from that tribute suggests, she called attention to Bengtson's keen ability to cultivate young scholars who explore new research terrains in aging, family, and intergenerational relations and who do so with "sociological imagination" (Mills, 1959). She also shared personal reflections about the exemplary training she received from Bengtson and about her early research collaborations with him on studies of grandparenthood (see Burton & Bengtson, 1985). Burton, a sociologist and ethnographer, indicated that Bengtson inspired her to investigate the impact of diverse family structures on intergenerational family dynamics in new and exciting ways. He always encouraged her to follow "her ethnographic research gut" and to pay particular attention to the intergenerational behaviors that were being played out in families just below the radar screen of what more traditional approaches to the study of generations would lead scientists to explore. It was Burton's experiences as Bengtson's student that motivated us to celebrate his career by writing a chapter about a central topic in his research, grandparenting, and to do so in ways that integrate the emergent science approach that he encourages his students to pursue in their work (see Bengtson, 2001). In this way, we see ourselves continuing the Bengtson legacy. It is not by happenstance that Burton coauthored this chapter with two of her graduate students, Whitney Welsh and Lane Destro, both of whom recently earned their PhDs in sociology from Duke University. Burton is following in her mentor's footsteps, seeking to inspire her students to explore new questions about families and generations with an emergent perspective and with "sociological imagination."

ACKNOWLEDGEMENTS

The authors thank the National Institute of Child Health and Human Development for providing core support to the FLP ethnography through grant number R01 HD51859-03 and the National Science Foundation for its support of their work on intergenerational resource allocation through grant SES-07-0396 and multiple partner fertility through grant SES-1061591. They also acknowledge the Administration on Children and Families for supporting their research on marriage and relationships among low-income families through grant 90OJ2020. Most importantly, they thank the families who graciously participated in the research reported in this article.

REFERENCES

Bengtson, V. L. (2001). Beyond the nuclear family: The increasing importance of multi-generational bonds. *Journal of Marriage and the Family, 63*, 1–16.
Bronte-Tinkew, J., Horowitz, A., & Scott, M. E. (2009). Fathering with multiple partners: Links to children's well-being in early childhood. *Journal of Marriage and Family, 71*, 608–631.

Brown, S.L., & Manning, W. D. (2009). Family boundary ambiguity and the measurement of family structure: The significance of cohabitation. *Demography, 46*(1), 85–101.

Burton, L. M. (2005). The scholar and the oak tree: A profile of Vern L. Bengtson. *Contemporary Gerontology, 11*, 91–94.

Burton, L. M., & Bengtson, V. L. (1985). Black grandmothers: Issues of timing and meaning in roles. In V. L. Bengtson & J. Robertson (Eds.), *Grandparenthood: Research and policy perspectives* (pp. 61–77). Beverly Hills, CA: Sage.

Burton, L. M., Cherlin, A. J., Skinner, D., & Destro, L. M. (2006). Multi-partner fertility patterns in low-income urban and rural families. *Paper presented at the annual meeting of the American Sociological Association.* Montreal, Canada.

Burton, L. M., Cherlin, A., Winn, D. M., Estacion, A., & Holder-Taylor, C. (2009). The role of trust in low-income mothers' intimate unions. *Journal of Marriage and Family, 71*, 1107–1127.

Burton, L.M. & Hardaway, C. R. (2012). Low-income mothers as "othermothers" to their romantic partners' children: Women's coparenting in multiple partner fertility relationships. *Family Process, 51*, 343–359.

Cancian, M., Meyer, D. R., & Cook, S. T. (2011). The evolution of family complexity from the perspective of nonmarital children. *Demography, 48*, 957–982.

Carlson, M. J., & Furstenberg, F.F. Jr. (2006). The prevalence and correlates of multi-partnered fertility among urban U.S. parents. *Journal of Marriage and the Family, 68*, 718–732.

Carlson, M., McLanahan, S., & England, P. (2004). Union formation in fragile families. *Demography, 41*, 237–261.

Charmaz, K. (2006). *Constructing grounded theory.* London: Sage.

Cherlin, A., & Furstenberg, F. (1994) Stepfamilies in the United States: A reconsideration. *Annual Review of Sociology, 20*, 359–381.

Cogswell, C., & Henry, C. S. (1995). Grandchildren's perceptions of grandparental support in divorced and intact families. *Journal of Divorce and Remarriage, 23*, 16–27.

Davidson, G. O. (1996). *Broken heartland: The rise of America's rural ghetto.* Iowa City, IA: University of Iowa Press.

Dill, B. T. (1999). *Poverty in the rural U.S.: Implications for children, families, and communities.* Literature review prepared for The Annie E. Casey Foundation.

Ehrenberg, M. F., & Smith, S. T. (2003). Grandmother-grandchild contacts before and after an adult daughter's divorce. *Journal of Divorce and Remarriage, 39*, 45–62.

Fingerman, K. L. (1998). The good, the bad, and the worrisome: Emotional complexities in grandparents' experiences with individual grandchildren. *Family Relations, 47*, 403–414.

Furstenberg, F. F. Jr. (1995). Changing roles of fathers. In P. L. Chase-Lansdale & J. Brooks-Gunn (Eds.), *Escape from poverty: What makes a difference for children* (pp. 189–210). Cambridge: Cambridge University Press.

Guzzo, K. B., & Furstenberg, F. F. Jr. (2007). Multipartnered fertility among young women with a nonmarital first birth: Prevalence and risk factors. *Perspectives on Sexual and Reproductive Health, 39,* 29–38.

Harknett, K., & Knabb, J. (2007). More kin, less support: Multipartnered fertility and perceived support among mothers. *Journal of Marriage and Family, 69,* 237–253.

King, V., & Elder, G. H. Jr. (1995). American children view their grandparents: Linked lives across three rural generations. *Journal of Marriage and the Family, 57,* 165–178.

Klerman, L. (2007). Multipartnered fertility: Can it be reduced? *Perspectives on Sexual and Reproductive Health, 39,* 56–59.

LaRossa, R. (2005). Grounded theory methods and qualitative family research. *Journal of Marriage and Family, 67,* 837–857.

Lichter, D. T., & Graefe, D. R. (2011). Rural economic restructuring: Implications for children, youth, and families. In K. Smith & A. Tickamyer (Eds.), *Economic restructuring and family wellbeing in rural America.* University Park, PA: Penn State University Press.

Lincoln, Y., & Guba, E. (1985). *Naturalistic inquiry.* Thousand Oaks, CA: Sage.

Maggard, S. W. (1984). From the farm to coal camp to back office and McDonalds's: Living in the midst of Appalachia's latest transformation. *Journal of the Appalachian Studies Association, 6,* 14–38.

McLanahan, S. & Beck, A. N. (2010). Parental relationships in fragile families. *The Future of Children, 20*(2), 17–37.

Manlove, J., Logan, C., Ikramullah, E., & Holcombe, E. (2008). Factors associated with multiple-partner fertility among fathers. *Journal of Marriage and Family, 70,* 536–548.

Manning, W .D., & Smock, P. J. (2000). "Swapping" families: Serial parenting and economic support for children. *Journal of Marriage and the Family, 62,* 111–122.

Meyer, D.R. & Cancian, M. (2011). "I'm not supporting his kids": Nonresident fathers' contributions given mothers' new fertility. *Journal of Marriage and Family, 74,* 132–151.

Meyer, D. R., Cancian, M. & Cook, S. T. (2005). Multiple-partner fertility: Incidence and implications for child support policy. *Social Service Review, 79,* 577–601.

Mills, C. W. (1959). *The sociological imagination.* London: Oxford University Press.

O'Conner, T. G., Dunn, J., Jenkins, J. M., & Rasbash, J. (2006). Predictors of between-family and within-family variation in parent-child relationships. *Journal of Child Psychology and Psychiatry, 47,* 498–510.

Roy, K., & Dyson, O. (2005). Gatekeeping in context: Babymama drama and the involvement of incarcerated fathers. *Fathering: A Journal of Theory, Research, and Practice about Men as Fathers, 3,* 289–310.

Snyder, A. R. & McLaughlin, D. K. (2004). Female-headed families and poverty in rural America. *Rural Sociology, 69,* 127–149.

Strauss, A. (1987). *Qualitative analysis for social scientists.* New York: Cambridge University Press.

Strauss, A., & Corbin, J. (1998). *Basics of qualitative research: Techniques and procedures for developing grounded theory* (2nd ed.). Thousand Oaks, CA: Sage.

Winston, P., Angel, R. J., Burton, L. M., Chase-Lansdale, P. L., Cherlin, A. J., Moffitt, R. A., & Wilson, W. J. (1999). Welfare, children, and families: Overview and design. Retrieved April 20, 2009 from Johns Hopkins University, *Welfare, Children, & Families: A Three-City Study* website (http://web.jhu.edu/threecitystudy/images/ overviewanddesign.pdf).

CHAPTER FIVE

The Role of Grandparents in the Transition to Adulthood

Grandparents as "Very Important" Adults in the Lives of Adolescents

Miles G. Taylor, Peter Uhlenberg, Glen H. Elder, Jr., and Steve McDonald

Demographic shifts over the past century have increased the percentage of grandchildren who have living grandparents, and these historical changes are especially impressive for young adults. For example, in 1900 about half of all 20-year-olds had at least one living grandparent; in 2000, 90% did. For 30-year-olds, these chances increased from 21% to 75% (Uhlenberg, 1996, 2004). Heterogeneity of the grandparenting role has notably increased across time and across age (Silverstein & Marenco, 2001). Reports on grandparent-grandchild interaction indicate that frequent contact is common, but substantial variation exists across individuals (Cherlin & Furstenberg, 1986; King & Elder, 1995; Uhlenberg & Hamill, 1998). Grandparent involvement has been seen as important both for the development of children and for the social support it provides for parents (McCluskey & McCluskey, 2000). Reciprocally, grandparent-grandchild contact tends to increase satisfaction with the grandparent role (Mueller & Elder, 2003; Peterson, 1999).

Research has mainly focused on the grandparent-grandchild relationship when grandchildren are under 18 (Connidis, 2001). Far less is known about how these relationships change as children transition into adulthood or whether predictors of relationship quality change during this transition. The increasing number of young adults with living grandparents and the previous research on the importance and variability of the grandparenting role suggests that more research is needed to understand this relationship as children become adults.

The importance of grandparents to children's well-being on the whole, and their role as custodians specifically, has gained attention in recent years (Fuller-Thompson & Minkler, 2001; Henly, 1997; Jendrek, 1993). Living in multigenerational households can benefit children from female-headed families so that their outcomes are no different from those of children who reside with both parents (Deleire & Kalil, 2002). In addition, the added social capital provided by grandparents to at-risk youth has been shown to be significant in predicting the well-being of this group (Furstenberg & Hughes, 1995).

The research surrounding grandparent and great-grandparent custodial or caregiving relationships has focused on African Americans in particular, since the increases in custodial relationships have occurred primarily in this group over the past decade (McDonald & Armstrong, 2001; Minkler & Fuller-Thompson, 2005; Ruiz, 2000). However, the majority of this research remains cursory or relies on small, racially homogeneous, qualitative samples. Little to no research has examined the grandparenting role for at-risk adolescents or for those who experience negative life events such as parental divorce or teen childbearing (Ruiz, 2000).

This project will study the relationship between grandparents and grandchildren during the time between adolescence and young adulthood. We focus on the role grandparents play as important adults or mentors. Previous research on relationship quality and closeness between grandparents and grandchildren of this age has relied on either small or homogeneous samples containing rich relationship information or larger samples with few measures of relationship quality or adolescent well-being. Using Add Health data, we recast questions on mentoring at Wave 3 to allow a novel approach to the study of grandparenting. The Add Health data pose a unique opportunity to study the roles grandparents play in the lives of adolescents who are making the transition to adulthood.

We proceed by discussing the background literature on the somewhat disparate literatures of mentoring and grandparenting used to address our research questions. Next, we discuss the Add Health data and the process of recasting variables on mentoring to examine grandparents in the transition to adulthood. We move on to descriptive findings and a discussion of future research.

We address three specific research questions in our larger project: (1) What are the characteristics of grandchildren who report grandparents as their primary mentors, and what roles do mentors play in their lives? (2) What role do grandparents play in the face of negative transitions in young lives, such as parental divorce or teen childbearing? (3) How do grandparent mentors increase the resiliency of young adults in terms of well-being outcomes?

Research Questions and Background Literature

Research Question 1: What are the characteristics of grandchildren who report grandparents as their primary mentors, and what roles do mentors play in their lives?

The themes outlined in Neugarten and Weinstein's (1964) classic work have persisted across decades of literature on grandparenting and intergenerational relationships. Bengtson (1985) notes the importance of two emergent themes in grandparenting research, diversity and symbolism. In studying diversity, gender, age, race and ethnicity, and family structure are important in examining the grandparent role or grandparent-grandchild relationships. Gender differences in grandparenting are known to generally follow what may be called a "matrifocal tilt" owing to a stronger investment in intergenerational relationships by women (Hagestad, 1985; Mueller, Wilhelm, & Elder, 2002; Rossi, 1993). This tilt predicts stronger connections between granddaughters and their grandparents, grandmothers and their grandchildren, and grandchildren and their maternal grandparents (Kivett, 1991; Tinsley & Parke, 1984).

Age of the grandparent is known to be important, especially for grandparents who think they are too young to be filling the role or who are very old and more likely to be ill or frail (Burton & Bengtson, 1985; Neugarten & Datan, 1973; Neugarten & Weinstein, 1964). Age of the grandchild is also an important factor, as previous research suggests that there are multiple overlapping stages of the grandparenting career. These stages correspond to the age of the grandchild (Cherlin & Furstenberg, 1986) and to grandchildren's perceptions of grandparents as they age (Creasey & Kaliher, 1994). However, the empirical findings on the ages between adolescence and parenthood for the grandchild are sparse and are based mostly on convenience samples of college students (see Mills, 1999).

Racial and ethnic diversity in the grandparenting role has been a focus of research in recent decades. African American and (less so) Hispanic children are more likely to grow up in a household headed by a grandparent (Saluter & Lugaila, 1998). It has been shown that among grandparents, African Americans have 83% higher odds of engaging in caregiving activities (Fuller-Thompson, Minkler, & Driver, 1997). Although much of this research is focused on coresidential grandparents or grandparent caregivers (see Kataoka-Yahiro, Ceria, & Caulfield, 2004, for review), there is some reason to believe that there are racial and ethnic variations in how grandparents view their roles and responsibilities (Brown et al., 2000; Burton & de Vries, 1992; Kivett, 1993) and the perceived burden associated with responsibilities (Minkler, Roe, & Price, 1992; Pruchno, 1999). The way grandchildren view their grandparents' roles has also been shown to vary (Kennedy, 1990). The findings of these studies are particularly hard to generalize, since much of the work on racial/ethnic differences utilizes homogeneous samples (for example, poor African American grandmother caregivers) and little work has been done on variations other than comparing White or European grandparents to African Americans (see Caldwell, Silverman, & Silver, 2004; Yi, Pan, Chang, & Chan, 2006, for exceptions). Therefore, the role of cultural differences and migration is vastly understudied.

Three primary mechanisms shape the grandparenting role. The first is proximity: grandchildren who live near their grandparents have greater frequency of contact and report closer relationships with their grandparents (Brussoni & Boon, 1998; Cherlin & Furstenberg, 1986; Uhlenberg & Hammill, 1998). The second is parent-grandparent closeness: the quality of the parent-grandparent relationship is directly related to the frequency of contact and closeness of the grandparent. The mediating role of the parent is often highlighted in this research (King & Elder, 1995; Reitzes & Mutran, 2004; Tinsley & Parke, 1987). In the case of divorced or widowed parents, family structure may both decrease the proximity of grandchildren to their grandparents and decrease the parental gateways though which grandchildren have contact with grandparents (Gravenish & Thompson, 1996). The third is socioeconomic status: single-parent households are likely to be lower in parental education and household income (Haurin, 1992; McLanahan, 1985; McLanahan & Sandefur, 1994), and this may work to decrease both contact with grandparents and parent-grandparent closeness (Bray & Berger, 1990; Clingempeel, Colyar, Brand, & Hetherington, 1992). Alternately, family instability may facilitate three-generation households and increase the financial, instrumental, or emotional support grandparents provide their grandchildren (Johnson, 1988).

The symbolism (Bengtson, 1985) of the grandparenting role emerges in the context of continuities in how grandparents influence the lives of grand-children. The concept of "being there" is important in considering the transitions of individuals in intergenerational context. When parents divorce, for example, a grandparent may step in to keep the family intact through instrumental or ideological means (Hagestad, 1984; Hagestad, Symer, & Stierman, 1984). In addition, grandparents may serve as an emotional anchor of stability and family continuity during difficult transitions in the lives of younger generations (Hagestad, 1982; Johnson, 1985). Further, it is possible that the perception of this role by the grandparent is more important than support that is actually given.

Along with "being there," Bengtson (1985) describes grandparents as primary in the family's social construction of history, in the "building of reasonable connections among our past, present, and future." Indeed, this facet of the intergenerational stake (Bengtson & Kuypers, 1971; Giarrusso, Stallings, & Bengtson, 1995) places on grandparents the greatest responsibility of embedding the current experiences of children in the context of the past. Neugarten and Weinstein (1964) touched on this theme, describing it as a "reservoir of family wisdom" confined to authoritarian, patriarchal grandparent-grandchild relationships. King, Elder, and Conger (2000) describe this function of the grandparent role as a "wisdom of the ages," which is more in line with Bengtson's arguments and less central to a certain restrictive type of intergenerational relationship. Among the grandparents King, Elder, and Conger studied in rural Iowa, the majority reported giving advice, sharing stories of their own childhoods, and serving as "voices of wisdom and experience on a troublesome issue." This type of active mentoring, or support, coincided closely with the theme of grandparents as family historians with a substantial stake in the future of the family and its identity. Further, the majority reported offering some tangible support through financial aid or teaching their grandchildren specific skills.

From this work, we would expect that the reasons for grandparents to be important in the lives of children as they age may be unique compared to other family and nonfamily mentors. Grandparents may be more likely to offer financial assets or a stable home during family or economic instability or to have time and resources to help in childcare (Guzman, 2004; Tinsley & Parke, 1987; Wandersman, Wandersman, & Kahn, 1980) when compared to younger family members such as aunts and uncles. In addition, grandparents are noted as having the highest intergenerational stake in their families and may invest more than other family members in imparting the morals, values, and principles they associate with the family. Further, they may serve as unique role models for coping with adversity across the life course.

Research Question 2: What role do grandparents play in the face of negative transitions in young lives, such as parental divorce, parental loss, or teen childbearing? Do adolescents report grandparents as mentors more often when these transitions occur, and what may be unique among grandparents that allows them to offset negative turning points in young lives? How do these effects vary by race and ethnicity?

The study of the grandparent role has been increasingly framed in terms of specific transitions or turning points in young lives. Two of the most salient such transitions are parental divorce or single parenthood and teen childbearing. The research surrounding marital disruption and single parenthood of the middle (parental) generation is multi-faceted, speaking to the positive and negative effects of and on grandparents during and after this transition (see Johnson, 1998). For example, grandparents are often conceptualized as a potential family resource to single parents, but the research has dually noted that marital disruption or single parenthood may have negative effects for grandparents who become ill or need support (Cicirelli, 1984). In addition, marital disruption in the middle generation often distances grandchildren from the parents of their nonresidential parent (Cherlin & Furstenberg, 1986).

The reciprocal pushes and pulls of intergenerational relationships are complex in conceptualizing the effects of family structure, so we limit our discussion here primarily to literature focused on the grandparent's positive involvement or potential support for the grandchild in the case of marital disruption or single parenthood. Studies have found that grandchildren may have increased contact with at least one grandparent following a divorce (Gladstone, 1988; Johnson, 1983). In addition, it is likely that grandparents view themselves as surrogate parents (Neugarten & Weinstein, 1964; Robertson, 1995) to a grandchild after a divorce when they report closeness with some degree of distance from the child prior to divorce or disruption (Johnson, 1998; Rosenmayr, 1972). Grandparents may act as surrogate parents in the short term after marital disruption, but more long-term support of this kind is less common (Johnson, 1998). However, children living with single mothers are three times as likely to live with a grandparent than are their counterparts with married mothers (U.S. Census Bureau, 2005).Grandparents may be in a uniquely stable position in the family to assist with children financially, by providing a stable home, or by caring for them. In addition, the intergenerational stake for grandparents may increase, at least temporarily, in grandchildren from a single-parent or divorced household since the potential ties to family history decrease with one parent not in residence.

Teen childbearing has also received attention in the literature, since it places both adolescent mothers and their children at risk of negative outcomes (Flaherty, Facteau, & Garver, 1987; Smith, 1975). Becoming a parent in adolescence is considered an especially salient turning point where identities and relationships transition (Musick, 1993). The literature on grandparenting has more recently focused on custodial grandparenting or grandparent childcare (see Guzman, 2004). There are roughly 2.4 million grandparents reporting they fill at least some of the basic needs of their grandchildren, and teen mothers receiving childcare from family members fare better on education and employment outcomes (Gordon, Chase-Lansdale, & Brooks-Gunn, 2004; Unger & Cooley, 1992; U.S. Census Bureau, 2005). Indeed, the literature on teen or adolescent parents heavily emphasizes the importance of family support and caregiving to the child (Dickerson, 1995; Wilson, 1984, 1986). However, with increases in longevity (Cherlin & Furstenberg, 1986; Uhlenberg & Kirby, 1998) or when there are multiple generations of teen childbearing (Burton & Bengtson, 1985), the great-grandmother of the child (grandmother of the adolescent mother) may become a strong source of support because she is at an age or position to do so (see also Burton, 1992). The notion that grandparents may play a mediating role between parents and children, especially when parents are divorced or grandparents are custodial (Gladstone, 1989; Goodman & Silverstein, 2001; Werner, Buchbinder, Lowenstein, & Livni, 2005) bolsters the argument that adolescent mothers may draw upon their grandparents for additional support.

Grandparents may act as important buffers to negative transitions in children's lives, offsetting negative outcomes thereafter. Because of their life experience and increased stake in the family, they may be more likely to provide emotional support in young lives during transitions. In addition, grandparents report at least some period of acting in a stronger parental role toward grandchildren after negative transitions (for grandmothers acting as mothers, see Burton, Welsh, & Destro, Chapter 4), such that their involvement in children's lives increases. The unique experience of racial and ethnic minorities undergoing negative life transitions is at the forefront of this line of inquiry, since grandparent involvement in the case of adversity has shown to vary by race and ethnicity.

Research Question 3: How do grandparent mentors increase the resiliency of young adults in terms of well-being outcomes? Are the benefits of grandparent involvement unique to those experiencing adversity (through parental divorce, parental loss, or adolescent childbearing) or universal?

There is reason to believe that although not all grandparent influence is positive (see Tomlin, 1998), grandparents may promote resiliency in disadvantaged children. For example, children raised by their grandparents have been found to fare as well as children with two parents on health and deviance outcomes (Solomon & Marx, 1995). Children from single-parent households are also likely to benefit behaviorally and emotionally from having a grandparent in the household (Dornbusch et al., 1985; Lussier, Deater-Deckard, Dunn, & Davies, 2002; Stolba & Amato, 1993). Some research also reports higher levels of grandparent closeness among children from blended families compared to single-parent or two-biological-parent households (Kennedy & Kennedy, 1993). There is also research showing that children more often report grandparents than other family members as their primary confidants when families split (Dunn & Deater-Deckard, 2001).

Although far less is known about the benefits of noncustodial or nonresident grandparents for grandchild outcomes, a few studies show that overall exposure to grandparents may benefit adolescents in reducing problem behaviors among children in poverty (see Pittman, 2007, for review). Grandparent financial resources may directly increase educational opportunities for children (see Shapiro, 2004), and educational attainment of extended family members, including grandparents, has been shown to affect education outcomes for children (Loury, 2006). Silverstein and Ruiz (2006) found that grandparents moderate the transmission of depression from mothers to children as they pass into adulthood. More specifically, strong levels of cohesiveness with grandparents (as reported by grandchildren) buffered the effects of maternal depression. Although the findings of these innovative studies suggest that grandparent involvement may be beneficial even when the grandparent is not coresidential, there is far more research needed on the nuanced picture of grandparent involvement in nonresidential or noncustodial situations. Further, it is unclear which components of grandparent-grandchild cohesiveness (frequency of contact, emotional closeness, or instrumental support) are most important or characteristic of the grandparent-grandchild relationship in predicting child outcomes.

Bridging research on resiliency, mentors, and grandparent effects in residential and nonresidential settings, there is reason to believe that grandparents may bolster the resiliency of adolescents in the face of adversity through numerous mechanisms. They may work to decrease internalizing processes such as depression, therefore moderating the effects of negative life conditions or transitions (Pittman, 2007; Silverstein & Ruiz, 2006). In addition, they may decrease externalizing processes such as problem behaviors or delinquency for children at risk of negative turning points (Caldwell, Silverman, & Silver, 2004; Solomon & Marx, 1995; Stolba & Amato, 1993). It is unclear whether the benefits of grandparent involvement are universal across families or whether they are increasingly mobilized in the face of adversity.

Data Source, Variables of Interest, and Analyses

Data are drawn from the first and third wave of the National Longitudinal Study of Adolescent Health (Add Health). Add Health is a nationally representative, school-based survey of adolescents in grades 7–12. The study was originally designed to monitor the health and health-related behaviors of adolescents with particular focus on multiple domains of context (family, school, peer, etc.). The baseline survey was collected in 1994 and 1995 with a follow-up wave in 1996. A third wave was administered in 2001 and 2002 to follow adolescents as they transitioned into adulthood. Aged 18–28 in this wave, the young adults were asked a series of retrospective questions on mentoring during their adolescence. The mentoring questions, along with other variables of interest, are listed in table 5.1.

Specifically, respondents were asked, "Other than your parents or stepparents, has an adult made a positive difference in your life at any time since you were 14 years old?" This variable was originally designed to capture any nonparent adult who was important to the adolescent emotionally, instrumentally, or in other ways. Roughly 75% of respondents answered that they had a mentor in their life. The mentoring module also includes questions about who the mentor was, the respondent's past and current relationship to the mentor, and the timing and duration of the relationship. Thus, it is possible to ascertain whether the mentor was a grandparent, some other family member, or some non-family member such as a teacher. In this way, the Add Health data pose a unique opportunity to study the roles grandparents play in the lives of adolescents and their transition to adulthood.

Our first research question aims at assessing which adolescents report grandparents as mentors. Since survey respondents could only report one adult (other than their parents or stepparents) as their "very important person," we

Table 5.1. Selected Study Variables

Adolescents
  Age, gender, race, number of siblings (Wave 1)
  School ability and achievement (standardized PVT score, highest degree) (Waves 1 & 3)

  Health, well-being
  Health behaviors, depressive symptoms, delinquency scale (Waves 1 & 3)

  Family (all Wave 1)
  Family of origin (mother's and father's educational attainment)
  Parental welfare receipt
  Family structure (living with two biological parents, step-parents, etc.)
  Parental closeness (mother and father)
  Live with grandparents in household

  Life events (Wave 3)
  Parental divorce/union dissolution and age at which dissolution occurred
  Pregnancy/childbearing and age at which pregnancy/childbearing occurred

Mentor (retrospective, Wave 3)
  Adult that has made a positive difference in your life since you were 14? (Yes/No)
  Mentor relationship to adolescent
  Gender of grandparent
  Matrilineal/patrilineal grandparent
  Whether grandparent is still living
  How old was respondent when mentor first became important (timing)
  Whether mentor is still important to respondent
  Relationship duration (how may years mentor was important)
  How often respondent sees and has contact with mentor (phone/e-mails)
  Closeness to mentor (relationship quality)
  Most recent visit/contact
  How mentor "helped" respondent—open-ended question, coding below:
    A. Behavior (guidance, emotional nurturance, instrumental/practical, like a parent, etc.)
    B. Domain of mentoring (development or direction, household, religion, finances, etc.)

Weights
  Probability weight: GSWGT3_2
  Cluster variable: SCID

---

study the characteristics of those most likely to report grandparents as opposed to other adults. Basic factors like gender, race, socioeconomic status, family structure, parental closeness, frequency of contact with grandparent, and school achievement have not yet been examined in this context or in nationally representative samples of children.

We are also interested in the specific role of the grandparent in the life of the adolescent or what role they played to be distinguished as a mentor. This is assessed though an open-ended question on the role the mentor played in the life of the adolescent. In the series of mentoring questions, the open-ended question "How did he or she help you?" allowed the respondent to list specific roles or actions undertaken by the mentor. This qualitative item has since been recoded into quantitative variables on the behavior and domain of mentoring, including whether the mentor provided emotional or instrumental support to the adolescent and whether the mentor was described more as another parent or as a friend or role model.

The coding of this variable is perhaps the most valuable item for the study of grandparenting, since it allows the respondents to voice the most important or salient aspects of the grandparenting role in their own development during adolescence and transition into adulthood. This recoded variable also provides invaluable insight into the grandparenting role in comparison to the roles of other important family and nonfamily adults in the lives of adolescents as they move into adulthood. Future research will address whether grandparents are comparable in their roles to other family members (like aunts and uncles) or if they are closer to teachers and coaches. The ability to utilize multiple counter-factuals in the grandparent-grandchild relationship has been absent in the grandparenting literature to date.

Next we are interested in what roles grandparents play when negative life events occur during childhood and adolescence. Parental divorce or death and teen childbearing are two life events that have been noted in previous literature, but the richness or generalizability of those studies has been limited. In determining whether grandparents take a parental role when marital dissolution or parental loss occurs, we first examine here whether those adolescents with alternative family structures report grandparents as mentors more frequently than their counterparts with two biological parents. We also address whether teen mothers report grandparents to be more salient than adolescent females with no children before the age of 19. Racial differences are especially important to this line of study, since previous literature has noted differences in the roles of extended family members for different races, especially Blacks and Whites (McDonald & Armstrong, 2001; Ruiz, 2000). Since the Add Health data were originally designed to measure health and well-being among adolescents, questions on family structure and childbearing are included at each wave. Here we use only family status at Wave 1 and a dichotomous indicator for childbearing before the age of 19, but future research may address the timing of grandparent involvement by calculating both the ages at these negative events and the age at which the mentor became important in the respondent's life. For these questions, cross-tabulations are presented, with significance from chi-square statistics noted on graphs.

Finally, we study how adolescents reporting grandparents as mentors fare on well-being outcomes. Although many physical and mental health questions are asked in the Add Health survey, we restrict our analyses here to depressive symptoms and delinquency, two outcomes of noted importance in previous literature. Here we present preliminary bivariate regressions of depression and delinquency at Wave 3 on reporting a grandparent as a mentor, controlling for depression and delinquency at Wave 1. The longitudinal nature of the data allows us to control for early levels of mental and physical health, assuming that mentor involvement occurred between Waves 1 and 3. Although this type of analysis handles some of the issues of temporal order, more stringent tests including the duration of mentor involvement will be undertaken in future analyses. Controls for socioeconomic status, family factors, and negative life events will also be important in addressing the well-being of respondents in early adulthood.

Results

First, we are interested in the characteristics of those young adults reporting grandparents as mentors during adolescence and the transition to adulthood. The nationally representative portion of the sample in Wave 3 is composed of 14,322 young adults, of which 14,272 reported on the mentoring question. Of those who responded, 10,803 (76%) reported some mentor. We delete anyone who responds that the mentor first became important after age 18, a loss of 2,107 individuals (n = 8,696). We also delete individuals not reporting on the relationship type variable (n = 8,682) and those reporting younger siblings as mentors, since our interest lies in adult-adolescent relationships (n = 8,549). Of this analytic sample, 12% of young adults report a grandparent as their mentor. Figure 5.1 presents findings on those reporting grandparents as mentor by gender, race/ethnicity, and parental education. Women are more likely than men and African Americans are more likely than Whites to report a grandparent, replicating previous literature on grandparenting. Interestingly, Hispanic individuals are less likely than Whites or African Americans to report a grandparent, a departure from previous literature on intergenerational relationships among Hispanics but possibly explained though migration or acculturation (Silverstein & Chen, 1999). Asian individuals report grandparents least frequently of all racial/ethnic groups in this sample,

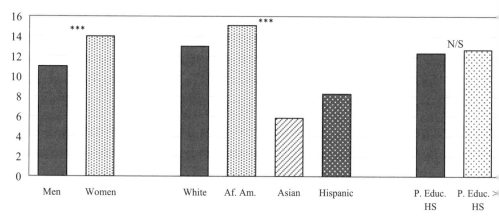

Figure 5.1. Percentage of respondents reporting a grandparent mentor, by key predictors. *Note:* *** *p* < .001; N/S = not significant

possibly also owing to migration. Interestingly, individuals whose highest level of parental education is greater than high school report grandparents as mentors at a proportion roughly the same as those with high school or less than high school parental education.

We are also interested in what role grandparent mentors may play in the lives of adolescents as they transition into adulthood. This exploration of the grandparent role is especially well captured through this use of counterfactual questions or comparisons to other important adults in the lives of adolescents, rather than a basic question about how important grandparents are to young people, because reports of closeness with grandparents may be inflated in comparison to frequency of contact. Results from the open-ended questions on the role mentors played in the lives of adolescents appear in figure 5.2. These qualitative responses have been coded into types of support. The percentages of adolescents reporting each type of support are presented for grandparent mentors as compared to other mentors. Although guidance and advice was the most frequently reported role played by mentors, young adults report receiving less guidance and advice from grandparent mentors during adolescence compared to other mentors. This may not be surprising when considering the other types of mentors commonly listed (older siblings, teachers, religious leaders, or employers). Respondents also reported that grandparent mentors were less "like a friend" in comparison to other mentors. Grandparents, however, provided more emotional and instrumental support. In addition, young adults report that grandparents served as surrogate parental figures more often than other mentors, suggesting that grandparents step into a sup-

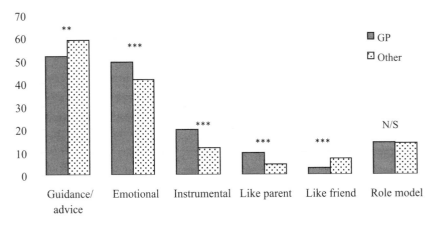

Figure 5.2. Role of mentors (grandparent vs. other). *Note:* ** *p* < .01, *** *p* < .001; N/S = not significant

plemental parenting role more often than other important adults. There was no significant difference, however, between grandparents and other mentors serving as role models to adolescents in the transition to adulthood.

Our second research question focuses on the roles grandparents play in the face of negative life events for children. We only present descriptive results here, so we focus on cross-sectional comparisons for two factors: family structure and teen childbearing. Figure 5.3 presents results for parental closeness and family structure at Wave 1. Although adolescents reporting parental closeness report grandparents as mentors more often, adolescents living with both biological parents at Wave 1 are less likely to report a grandparent as a mentor than are respondents living in stepparent households or single-parent households. This suggests that although previous literature has found grandparents to be most important to children with strong parental bonds, grandparents may play an important role when parents divorce or separate or when a parent dies.

Findings on teenage childbearing are shown in figure 5.4. Among both Black and White women, those reporting a live birth occurring before the age of 19 were not significantly more likely than their counterparts without births to report grandparents as mentors. Notably, grandparents also seem to be as important to White women reporting teen childbearing as they are to African American women. This is an important finding, since the literature focuses on the role of grandparents among African American teen mothers, assuming the supportive roles are different or stronger compared to Whites (McDonald & Armstrong, 2001).

Our third research question focuses on the effects of grandparents on

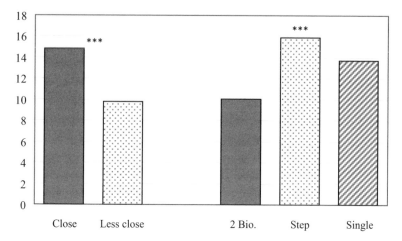

Figure 5.3. Percentage reporting a grandparent mentor, by parental closeness and family type. *Note:* *** *p* < .001

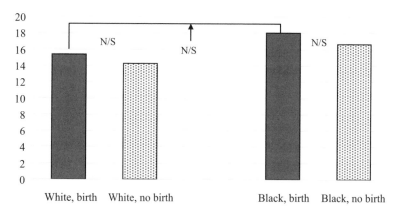

Figure 5.4. Percentage reporting a grandparent mentor, by teen birth (White and Black). *Note:* N/S = not significant

young adult well-being. In figure 5.5, we present regression estimates of depression and delinquency outcomes at Wave 3 on reports of grandparent mentors, controlling for depression and delinquency (respectively) at Wave 1. Adolescents who report grandparents as mentors during adolescence fare significantly better on measures of well-being in young adulthood, reporting lower rates of both depressive symptoms and delinquency on average compared to respondents reporting other mentors. Although temporal order of

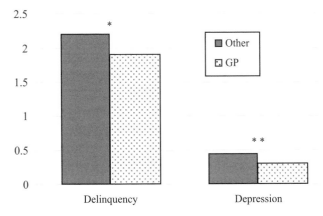

Figure 5.5. Wave 3 estimates of depressive symptoms and delinquency (grandparent vs. other). *Note:* * *p* < .05, ** *p* < .01

well-being and mentor involvement cannot be completely distinguished here (since relationships are likely to be longer with grandparent mentors than other mentors), it may be tested in future analyses using the timing of mentor relationship and age at Wave 1.

Conclusions and Next Steps

In this chapter, we have introduced a novel way of examining the grandparenting role as adolescents transition into adulthood. This topic becomes increasingly important when considering the percentage of adolescents expected to have living grandparents well into adulthood and in conceptualizing grandparents as a potential source of support for adolescents as they age. Understanding what is unique to the grandparenting role, both in comparing it to the role of other important adults, and in terms of what is most valuable to adolescents transitioning into adulthood as compared to young children, is an understudied and significant line of research.

We use a nationally representative sample of adolescents, unlike previous research that has primarily utilized small or homogeneous samples, to study diversity and symbolism in the grandparenting role. As part of a larger project, we outline three major research questions and discuss the life course concepts that help root them in the broader framework of the life course. We discuss the literatures on grandparenting and mentoring in order to build hypotheses.

As a first step, we present descriptive analyses. Our findings are both consistent with and in contrast to previous work on grandparenting and its importance to young lives.

As in previous literature, we find that women are more likely to report grandparents as mentors compared to men, supporting the matrifocal tilt of intergenerational relationships. African American young adults are the most likely of any racial/ethnic group to report grandparents as mentors. Further, we find that young adults reporting very high levels of parental closeness are more likely to report grandparents as mentors, as is consistent with the literature on the parental generation as mediators of the grandparent-grandchild relationship.

In terms of the roles grandparents play in young lives, we found that, as is consistent with previous literature on grandparental support of children, young adults report that grandparents offer more emotional and instrumental support than do other important adults in the transition to adulthood. Far less frequent, but of considerable importance, are greater reports of grandparents as surrogate parents in comparison with other adult mentors. These findings are consistent with research conducted more than 30 years before the Add Health data were collected by Neugarten and Weinstein (1964), who found that 14% of grandmothers reported surrogate parenting as part of the grandparenting role. This finding is even more interesting considering the changes in divorce rates and single-parent households occurring between the mid-1960s and the 1990s.

Also consistent with some previous literature is our finding that young people who report grandparents as mentors fare better on well-being outcomes during young adulthood. However, the descriptive analyses presented here do not allow the temporal order of these effects to be established. It is possible that other factors select healthier children to report grandparents as important adults in their lives (e.g., strong family bonds).

In addition to results replicating previous findings, there were a number of interesting contrasts to what has been previously emphasized in the literature on grandparenting. For example, although African Americans and Hispanics are more likely than Whites to grow up in a home with a grandparent, Hispanic young adults reported grandparents as mentors much less frequently than African Americans or Whites. Although this finding may be due to migration (grandparents living outside of the United States), it is also possible that it is due to acculturation or the way Hispanic youths view the significance of their grandparents in contrast to other adults in their lives (for more information about Hispanics, see Markides, Angel, & Peck, Chapter 15).

Our findings on family closeness and family structure are counterintuitive. We find that young adults reporting close parental bonds describe grandparents as mentors more often. Therefore, we would expect that adolescents living with two biological parents would also be more likely to report grandparents as mentors. However, adolescents with single-parent or stepparent family structures report grandparents more often. In models not shown, we drop adolescents who report living with a grandparent at some point prior to Wave 3 (8% of the working sample) with similar results to those presented here. This finding lends support to the idea that grandparents are an important source of support in families where one biological parent is missing from the household, even if parents are the gateway through which the grandparent-grandchild relationship occurs. Further, the push and pull of family structure is supported in these results, since adolescents from stepparent families are most likely to report grandparents. Here, it is likely that children in single-parent households (although having fewer adults in the household and more need for grandparents) have reduced contact or proximity to grandparents compared to those in stepparent families. In addition, the intergenerational stake may be higher for a paternal grandparent, for example, in regard to a child in a home where a stepfather is present compared to a household headed by a single mother. Future analyses may address these possibilities along with differences by race or socioeconomic status.

Further, the findings on teen childbearing are very interesting, since much of the literature on early or out-of-wedlock childbirth and intergenerational relationships is focused on African American families. Here, we find that among both White and African American young women, there is no significant difference in reporting a grandparent mentor by teen childbearing. Further, there is no significant difference between White and African American teen mothers in reporting a grandparent mentor. Although factors such as socioeconomic status and the outcome of the birth (who raises the baby) cannot be controlled for here, these findings lead to further questions, such as whether African American teen mothers report similar or different roles (e.g. instrumental support) provided by grandparent mentors compared to their White counterparts. Regardless, these findings lead us to suspect that racial/ethnic differences in the support systems for teen mothers and their intergenerational relationships are more nuanced than previously suspected.

Finally, we find that although young adults report higher levels of emotional and instrumental support among grandparent mentors, they report less friend-like relationships and less guidance and advice compared to other important adults. Although the "fun seeker" and "reservoir of wisdom" are re-current themes in the grandparenting literature, we find that these aspects of the grandparenting role are not as important to adolescents as they transition into adulthood. There are numerous possible causes of this. First, what children report as the most important features of the grandparenting role may not be the same as what would be reported by the grandparents themselves. Second, since adolescents were asked to report the single most important nonparental adult in their life, they may have chosen adults who had contributed more tangible or substantial forms of support than friendship or general advice. Third, the most salient forms of the grandparenting role may change as children transition into adulthood, where advice and friendship are solicited from peers or adults closer in age or daily proximity (e.g. at school or work) rather than grandparents.

Although we think these findings are telling, they are descriptive only. Temporal order cannot be established and is relegated to future research on this topic. Further, we cannot control for other confounding factors in these analyses. In addition, we do not distinguish here between family and nonfamily mentors (is the grandparenting role distinct from the roles of aunts and uncles or just distinct from that of teachers and coaches?). Rather, we present these results as a first step in understanding grandparents as mentors in a nationally representative sample of adolescents as they transition into adulthood. Although we claim this is a unique opportunity to address these research questions in a creative and stringent manner, there are a number of general limitations inherent in these and future analyses using these data. First, although the Add Health data are nationally representative of adolescents in grades 7–12 in 1994 and 1995, the mentoring variables are retrospective, asked of young adults about who was most important in their adolescent lives. Further, the analyses are confined to one mentor viewed as the most important, so although grandparents can be compared to other mentors, young adults were not directly asked about their grandparent-grandchild relationships. In other words, these analyses are biased in terms of positive relationships (negative relationships with grandparents or other nonparent adults would not be reported). In addition, it is possible that adolescents with strong grandparent relationships are not represented here because they reported as a mentor some other adult who made a substantial or easily definable impact on their lives. It is also possible that children living with or otherwise dependent on a grandparent think of them as parents and thus do not report them as important nonparental adults.

In addition, the distinction between custodial and noncustodial grandparent mentors is difficult to establish. Although we have reports in the data of living with a grandparent at some point during childhood, we cannot determine whether it is the same grandparent a young adult lists as a mentor. Rather, we may control for residence with any grandparent in subsequent analyses. Selection effects are also difficult to pin down in these analyses, but they can be handled more stringently in subsequent work. Certain characteristics may select adolescents into reporting a grandparent as a mentor, and although we cannot directly test those here, controlling for characteristics of the adolescent at Wave 1 could tease out at least some of the selection bias in estimating the positive effects of grandparent mentors in the future.

Given these limitations, we outline here a larger project with a great deal of room for research and many unanswered questions. Although we present some interesting findings, these analyses serve as a first step in a broader research plan. Future work will address these research questions in more detail, especially those seemingly counterintuitive findings. Further, we are interested in the unique nature of the grandparent role in comparison to other important adults in young lives. It is very possible that grandparents may have substantially different impacts on an adolescent's transition to adulthood compared to nonfamily mentors but that their contributions are similar to those of other family members. We are also interested specifically in those youth most at risk. For example, how do grandparents fill in in the case of a parental divorce or loss? The ability to separate out those adolescents with histories of marital disruption, parental loss, or single parenthood allow a much more in-depth analyses of this kind using nationally representative data.

ACKNOWLEDGMENT

Miles G. Taylor was supported by the National Institute on Aging (grants no. F32AG026926 and K99AG030471).

REFERENCES

Bengtson, V. L. (1985). Diversity and symbolism in grandparental roles. In V. L. Bengtson & J. F. Robertson (Eds.), *Grandparenthood* (pp. 11–25). Beverly Hills, CA: Sage.
Bengtson, V. L., & Kuypers, J. A. (1971). Generational difference and the generational stake. *Aging and Human Development, 2,* 249–260.

Bray, J. H., & Berger, S. H. (1990). Noncustodial father and paternal grandparent relationships in stepfamilies. *Family Relations, 39,* 414–419.

Brown, E. J., Sweet-Jemmott, L., Outlaw, F. H., Wilson, G., Howard, M., & Curtis, S. (2000). African American grandmothers' perceptions of caregiver concerns associated with rearing adolescent grandchildren. *Archives of Psychiatric Nursing, 14,* 73–80.

Brussoni, M. J., & Boon, S. D. (1998). Grandparental impact in young adults' relationships with their closest grandparents: The role of relationship strength and emotional closeness. *International Journal of Aging and Human Development, 46,* 267–286.

Burton, L. M. (1992). Black grandparents rearing children of drug-addicted parents: Stressors, outcomes, and social service needs. *The* Gerontologist, *32,* 744–751.

Burton, L. M., & Bengtson, V. L. (1985). Black grandmothers: Issues on timing and continuity of roles. In L. M. Burton & V. L. Bengtson (Eds.), *Grandparenthood* (pp. 61–77). Beverly Hills, CA: Sage.

Burton, L. M., & deVries, C. (1992). Challenges and rewards: African American grandparents as surrogate parents. *Generations, 16,* 51–54.

Caldwell, J., Silverman, N. L., & Silver, N. C. (2004). Adjudicated Mexican American adolescents: The effects of familial emotional support on self-esteem, emotional well-being, and delinquency. *The American Journal of Family Therapy, 32,* 55–69.

Cherlin, A. J., & Furstenberg, F. F. (1986). *The new American grandparent: A place in the family, a life apart.* New York: Basic Books.

Cicirelli, V. (1984). Marital disruption and adult children's perception of their siblings' help to elderly parents. *Family Relations, 33,* 613–621.

Clingempeel, W., Colyar, J., Brand, E., & Hetherington, M. (1992). Children's relationships with maternal grandparents: A longitudinal study of family structure and pubertal status effects. *Child Development, 63*(6), 1404–1422

Connidis, I. A. (2001). *Family ties and aging.* Thousand Oaks, CA: Sage.

Creasey, G. L., & Kaliher, G. (1994). Age differences in grandchildren's perceptions of relations with grandparents. *Journal of Adolescence, 17,* 411–426.

Deleire, T., & Kalil, A. (2002). Good things come in threes: Single-parent multigenerational family structure and adolescent adjustment. *Demography, 39,* 393–413.

Dickerson, B. J. (1995). African-American single mothers: Understanding their lives and families. Sage Series on Race and Ethnic Relations, Vol. 10. Thousand Oaks, CA: Sage.

Dornbusch, S. M., Carlsmith, M., Bushwall, S., Ritter, P., Liederman, H., Hastorf, A., & Gross, R. (1985). Single parents, extended households, and the control adolescents. *Child Development, 56,* 326–341.

Dunn, J., & Deater-Deckard, K. (2001). *Children's views of their changing families.* New York: York Publishing/Joseph Rowntree Foundation.

Flaherty, M. J., Facteau, L., & Garver, P. (1987). Grandmother functions in multigenerational families: An exploratory study of Black adolescent mothers and their infants. *Maternal-Child Nursing Journal, 16,* 61–73.

Fuller-Thomson, E., & Minkler, M. (2001). American grandparents providing extensive child care to their grandchildren: Prevalence and profile. *The Gerontologist,* *41,* 201–209.

Fuller-Thomson, E., Minkler, M., & Driver, D. (1997). A profile of grandparents raising grandchildren in the United States. *The Gerontologist, 37,* 406–411.

Furstenberg, F. F., & Hughes, M. E. (1995). Social capital and successful development among at-risk youth. *Journal of Marriage and the Family, 57,* 580–592.

Giarrusso, R., Stallings, M., & Bengtson, V. L. (1995). The "intergenerational stake" hypothesis revisited: Parent-child differences in perceptions of relationships 20 years later. In V. L. Bengtson, W. K. Schaie, & L. M. Burton (Eds.), *Adult intergenerational relations: Effects of societal changes* (pp. 229–296). New York: Springer.

Gladstone, J. W. (1988). Perceived changes in grandmother-grandchild relations following a child's separation or divorce. *The Gerontologist, 28,* 66–72.

Gladstone, J. W. (1989). Grandmother-grandchild contact: The mediating influence of the middle generation following marriage breakdown and remarriage. *Canadian Journal on Aging, 8*(4), 355–365.

Goodman, C. C., & Silverstein, M. (2001). Grandmothers who parent their grandchildren: An exploratory case of close relations across three generations. *Journal of Family Issues, 22,* 557–578.

Gordon, R. A., Chase-Lansdale, P. L., & Brooks-Gunn, J. (2004). Extended households and the life course of young mothers: Understanding the associations using a sample of mothers with premature, low birth weight babies. *Child Development 75*(4), 1013–1038.

Gravenish, B. A., & Thompson, E. (1996). *Marital disruptions and grandparent relationships* (working paper). Madison, WI: University of Wisconsin Center for Demography and Ecology.

Guzman, L. (2004). Grandma and grandpa taking care of the kids: Patterns of involvement. *Child Trends Research Brief,* Publication No. 2004–17. Washington, DC: Child Trends.

Hagestad, G. O. (1982, Winter). Divorce: The family ripple effect. *Generations: The Journal of the Western Gerontological Society,* 24–31.

Hagestad, G. O. (1984). The continuous bond: A dynamic multigenerational perspective on parent-child relations between adults. In M. Perlmutter (Ed.), *Parent-child relations in child development* (pp. 129–158). The Minnesota Symposium on Child Psychology (Vol. 17).

Hagestad, G. O. (1985). Continuity and connectedness. In V. L. Bengtson & J. F. Robertson (Eds.), *Grandparenthood* (pp. 31–48). Beverly Hills, CA: Sage.

Hagestad, G. O. Symer, M. A., & Stierman, K. L. (1984). Parent-child relations in adulthood: The impact of divorce in middle age. In R. Cohen, S. Weissman, & B. Cohler (Eds.), *Parenthood: Psychodynamic perspectives* (pp. 247–262). New York: Guilford.

Haurin, R. J. (1992). Patterns of childhood residence and the relationship to young adult outcomes. *Journal of Marriage and the Family, 54,* 846–860.

Henly, J. R. (1997). The complexity of support: The impact of family structure and provisional support on African American and White adolescent mothers' well-being. *American Journal of Community Psychology, 25,* 629–655.

Jendrek, M. P. (1993). Grandparents who parent their grandchildren: Effects on life-style. *Journal of Marriage and Family, 55,* 609–621.

Johnson, C. L. (1983). A cultural analysis of the grandmother. *Research in Aging, 5,* 547–567.

Johnson, C. L. (1985). Grandparenting options in divorcing families. In V. Bengtson & J. Robertson (Eds.), *Grandparenthood* (pp. 81–96). Beverly Hills, CA: Sage.

Johnson, C. L. (1988). Active and latent functions of grandparenting during the divorce process. *The Gerontologist, 28,* 185–191.

Johnson, C. L. (1998). Effects of adult children's divorces on grandparenthood. In M. Szinovacz (Ed.), *Handbook on grandparenthood* (pp. 184–199). Westport, CT: Greenwood.

Kataoka-Yahiro, M., Ceria, C., & Caulfield, R. (2004). Grandparent caregiving role in ethnically diverse families. *Journal of Pediatric Nursing, 19,* 315–328.

Kennedy, G. E. (1990). College students' expectations of grandparent and grandchild role behaviors. *The Gerontologist, 30*(1), 43–48.

Kennedy, G. E., & Kennedy, C. E. (1993). Grandparents: A special resource for children in stepfamilies. *Journal of Divorce and Remarriage, 19,* 45–68.

King, V., & Elder, G. H., Jr. (1995). American grandchildren view their grandparents: Linked lives across three rural generations. *Journal of Marriage and the Family, 57,* 165–178.

King, V., Elder, G. H., & Conger, R. D. (2000). Wisdom of ages. In G. H. Elder & R. D. Conger (Eds.), *Children of the land: Adversity and success in rural America.* Chicago, IL: University of Chicago Press.

Kivett, V. R. (1991). The grandparent-grandchild connection. *Marriage and Family Review, 16,* 267–290.

Kivett, V. (1993). Grandparenting: Racial comparisons of the grandmother role: Implications for strengthening the family support system of older Black women. *Family Relations, 42,* 165–172.

Loury, L. (2006). All in the extended family: Effects of grandparents, aunts, and uncles on educational attainment. *American Economic Review Papers and Proceedings, 96,* 275–278.

Lussier, G., Deater-Deckard, K., Dunn, J., & Davies, L. (2002). Support across two generations: Children's closeness to grandparents following parental divorce and remarriage. *Journal of Family Psychology, 16,* 363–376.

McCluskey, K., & McCluskey, A. (2000). Gray matters: The power of grandparent involvement. *Reclaiming Children and Youth, 9,* 111–115.

McDonald, K. B., & Armstrong, E. M. (2001). De-romanticizing Black intergenerational support: The questionable expectations of welfare reform. *Journal of Marriage and the Family, 63,* 213–223.

McLanahan, S. S. (1985). Family structure and the reproduction of poverty. *American Journal of Sociology, 90,* 873–901.

McLanahan, S., & Sandefur, G. (1994). *Growing up with a single parent.* Cambridge, MA: Harvard University Press.

Mills, T. L. (1999). When grandchildren grow up: Role transition and family solidarity among baby boomer grandchildren and their grandparents. *Journal of Aging Studies, 13,* 1–20.

Minkler, M., & Fuller-Thompson, E. (2005). African American grandparents raising grandchildren: A national study using the Census 2000 American Community Survey. *Journal of Gerontology: Social Sciences, 60B,* S82–S92.

Minkler, M., Roe, K. M., & Price, M. (1992). The physical and emotional health of grandmothers raising grandchildren in the crack cocaine epidemic. *The Gerontologist, 32*(6), 752–761.

Mueller, M., & Elder, G. H. (2003). Family contingencies across the generations: Grandparent-grandchild relationships in holistic perspective. *Journal of Marriage and the Family, 65,* 404–417.

Mueller, M. M., Wilhelm, B., & Elder, G. H. Jr. (2002). Variations in grandparenting. *Research on Aging, 24,* 360–388.

Musick, J. S. (1993). *Young, poor, and pregnant: The psychology of teenage motherhood.* New Haven, CT: Yale University Press.

Neugarten, B. J., & Datan, N. (1973). Sociological respectives of the life cycle. In P. B. Baltes & K. W. Schaie (Eds.), *Life-span development psychology: Personality and socialization* (pp. 53–69). New York: Academic Press.

Neugarten, B. L., & Weinstein, K. K. (1964). The changing American grandparent. *Journal of Marriage and the Family, 26,* 199–204.

Peterson, C. C. (1999). Grandfathers' and grandmothers' satisfaction with the grandparenting role: Seeking new answers to old questions. *International Journal of Aging and Human Development, 49,* 61–78.

Pittman, L. D. (2007). Grandmothers' involvement among young adolescents growing up in poverty. *Journal of Research on Adolescence, 17,* 89–116.

Pruchno, R. (1999). Raising grandchildren: The experiences of Black and White grandmothers. *The Gerontologist, 39,* 209–221.

Reitzes, D. C., & Mutran, E. J. (2004). Grandparent identity, intergenerational family identity, and well-being. *Journal of Gerontology: Social Sciences, 59B,* S213–S219.

Robertson, J. (1995). Grandparenting in an era of rapid change. In R. Blieszner & V. H. Bedford (Eds.), *Aging and the family: Theory and research* (pp. 243–260). Westport, CT: Greenwood.

Rosenmayr, L. (1972). The elderly in Austrian society. In D. Cogwill & L. Holmes (Eds.), *Aging and modernization* (pp. 183–196). New York: Appleton-Century-Crofts.

Rossi, A. S. (1993). Intergenerational relations: Gender, norms, and behavior. In V. L. Bengtson & W. A. Achenbaum (Eds.), *The changing contract across generations* (pp. 191–212). New York: Aldine.

Ruiz, D. S. (2000). Guardian and caretakers: African American grandmothers as primary caregivers in intergenerational families. *African American Research, 6,* 1–12.

Saluter, A. F. & Lugaila, T. A. (1996). *Marital status and living arrangements: March 1996 (update).* Current Population Reports, Series P-20: Population Characteristics, No. 496. Washington, DC: U.S. Bureau of the Census.

Shapiro, T. M. (2004). *The hidden cost of being African American: How wealth perpetuates inequality.* New York: Oxford University Press.

Silverstein, M., & Chen, X. (1999). The impact of acculturation in Mexican American families on the quality of adult grandchild-grandparent relationships. *Journal of Marriage and the Family, 61,* 188–198.

Silverstein, M., & Marenco, A. (2001). How Americans enact the grandparent role across the family life course. *Journal of Family Issues, 22,* 493–522.

Silverstein, M., & Ruiz, S. (2006). Breaking the chain: How grandparents moderate the transmission of maternal depression to their grandchildren. *Family Relations, 55,* 601–612.

Smith, E. W. (1975). The role of the grandmother in adolescent pregnancy and parenting. *Journal of School Health, 45,* 278–283.

Solomon, J. C., & Marx, J. (1995). To grandmother's house we go: Health and school adjustment of children raised solely by grandparents. *The Gerontologist, 35,* 386–394.

Stolba, A., & Amato, P. R. (1993). Extended single-parent households and children's behavior. *Sociological Quarterly, 34,* 543–549.

Tinsley, B. R., & Parke, R. D. (1984). Grandparents as support and socialization agents. In M. Lewis (Ed.), *Beyond the dyad* (pp. 161–194). New York: Plenum Press.

Tinsley, B. J., & Parke, R. D. (1987). Grandparents as interactive and social support agents for families with young infants. *International Journal of Aging and Human Development, 25,* 259–278.

Tomlin, A. M. (1998). Grandparents' influence on grandchildren. In M. Szinovacz (Ed.), *Handbook on grandparenthood* (pp. 159–170). Westport, CT: Greenwood.

Uhlenberg, P. (1996). Mortality decline in the twentieth century and supply of kin over the life course. *The Gerontologist, 36,* 681–685.

Uhlenberg, P. (2004). Historical forces shaping grandparent-grandchild relationships: Demography and beyond. In M. Silverstein (Ed.), *Annual review of gerontology and geriatrics: Intergenerational relations across time and place.* New York: Springer.

Uhlenberg, P., & Hammill, J. G. (1998). Frequency of grandparent contact with grandchild sets: Six factors that make a difference. *The Gerontologist, 38,* 276–285.

Uhlenberg, P., & Kirby, J. B. (1998). Grandparenthood over time: Historical and demographic trends. In M.E. Szinovacz (Ed.), *Handbook on grandparenthood* (pp. 24–39). Westport, CT: Greenwood.

Unger, D., & Cooley, M. (1992). Partner and grandmother contact in Black and White teen parent families. *Journal of Adolescent Health,13,* 546–552.

U.S. Census Bureau. (2005). America's families and living arrangements, detailed tables. Retrieved July 1. 2008 (http://www.census.gov/population/www/socdemo/hh-fam/cps2005.html).

Wandersman, L. P., Wandersman, A., & Kahn, S. (1980).Social support in the transition to parenthood. *Journal of Community Psychology, 8,* 332–342.

Werner, P., Buchbinder, E., Lowenstein, A., & Livni, T. (2005). Mediation across generations: A tri-generational perspective. *Journal of Aging Studies, 19,* 489–502.

Wilson, M. N. (1984). Mothers' and grandmothers' perceptions of parental behavior in three-generational Black families. *Child Development, 55,* 1333–1339.

Wilson, M. N. (1986). The Black extended family: An analytical consideration. *Developmental Psychology, 22,* 246–258.

Yi, C., Pan, E., Chang, Y., & Chan, C. (2006). Grandparents, adolescents, and parents: Intergenerational relations of Taiwanese youth. *Journal of Family Issues, 27,* 1042–1067.

PART III / Of Generations and Cohorts

Micro-Macro Dialectics

One of the most vexing methodological problems in the study of aging and the life course is trying to tease apart age, period, and cohort effects. An age effect is change that occurs as a result of advancing age; a period effect is the impact of a historical event on an entire society; and a cohort effect is social change that occurs as one cohort replaces another. It is not possible to disentangle all three effects. Adding to this conundrum is that researchers often use the terms "cohort" and "generation"—the latter of which, some argue, should be reserved for the study of families—interchangeably.

The chapter by Alwin disaggregates the term "generation" to distinguish its various meanings along social, demographic, and family dimensions. Drawing on the voting behavior data from the Bennington study, he shows how all three generational elements—participation in social movements, historical location, and kinship position—converge to produce social change and unique life course pathways. Along similar lines, Biggs and Lowenstein develop "generational intelligence" as concept that integrates self-conscious notions of generational identity—as a temporally located cultural field—with intergenerational interactions that occur in the family. In the authors' view, generational intelligence provides key insights about cohort differences that may lead to greater intergenerational empathy in the family. The chapter by Johnson, which deals with end-of-life issues he calls "biographical pain," highlights the importance of cohort placement. Cohorts born between 1900 and 1935, unlike their baby boom successors born between 1946 and 1964, cannot necessarily assuage their biographical pain with spirituality, religion, and faith communities; rather, they must come to understand how their unique individual (micro) biographies were influenced by the (macro) sociohistorical conditions into which they were born

CHAPTER SIX

Who's Talking about My Generation?

Duane F. Alwin

> The problem of generations, from mankind's earliest writings down to con-
> temporary mass media accounts, involves the tension between continuity
> and change among age groups in the succession of social order.
>
> VERN BENGTSON (1989, P. 48)

Following one of the key themes of Vern Bengtson's long scholarly career, this chapter considers the theoretical concept of "generation" as it has been used in the social and behavioral sciences (see Bengtson, 1989). A lot has been written using the concept(s) of generations, and nearly everyone agrees that it is, or they are, critical for linking the individual and society. What is significant, however, is that there is no single meaning of the term. Because of this, Kertzer (1983, p. 135) stated that although "the concept of generation is important to future [social science] research . . . progress can only be made if an acceptable definition of generation is employed and *other usages are abandoned* (emphasis added)." Consistent with this position, many scholars suggest restricting the word's meaning or doing away with the concept altogether (e.g. Elder, Johnson, & Crosnoe, 2003).

I argue, along with Bengtson (1989), that a broader assessment of the concept of generation is desirable. The term has several legitimate scientific meanings, and there is not one single correct meaning but rather at least three legitimate uses of the concept in research on human development. These meanings are distinct from one another, but they are united, not only by a common terminology but by the fact that many different factors involving generational influences converge upon the developing individual. That the same term is used in different ways does not render any one of these uses inadequate or imprecise. Taking a broad perspective, in this chapter I focus on the nature of generational accounts appearing both in the social science scholarly literature and also the writings of journalists and others. I consider the ways in which the concept is used, some of the convergences across perspectives, and the utility of the concept for present-day research on human development that can ultimately lead to a more profound understanding of the linkage between the individual and society.

To illustrate the distinctions among these various "generational" concepts and how all three are important to studying human development, I present data from our well-known Bennington longitudinal study and the National Election Study of 1984, both dealing with political beliefs and attitudes (see Alwin, Cohen, & Newcomb, 1991). Via an analysis of these data, I show how an understanding of the development of political beliefs and attitudes can be informed by all three types of generational concepts, which are (1) the influence of socialization of young people by prior generations, a type of lineage effect as described by Bengtson (1989); (2) a generational effect due to historical location; and (3) generations (or what I have elsewhere called "big G" Generations, see Alwin & McCammon, 2003) as historical participation. Following this discussion, I briefly examine some examples of how the concept is used in public discourse by journalistic narratives about age differences in society and how these treatments compare to the generational logics employed by social scientists.

Logics of Generations

In this section I examine the richness of the concept of generation with respect to its historical roots and the classical writings on the subject. Through my research, I have uncovered three distinct concepts of generation in the sense that each deals with a unique set of differences and a different logic for the role of generational influences—(1) generations as positions in family lineages, (2) generations as birth cohorts or historical locations, and (3) generations as historical participation—and all are useful (see also Alwin & McCammon, 2003, 2007). Unfortunately, there is a great deal of confusion about the adequacy of these concepts, due to a failure to appreciate their differences and the key underlying theoretical principles governing their relevance to human development.

I begin with a discussion of the distinctiveness of the phenomena to which these three different concepts of generation apply—in one case to families, in another to the historical location of birth cohorts, and in the third to social movements or organizations in which participation and identification is involved. These three critical levels of analysis—families, cohorts, and social movements or organizations—converge within the life history of the individual. Given this convergence, their influences are often confounded with one another, and the use of the same word for three distinct concepts invites confusion. Some argue that the concept of generation is inadequate for understanding individual life course analysis (see Elder, Johnson, & Crosnoe, 2003, pp. 8–9); others say that a life course perspective on families specifies an interdependence of lives across at least three levels: "the interdependence of cohorts in societies, of generations in the family (members of which also belong to different cohorts), and of individual life paths in connection to these and other social relationships" (Settersten, 2006, p. 7). Hence, I discuss three distinct concepts that go by the same name—generation—and will argue that all three are important for understanding generational phenomena.

Generations as Kinship Positions

Again, as articulated in the work of Vern Bengtson and his colleagues, the concept of generations as positions in the family is critical to the understanding of family relationships across the life span from many disciplinary perspectives. Social scientists who study families have long considered the relationships among generations, defined in these kinship terms, and this is perhaps the most fundamental use of the concept. In this sense, generations are nested within families, and they are linked through the life cycle. Later on, I will consider the relationship of this concept to other concepts of generation, but for now I want to focus specially on the family, which is the primary unit of analysis pursued by Bengtson's long line of research.

From the point of view of what sociologists consider primary and secondary socialization processes, intergenerational relations are critical to the transmission of culture and human development. As with all species, this usage rests on the presumption that evolution and survival of the human species is furthered by reproduction—within families each new generation completes the cycle of life and another one takes over. "The problem of generations," wrote Vern Bengtson (1989, p. 48), "from mankind's earliest writings down to contemporary mass media accounts, involves the tension between continuity and change among age groups in the succession of social order." The earlier generation attempts to pass along cultural heritage while at the same time preparing its children for a life in a future world. Elsewhere I have argued (Alwin, 2001, pp. 111–113) that parents are motivated to prepare their children for a future life and that they make their child-rearing choices within the framework of the constraints and opportunities posed by history, culture, and social structure. The parental generation is motivated jointly by the desire to preserve elements of the social environment and the need to adapt to prepare children for the future. Given this *motivational assumption*, there is, thus, a strong reason to expect parents to adapt their values to their beliefs about the kind of qualities that will be required of their children in a future world. And thus there is strong justification for looking at adult orientations toward children as one important indicator of social change (see Alwin, 2001).

This line of argument fits well with Alex Inkeles's (1983 [1955]) observation that the family is an important mechanism for the mediation of social change and that parental approaches to child-rearing are as much an effort to prepare children for a life in society's future as they are reflections of current life circumstances. One can only speculate about the motivational basis for parental behavior, as it is no doubt strongly affected by "current" conditions of life (Elder, 1974), but it is also clearly the case that in theory parents would prefer their children to survive in the future society as well as the present one. Thus, what parents perceive the future to be has a direct bearing on their approaches to the socialization of children and their perceptions of desirable qualities of children. Parents are, thus, motivated to transmit both the values of the past and the values that may be required for successful behavior in the future.

Elder (1974, p. 13) suggests a different perspective, arguing that we assume too great a degree of "future awareness, rationality, and choice in parental behavior" and that this may not be relevant in all situations. He argues specifically that during times when family survival is at stake, the parental generation focuses on the immediate needs of children, not on "future adult roles." Elder's research into the impact of the economic deprivation experiences connected to the Depression suggests that "the socialization environment and the response of parents to children in deprived situations during the 1930s [in America] had much less to do with their anticipation of life in the future than with the immediacy of survival requirements" (Elder, 1974, p. 13). These are points well taken.

However, if only from the point of view of self-preservation of the family grouping (and its genetic material), one can assume that parents have considerable motivation to prepare their children for the future, as well as the present. So, in a very real sense, parents contribute to both social stability and so-cial change through the socialization of their children. Presumably, in addition to the conditions of life they face during their parental years, parents are also affected by their own experiences as children, as adolescents, or as young adults. Thus, their past experiences contribute greatly to their present orien-tations to children. Parental experiences, thus, reflect changes carried for-ward by previous generations, and given that with "biographic" time, the most basic of human orientations (e.g., beliefs and values) tend to stabilize over in-dividual life-course trajectories (see Alwin, Cohen, & Newcomb, 1991; Alwin, 1994, 1995, 1996), we would expect that parental orientations to children will reflect something stable about the individual. That is to say, while we normally assume that parents are relatively adaptive and orient themselves toward pre-paring their children for a future life in the society, there may be a point at which parents are unable to adapt to change because of the crystallization of beliefs and values in their own cognitive organization and world view.

Thus, generational succession and its impact on later generations involves some combination of the preservation of the past and an orientation to the fu-ture. The theoretical question posed by Bengtson (1989, p. 48) that asks "How does generational succession relate to the balance between change (and sta-bility) in human societies?" can be cast within a developmental framework. How do individual orientations (of children or otherwise developing individu-als) simultaneously depend upon the parental generation and on contempo-rary factors linked to historical location and historical participation? Within this context, Bengtson's (1989) analysis introduced the notion of a "lineage effect," that is, the association of individual differences in the parental gener-ation to individual differences among children. He distinguished this from cohort effects (due to historical location) and period effects (which potentially affect multiple familial generations). I return subsequently to a consideration of a lineage effect within the Bennington study (see Alwin, Cohen, & New-comb, 1991).

Generations as Historical Location

A second important aspect of the concept of generation is that of "genera-tion as historical location," that is, birth cohorts. Indeed, one of the most com-mon uses of the idea of generations is "a group of individuals born and living at about the same time." This meaning of generation is critical to the scientific study of social change in sociology and demography, where the goal is to sepa-rate cohort replacement effects from intra-cohort change in accounting for social change (see Firebaugh, 1992). Demographers tend to refer to those persons born during the same calendar year as members of the same birth cohort (Alwin, McCammon, & Hofer, 2006).

In the words of Norman Ryder (1965, p. 845), "a cohort may be defined as the aggregate of individuals (within some population definition) who experienced the same event within the same time interval." He notes that in almost all cohort research to date, the defining event has been birth, but this is only a special case of the more general approach. The work of Karl Mannheim (1952 [1927]) can be credited with bringing the concept of cohorts into modern social science as well as introducing ideas related to mechanisms of cohort replacement as a tool for understanding social change (see Ryder, 1965, p. 849).

Mannheim's (1952 [1927], pp. 292–300) analysis of how social change occurs via a succession of cohorts can be summarized by the following principles: 1) the continuous emergence of new participants in the cultural process; 2) the continuous withdrawal of previous participants in the process of culture; 3) members of any one generation [cohort] can only participate in a temporally limited section of the historical process; and 4) a necessity for constant transmission of the cultural heritage. Mannheim uses the term "generation" to describe what he refers to as a group that shares "a common location in the social and historical process . . . [which exposes them] to a specific range of *potential experience* [emphasis added], predisposing them for a certain characteristic model of thought and experience, and a characteristic type of historically-relevant action" (Mannheim, 1952 [1927], p. 291).[1] His argument is that these early formative influences contributing to a particular *Zeitgeist* (or worldview) are strong, and that youth is a particularly impressionable period in the life span, with considerably more openness to change compared to other stages in life. Youth is a period of "plasticity," and these early experiences are the most lastingly influential on human tendencies. In Mannheim's words,

> Early impressions tend to coalesce into a *natural view* of the world. All later experiences then tend to receive their meaning from this original set . . . (and) even if the rest of one's life consisted of one long process of negation and destruction of the natural world view acquired in youth, the determining influence of these early impressions would still be predominant.

As we noted earlier, in the social circles inhabited by demographers there is often a great deal of pressure to use the concept of "birth cohort" rather than that of "generation," although in many social science fields they are used as equivalent ideas (e.g., Amato & Booth, 1997; McCluskey & Reese, 1984). Indeed,

Ryder (1965, p. 853) argues that "for the sake of conceptual clarity, 'generation' should be used solely in its original and unambiguous meaning as the temporal unit of kinship structure. . . ." At the same time, neither should this idea of "generation as cohort" be confused with Mannheim's (1952 [1927]) concept of the "generational unit" (discussed below), meaning a group of people identified by themselves and others as part of a social movement or organizational unit that produces social changes in culture, norms, and behavior.

Much writing on the subject of what we here call "cohort" enlists the concept of "generation" as a coequal term. Ryder (1965, p. 853) suggests that we reserve the term "generation" solely for purposes of designated stages in the natural line of descent within families, a position with which I basically agree. In his words:

> "Generation" may be a fitting general temporal reference in societies where the dominant mode of role allocation is ascription on the basis of kinship. . . . But societies undergoing cultural revolution . . . diminish the social significance of "generation," in both its kinship and relative age connotations, and produce the kind of social milieu in which the cohort is the most appropriate unit of temporal analysis.

While I tend to agree with Ryder regarding a preference for the use of the concept of cohort here, there is more to it, and we would also urge the reader to consider a degree of flexibility in the use of generation concepts. Any use of generational ideas should clarify the meaning it intends for any particular application, but to claim there is just one appropriate meaning of the term is somewhat short-sighted.

The record of a particular cohort is, according to Ryder (1965, p. 845), "not merely a summation of a set of individual histories." Rather, each cohort "has a distinctive composition and character reflecting the circumstances of its unique origination and history." Because members of a birth cohort share the experience of the life cycle, it is possible that the unique intersection of biography and history produce what are referred to as "cohort effects," effects that contribute to social change through processes of "cohort replacement." A cohort effect, thus, is a distinctive, formative experience that members of a birth cohort (or set of birth cohorts) share that indelibly marks them for the remainder of their lives.

Whatever terms one uses to describe the phenomenon of temporal location in the historical process, the basic idea is that historical events and processes influence the composition of populations via differences in (birth) cohort experiences, and this has been a prominent theoretical tool in the disciplines of economics, demography, sociology, political science, and psychology over at least the past 50 years. There are many examples of how these ideas have usefully advanced the understanding of social change and its components. Several factors connected to the lives of individuals have a bearing on how society changes, and thus there is a linkage between individuals and social change. Society changes, paradoxically, both because individuals change and because they remain stable or unchanged after an early period of socialization. Popular theories of social change rest on the idea that culture, social norms, and social behavior change through two main mechanisms: (1) through changes undergone by individuals (due to aging or period effects), and (2) through the succession of cohorts (Ryder, 1965; Firebaugh, 1992; Glenn, 2003).

The existence of cohort effects, and their ability to influence social change via cohort replacement, depends critically on the nature of processes at the individual level. As Ryder (1965, p. 861) observes, "the case of the cohort as a temporal unit in the analysis of social change" rests on a set of three primitive assumptions: that (1) persons of age *a* in time *t* are those who are age *a-1* in time *t-1*; (2) transformations of the social world modify people of different ages in different ways; and (3) the effects of these transformations are persistent. The first of these refers to the inevitability of cohort replacement emphasized in the writings (mentioned above) of Mannheim (1952 [1927], pp. 292–300)— the emergence of new participants in the social and historical process and the withdrawal of others. The second and third so-called "primitive" assumptions are empirically testable, and they refer to the dual tendencies of individuals to be open to change in young adulthood, but relatively inflexible thereafter (Ryder, 1965, pp. 854–861). There is a substantial literature that has investigated these matters (see, e.g., Alwin, 1994, 1997; Alwin, Cohen, & Newcomb, 1991; Alwin & McCammon, 2003; Ardelt, 2000; Costa and McCrae, 1994; Heatherton & Weinberger, 1994).

Generations as Historical Participation

If we could understand generational phenomena solely in biological and life cycle terms, or, alternatively, understand their existence merely in terms of historical location, we would need to go no farther. However, there is a need for a third concept of generation. So, finally, I discuss the least well understood of these generational concepts. This meaning of the concept is "generations as historical participation," a concept that is prominent in the writings of sociologist Karl Mannheim. As noted above, for Karl Mannheim (1952 [1927], pp. 302–312) and others, Generation may be something quite different from birth cohort. Mannheim considered Generations (we use capital "G" for this type of generation concept—see Alwin & McCammon, 2003) to be situated at the confluence of birth cohort and what he calls the "stratification of experience." This use of the concept of Generation, which Mannheim referred to as "generational unit," develops the idea of the participation of individuals in the social and historical process at a given point in time—not simply their temporal placement in historical time, but their participation in the social movements of their time.

Mannheim (1952 [1927], p. 303) indicates that "a generation in the sense of a location phenomenon" falls short of fully encompassing generation phenomena. He distinguishes between "generation location" and "generation in actuality" and argues that Generation as an actuality "involves more than mere co-presence in such historical and social region." Many young people living in a society at a given time are unaffected by its significant social movements and events; even though they share the same temporal location, they are not members of the same "generation as an actuality." They are similarly located insofar as they are potentially capable of being impelled into the vortex of social change, but temporal location is not enough; they must participate in the movements linked to social transformation. He uses the term "generation unit" to distinguish this aspect of participation as follows:

> The *generation unit* represents a much more concrete bond than the actual generation as such. *Youth experiencing the same concrete historical problems may be said to be part of the same actual generation; while those groups within the same actual generation which work up the material of their common experiences in different specific ways, constitute separate generation units.*

By invoking this definition of Generation, Mannheim is being completely consistent with the view that the term "generation" should *not* be used when we mean birth cohort (Kertzer, 1983; Ryder, 1965).

In other words, cohort effects, or generation effects in the sense of historical location, do not automatically imply the existence of Generations. According to White (1992), cohorts only become "actors" when they cohere enough around historical events, in both their own and others' eyes, to be called "Generations." Roscow (1978) suggests that incisive historical events may distinguish Generations, but when such events "are soft and indistinct, [Generations] . . . may be clearest at their centers, but blurred and fuzzy at the edges. They may remain so as long as transitional events are still gathering force, but a new [Generation] . . . has not yet blossomed" (p. 69). White (1992, p. 32), argues that "Cohort can turn into [G]eneration only if there is some previous [G]eneration, and then only as previous [G]enerations—and the concerns they wrap around—are moved out of the way." Thus, Generations are frequently formed through identification with and participation in youth-based social movements that cohere around a particular event or the conditions left to them by a previous generation. While this seems a compelling enough mechanism for the formation of Generations, there is also the potential for Generational units to influence their cohort contemporaries in ways that may manifest themselves as cohort effects, or, more importantly, as period effects. The effects of the civil rights activists of the early 1960s on their contemporaries and the country as a whole provide an excellent example of this (see McAdam, 1988).

In this sense, we would distinguish between cohorts and Generations—the former refers to the effects attributable to having been placed by one's birth in a particular historical period, whereas a Generation is (in White's words) a "joint interpretive construction which insists upon and builds among tangible cohorts in defining a style recognized from outside and from within" (p. 31). Cohort effects are given life through these interpretive and behavioral aspects. There is an identity component to Generations, made explicit in the work of Mannheim (1952 [1927]) and Ortega y Gasset (1933), that may be difficult to pin down when simply studying cohort differences and their tendencies to persevere. The existence of cohort effects and the existence of Generations are two different, albeit related, questions (Modell, 1989).

If we define Generations, following Mannheim (1952 [1927]), as groups of people sharing a distinctive subcultural identity by virtue of having experienced the same historical events in the same ways at approximately the same time in their lives, that is, as generation units, we can see that this third meaning of Generations refers to distinct historical phenomena. These phenomena do not map neatly to birth cohort, or even to a fixed number of birth cohorts. Unlike cohorts, Generations do not enjoy a fixed metric that easily lends itself to statistical analysis. Rather, the distinctions between Generations are a matter of quality, not degree, and the temporal location of their boundaries cannot be easily identified, particularly without the context of a set of particular analytic questions (see Alwin & McCammon, 2003).

Mannheim (1952 [1927]) suggests that distinctive Generations may fail to materialize for long periods of time should economic and social conditions remain stable, such that "largely static . . . communities like the peasantry display no such phenomenon as new generation units sharply set off from their predecessors . . . the tempo of change is so gradual that new generations evolve . . . without any visible break" (Mannheim, 1952 [1927], p. 309). Further complicating the study of Generations is the fact that they are not monolithic, homogeneous groupings of all members of a set of birth cohorts but instead are divided into what Mannheim called "generational units" by social position and level of involvement in the events of the day. How these subgroupings are identified and understood is again contingent on the substantive questions at hand, as Generations do not exist in a vacuum, operating in the same way at all times for all members. Rather, like all good sociological variables, Generational experiences differ by social position and the corresponding differential experience of events based on those contexts. The civil rights movement in the United States was largely carried out by a particular subset of the youth of the era, and there are clear Generational identities associated with the movement, but the content of this identity obviously varies along geographic and racial dimensions. Similarly, the Vietnam War was a defining experience for the so-called Baby Boom cohorts, but the imprint of the war on identity for a conscientious objector who fled the country was vastly different than that for his shared cohort counterpart who experienced the war as a soldier in Hanoi (Hagan, 2001). John Kerry's Veterans against the Vietnam War and the Swift Boat Veterans are all members of the same cohorts, but they are members of very different Generations. Both may have Generational identities linked to the war, but those identities are far from uniform. In contrast to the concept of "cohorts," which have extremely broad coverage and precise boundaries but lack specific explanations for the phenomena to which they are related, Generations lack specific boundaries and are meaningful in their distinctiveness largely as subpopulations, but they offer the potential of being used as powerful explanations in and of themselves for distinctive patterns of attitudes, beliefs, and behaviors.

In keeping with this line of thought, I would argue that the unique historical and social events happening during the period of youth undoubtedly play a strong role in shaping human lives. Certainly, some eras and social movements provide particularly distinctive experiences for youth during particular times. The political ideologies formed during Roosevelt's New Deal in the 1930s and 1940s, the civil rights and feminist movements of the 1960s and 1970s, the 1973 pro-choice Supreme Court decision in Roe vs. Wade, or the environmentalist movement of the 1970s and 1980s are all examples of particular historical stimuli to the development of such worldviews during specific historical periods (see Alwin & McCammon, 2003, pp. 40–41). It is not, however, simply the influence of these historical and social events on society that interests us here—it is their distinctive impact on the youth of the period. As Ryder (1965, p. 848) put it, "the potential for change is concentrated in the cohorts of young adults who are old enough to participate directly in the movements impelled by change, but not old enough to have become committed to an occupation, a residence, a family of procreation, or a way of life."

The Bennington Study

In order to illustrate these distinctions between various "generational" concepts and demonstrate how all three are important from the perspective of studying human development, I rely upon data from the well-known Bennington longitudinal study (see Alwin, Cohen, & Newcomb, 1991) and the National Election Study of 1984, having to do with political beliefs and attitudes of the American public. By analyzing these data, I can show the power of all three types of "generational" influence discussed above: (1) the influence of socialization of young people by prior generations, (2) the effects of historical location, and (3) the effects of historical participation on the development of political identities.

Bennington College was the site of one of the early experiments in liberal arts education as well as the subject of one of the best-known early studies of the effects of college attendance on the development of students' political orientations. Bennington College, founded as a women's college in 1932, was one of many colleges founded in the nineteenth and twentieth centuries to provide women access to education that had been previously denied them. Although similar to many other women's colleges in providing areas of the curriculum that were underrepresented in more traditional liberal arts colleges, Bennington was unique in its emphasis on the progressive ideals of fostering students' autonomous personal and academic development. Situated in rural Vermont, Bennington of the 1930s was a largely self-contained, geographically isolated, and highly integrated community of young women and their teachers.

The women who attended Bennington in the 1930s were largely, although not exclusively, from relatively established, conservatively oriented families. At the time, Newcomb described the family orientations of most students with respect to contemporary social issues as "definitely conservative," noting that "both home and school influences [were] such that there was little or no necessity for [the students] to come to very definite terms with public issues"

(Newcomb, 1943, pp. 10–11). By contrast, the college had recruited for its faculty persons who were open to the kind of educational innovation emphasized by the administration. These faculty members surprised the administration by being much more liberal and progressive in their political orientations than the student body. No one possibly predicted what would follow from the admixture of young, impressionable women from sheltered conservative backgrounds and an intense young faculty that was on the vanguard of social change, aware of the problems facing society, and committed to a particular set of ideological positions regarding their solution.

In the historical context of the 1930s, members of the Bennington faculty were determined not only to expose their young students to the public issues of the day but to also to get them to appreciate how a more progressive understanding of these matters would interpret them. On hand for this "natural experiment" of these women confronting the public issues of the period—worldwide economic depression, the development of fascism in Europe, and the growing popularity of the social policies of Roosevelt's New Deal—in the context of the liberal climate of faculty orientations, Newcomb decided to study the processes of attitude development among the students as they spent more time in the Bennington environment. Between 1935 and 1939, Newcomb (1943) collected data from a sample of Bennington students (n = 527) on their own political orientations and those of their parents as well as on their experiences at Bennington. Newcomb's research demonstrated that political attitudes and identities of college-aged adults can be quite malleable and open to change (see Alwin, Cohen, & Newcomb, 1991, Chapter 2).

Newcomb's (1943) research documented systematic and meaningful changes in attitudes over the collegiate years in this sample of women, finding that their attitudes moved in the direction of the Bennington faculty's and away from the orientations of their parents. His research provided support for the notion that parental influences are attenuated as a young person comes into contact with new informational environments and normative influences (see Alwin, Cohen, & Newcomb, 1991, p. 52). These results are reproduced in table 6.1, where a common factor underlying student political orientations—a political and economic progressivism scale (PEP30) and political party identity (PID30)—is predicted from three variables: (1) the year the student entered Bennington, (2) the number of years at Bennington, and (3) parental political orientations. The details of this analysis are presented elsewhere (see Alwin, Cohen, & Newcomb, 1991, pp. 145–149), and we cannot present here all of the methodological information necessary to completely understand the

Table 6.1. Parameter estimates for a linear structural equations model for early sociopolitical orientation

	Dependent variable		
Predictor variable	(1) PEP30	(2) PID30	(3) SPO30
1930s sociopolitical factor	.677**	.814**	—
Year entered Bennington	—	—	.190**
Number of years at Bennington	—	—	-.101
Parental orientations	—	—	.628**
R-squared	.458	.662	.473

Source: Alwin, Cohen, and Newcomb (1991), table 7.3
Note: Based on a model with 2 *df* and χ^2 of 2.10 (p = .350)
*p < .05, **p < .01

analysis. Suffice it to say that the observed variables in this analysis are scored so that a high score is more conservative. It is clear from these results that there is a strong relationship between the liberal-conservative direction of parents and that of their offspring. At the same time, the timing of a student's stay at Bennington, as measured both in terms of her year of entry and in terms of the number of years she remained at Bennington, is significant. Those who entered Bennington later were more conservative, and (although it is not statistically significant) the longer students remained at Bennington, the more liberal were their political views. This is a relatively strong model for the prediction of variation in political orientations: nearly one-half of the variance in early sociopolitical orientations can be accounted for by knowing parental orientations and these few indicators of the Bennington experience.

These results illustrate the kind of tension Bengtson (1989) noted between the desire of families to transmit their own values and orientations in an effort to preserve past patterns and to prepare children for the future, on one hand, and the process of change, which involves secondary socialization institutions, on the other. The dependence of student political orientations on parental orientations is what Bengtson (1989) referred to as a "lineage" effect, or the tendency of families to transmit their values and orientations to their children. The power of this "kinship structure of families" is clearly an essential component for understanding the unfolding of the life cycle, the progression of biological development (ontogeny), and the succession of roles and relationships. These results illustrate the concept of generation in the sense that they permit the understanding of the critical socialization function performed by the parental generation in all known societies. In addition, intergenerational relationships continue across the entire life span, including intergenerational relations in old age as well as intergenerational relations during childhood and other phases of the life span. I suggest that from the point of view of studying families, it is therefore important to study the nature of intergenerational relationships, regardless of life stage, as well as the differences among generations.

Persistence of the Bennington Effect

Despite the obvious strength of the pull of parental orientations on the political orientations of the Bennington women, it is clear that there was also a "Bennington effect," as observed in Newcomb's early work (see table 6.1). Although Newcomb's Bennington research provided evidence for the conclusion that under certain conditions the divergence from parental orientations could be quite dramatic, it was less clear whether these newly formed attitudes would persist or whether this kind of attitudinal flexibility would continue throughout life. Hence, in an effort to investigate the extent to which the "Bennington effect" persisted in the early 1960s, Newcomb and his students followed up on the Bennington women some 25 years following the first set of studies (Newcomb, Koenig, Flacks, & Warwick, 1967). And, in 1984, Newcomb, along with Ron Cohen and me, returned to these women to inquire of their political attitudes in later life (Alwin, Cohen, & Newcomb, 1991). We found that the political identities Newcomb had witnessed in the young lives of these women gained considerable strength and continued with a rather high degree of stability into old age. Identities, once formed, are highly stable structures (Alwin, 1994). The results of this follow-up revealed what we elsewhere referred to as "dynamic stability" (Alwin, Cohen, & Newcomb, 1991, p. 252), in which the persistence of sociopolitical orientations was the result of an organization of one's social environment in ways that are compatible with one's own orientations. Newcomb, Koenig, Flacks, and Warwick (1967) argued that the Bennington women were led to create "a social environment which would nurture and reinforce the value systems with which they left college" (p. 53).

The results in figure 6.1 indicate that roughly two-thirds of the Bennington women voted for Democratic or liberal candidates in all elections from 1940. Although there are important exceptions, this is a highly consistent pattern. The Bennington women were strongly supportive of the liberal political party, the Democrats, throughout their lives. During the 1950s, there was some weak-

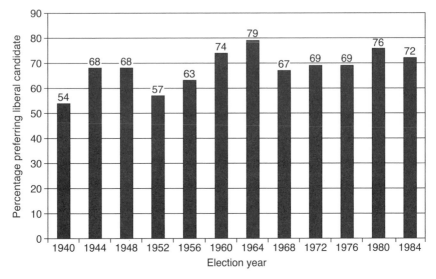

Figure 6.1. Retrospective reports of candidate preferences obtained in 1984.
Source: Alwin, Cohen, and Newcomb (1991), table 5.5.

ening of this support, but the data shown here are highly consistent with the idea that there was a "Bennington effect" resulting either from their histori-cal location or their historical participation, or both. Arguing for both co-hort and Generation effects in this instance, when coupled with the evidence provided earlier on "lineage effects," shows that the experiences of the Bennington women are consistent with all three types of effects: generation as kinship, generation as historical location, and generation as historical participation.

Generations and Cohorts

One of the issues we raised in the third Bennington study was whether the Bennington effect (see table 6.1) was possibly due to the effects of the larger historical context. Perhaps, we suggested, the distinctiveness of the Benning-ton women was due to historical location, that is, a cohort effect (Alwin, Cohen, & Newcomb, 1991, pp. 88–119). To explore this question, figure 6.2 presents patterns of candidate preference to illustrate the distinctiveness of the Bennington women during the 1984 election campaign. There is some slight support for a cohort effect: NES women born between 1910 and 1924, and especially those with college experience, move in a more liberal direc-tion, like the Bennington women. The overwhelming result here involves the

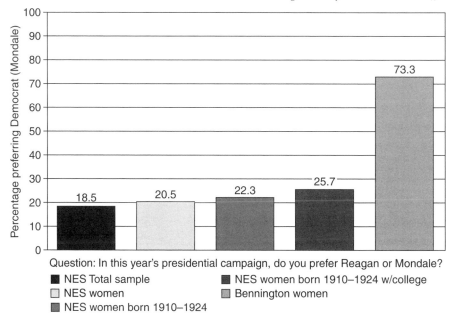

Figure 6.2. Comparison of the Bennington respondents and the 1984 National Election Study respondents: candidate preference (C11). *Source:* Alwin, Cohen, and Newcomb (1991), Appendix D.

huge difference between the Bennington women and other segments of the population—in the 1984 election, nearly three-fourths of the Bennington women supported the liberal candidate. In the population as a whole, this figure was 18.5 percent.

The Bennington women reflect social processes that are clearly more than just a cohort effect. The entire experience of attending college at Bennington during the 1930s was a type of Generation effect. That is, what we have been calling a "Bennington effect" might just as well be thought of in terms of the kinds of social movements that were propelling young people in the direction of progressive politics. The Bennington women were babies during the era of women's suffrage, they were children of the Depression, they were mothers of the Vietnam and civil rights generations, and they are the heirs to the Gray Panthers of the 1970s. Franklin Delano Roosevelt's New Deal program heightened the political awareness and involvement of these women in political affairs during their youth. As noted earlier, the concept of generation as historical location—that is, what we often think of as cohort effects—gives way to a more nuanced understanding of the impact of history, which we have here

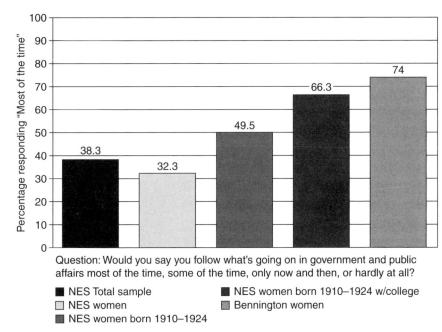

Question: Would you say you follow what's going on in government and public affairs most of the time, some of the time, only now and then, or hardly at all?

■ NES Total sample   ■ NES women born 1910–1924 w/college
☐ NES women   ▨ Bennington women
■ NES women born 1910–1924

Figure 6.3. Comparison of the Bennington respondents and the 1984 National Election Study respondents: follow government affairs (C9). *Source:* Alwin, Cohen, and Newcomb (1991), Appendix D.

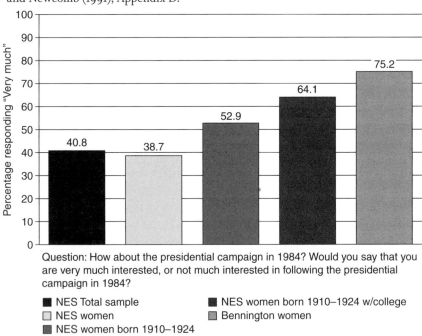

Question: How about the presidential campaign in 1984? Would you say that you are very much interested, or not much interested in following the presidential campaign in 1984?

■ NES Total sample   ■ NES women born 1910–1924 w/college
☐ NES women   ▨ Bennington women
■ NES women born 1910–1924

Figure 6.4. Comparison of the Bennington respondents and the 1984 National Election Study respondents: interest in election campaigns (C10). *Source:* Alwin, Cohen, and Newcomb (1991), Appendix D.

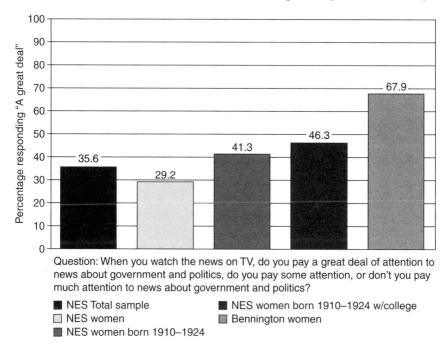

Question: When you watch the news on TV, do you pay a great deal of attention to news about government and politics, do you pay some attention, or don't you pay much attention to news about government and politics?

■ NES Total sample   ■ NES women born 1910–1924 w/college
☐ NES women   ▨ Bennington women
■ NES women born 1910–1924

Figure 6.5. Comparison of the Bennington respondents and the 1984 National Election Study respondents: attention to political news (C14). *Source:* Alwin, Cohen, and Newcomb (1991), Appendix D.

called Generation as historical participation. Beginning with Mannheim (1952 [1927]), many scholars have observed that individuals vary in their level of participation in the movements and social organizations that shape the historical process. While individuals are simultaneously nested within families and within birth cohorts, they are also nested with the social environments that are defined by historical events (see Sewell, 2005). Individuals are nested within the social movements and organizations in which they participate at the point of their intersection of biographical and historical time.

This third component of generational thinking as an important factor in understanding the Bennington case can be seen in figures 6.3, 6.4, and 6.5. These reveal both the effects of cohort and the effects of Generations, the latter of which in some cases may be even more important to understanding patterns of human growth and development. Our Bennington results clearly point to a conclusion of a heightened level of participation in public affairs, certainly in terms of the respondents' self-perceptions (Cohen & Alwin, 1993). The Bennington women were more likely to follow government affairs (see figure 6.3), were more likely to have an interest in election campaigns (see figure 6.4), and are more likely to pay attention to political news (see figure 6.5) than are comparable women in their birth cohorts. Notice in all three cases that there appears to also be a cohort effect in the sense that the Bennington women, and the cohorts of which they were a part (i.e., those born 1910 to 1924), all have stronger tendencies toward attention to public affairs, but the Bennington women are even more extreme.

Hence, it appears that the so -called "Bennington effect" may in fact reflect the participation in the social movements brought to life in the collegiate environment of Bennington College, and the Bennington environment may have sown the seeds for participating in the issues of the times. In the words of Theodore Newcomb (1943, p. 12):

> whatever the manner in which public issues come to be related to individual values, the relationship will be established through the medium of whatever group or groups of which the individual is a member.

The Bennington College environment required its students to come to terms with the social and political issues of the day. These young women came into a setting where community life was intense, and

> where there (was) much more pressure to come to terms with public issues, and where there (were) people of intelligence and good breeding (upper class students and faculty, in the main) who do not agree with their families and their families' friends regarding contemporary public affairs (Newcomb, 1943, pp. 10–11).

These factors not only gave shape to the young lives of the Bennington women but were indicative of how Generation effects emerge out of historical participation (see Alwin, Cohen, & Newcomb, 1991, pp. 31–34, for a detailed discussion of the nature of the Bennington College environment at that time).

Talking about Generations

In this chapter I have attempted to highlight the differences among three different conceptions of generations and have illustrated the importance of retaining these conceptual distinctions. "Generation as kinship position" captures the critical genealogical distinction about the passage of biographical time within families. "Generation as cohort" refers to the location of groups of individuals in historical time (for other uses of the term "cohort," see Biggs and Lowenstein, Chapter 7, and Johnson, Chapter 8). In contrast to defining generation as kinship position, conceiving of generations in terms of those people who are born and who lived at about the same time captures the influence of historical events and processes on human development. Imagining generations as cohorts captures the effects of historical placement in ways that other notions of generation cannot. In the words of Elder, Johnson, and Crosnoe (2003, p. 9), "locating people in (birth) cohorts provides more precise historical placement" than do other concepts of generation. If the goal is to entertain the ideas of cohort effects and cohort replacement to understand measured social change, there is no better conception of generational influences, but the fact that individuals are nested within birth cohorts does not deny the relevance of the fact that they are also nested within families as well as within other historically relevant social locations that very clearly influence their development. And, finally, defining generation as historical participation specifies another important dimension of generational influences, namely, the consequences for individuals of participation in the social movements of their youth and the resultant effects on their identities, attitudes, and beliefs.

Another aspect of the problem is that popular conceptions and "scientific" concepts may not perfectly coincide, and nonspecialists often rely on the same terms as do social scientists without necessarily employing the conceptual and empirical rigor that would accompany their use in a social science context. For example, journalists are frequently content with labeling entire groups of people who share a particular historical location as "generations" and therein attempting to explain social differences among age groups by capturing in a word or phrase the essential differences in historical experiences across lengthy periods of time. One of the best recent examples of this kind of approach to interpreting social history is Tom Brokaw's *The Greatest Generation* (1998), which has become a quite popular descriptor for those people who came of age during the Depression and World War II and experienced the years of prosperity that followed. They are often contrasted with those who grew to maturity during the 1960s and 1970s (their children), who ushered in an era of rebellion and tolerance. There is nothing inherently wrong with the journalist's use of the term "generation" to describe what appear to be differences in participation in the unique "slices of history" experienced by young people during a particular period of time. In some quarters, however, there is a substantial degree of skepticism about the source of their data. Rosenberg

(1959, pp. 241–258), for example, suggested that journalistic accounts of generations are often "concocted . . . out of trivial or ephemeral data." As I argue elsewhere, while I largely share Rosenberg's sentiment, Brokaw's usage may in fact be viewed as a good example of what Karl Mannheim referred to as a "generational unit" (see Alwin & McCammon, 2007).

Closing

I hope this chapter has clarified the fact that there are several legitimate uses of the term "generation," each separately conceptualizing a unique aspect of life experiences and influences. Consistent with Vern Bengtson's work on this subject (e.g., Bengtson, 1989), I argued there are three common uses of the concept of generation: generation as kinship position, generation as historical location, and generation as historical participation. One of these three concepts of generation is linked to each of the three critical levels of analysis—families, cohorts, and social movements or organizations—which converge within the life history of the individual. My discussion earlier suggested that it is understandable, given this convergence, that their influences are often confounded with one another, and the use of the same word for three distinct concepts invites confusion. It has been my intention to reduce the level of confusion surrounding the concepts of generation and further explore their utility for the analysis of human behavior.

My discussion of these various generational concepts goes well beyond clarifying the distinctions among these three concepts and reducing the confusion among them. It also makes a case for why all three are important for the study of human development. My examples from the Bennington research reinforce this conclusion. I was able to show that the political development of these women was dependent upon three discernible sets of influences—family, cohort, and historical participation. Importantly, the subjects were influenced by their parents, with there being a strong dependence of the young person's liberal-conservative orientation on that of their parents. At the same time, examination of the 1984 National Election Study data suggests there were cohort (i.e., historical location) factors at work as well as what appears to be a New Deal Generation effect in these data. The latter effect is reflected in the differences of the Bennington women in the extent to which they follow government affairs, the amount of interest they have in election campaigns, and their attention to political news (see also Cohen & Alwin, 1993).

Finally, with respect to laying claim on the concept of generation, I do not see the importance of phrasing the terminological issue as a competition among historical theorists on the one hand and life course analysts on the other (e.g., Kertzer, 1983). Neither meaning of the concept of generation should be confused with the ideas of cohorts and cohort effects. However, despite the potential confusion in terminology, it seems plausible to tolerate all meanings given above for generation, using each sense as appropriate.

The concept of Generation found in the work of Mannheim and Ortega y Gasset is not intended to be synonymous with "cohort," and when one appreciates the meaning of the concept as used in their writings it will become obvious that the concept of Generation entails much more than simply cohort differences. The latter may be suggestive of Generational differences, but although cohort differentiation may be thought to be a necessary condition for Generational differences, it may not be sufficient for saying that Generations truly exist in the sense of having a distinctive culture and shared identity. It is participation in the social movements of the day, during youth and the period of attitude development, which is critical to the production of a unique sense of Generational identity. I believe the Bennington women reflect such a case.

ACKNOWLEDGMENTS

Research reported here was supported by a grant from the National Institute on Aging (R01-AG04743). During the writing of this chapter, the author was supported by his current NIA grant (R01-AG-021203). He acknowledges the valuable assistance of Alyson Otto in the preparation of this chapter.

NOTES

The inspiration for the title of this chapter comes from the words of a 1960s hit song by the British rock group *The Who* (Roger Daltrey, Peter Townshend, John Entwistle, and Keith Moon) titled "Talkin' 'bout my GENeration," which was recorded on their 1965 debut album *My Generation* (in the United States, *The Who Sings My Generation*). The song, written by Townshend, has an angry motif reflecting sentiments of the youthful rebellion of the period. Some of the original performances by *The Who* can be found on YouTube: http://www.youtube.com. A remake of the song by *The Zimmers*, released in May 2007, can also be found on YouTube.

1. Ryder's (1965, p. 849) presidential address to the American Sociological Association credited Mannheim's work with the introduction of the concept of "cohort" to the analysis of social change and the fact that social change occurs in part via processes of cohort replacement.

REFERENCES

Alwin, D. F. (1994). Aging, personality and social change: The stability of individual differences over the adult life-span. In D. L. Featherman, R. M. Lerner, & M. Perl-mutter (Eds.), *Life-span development and behavior* (Vol. 12, pp. 135–185). Hillsdale, NJ: Lawrence Erlbaum Associates.

Alwin, D. F. (1995). Taking time seriously: Social change, social structure and human lives. In P. Moen, G. H. Elder, Jr., & K. Lüscher (Eds.), *Linking lives and contexts: Perspectives on the ecology of human development* (pp. 211–262). Washington, DC: American Psychological Association.

Alwin, D. F. (1996). Parental socialization in historical perspective. In C. Ryff & M. M. Seltzer (Eds.), *The parental experience at midlife* (pp. 105–167). Chicago, IL: University of Chicago Press.

Alwin, D. F. (1997). Aging, social change and conservatism: Linking aging and social change in the study of political identities. In M. Hardy (Ed.), *Conceptual and methodological issues in the study of aging and social change* (pp. 164–190). Beverly Hills, CA: Sage.

Alwin, D. F. (2001). Parental values, beliefs, and behavior: A review and promulga for research into the new century. In S. L. Hofferth & T. J. Owens (Eds.), *Children at the millennium: Where have we come from, where are we going?* (pp. 97–139). New York: Elsevier Science.

Alwin, D. F., Cohen, R. L., & Newcomb, T. M. (1991). *Political attitudes over the life span: The Bennington women after fifty years.* Madison, WI: University of Wisconsin Press.

Alwin, D. F., & McCammon, R. (2003). Generations, cohorts and social change. In J. T. Mortimer & M. J. Shanahan (Eds.), *Handbook of the life course* (pp. 23–49). New York: Kluwer Academic/Plenum Publishers.

Alwin, D. F., & McCammon, R. (2007). Rethinking generations. *Research in Human Development, 4,* 219–237.

Alwin, D. F., McCammon, R. J., & Hofer, S. M. (2006). Studying baby boom cohorts within a demographic and developmental context: Conceptual and methodological issues. In S. K. Whitbourne & S. L. Willis (Eds.), *The baby boomers grow up: Contemporary perspectives on midlife.* Mahwah, NJ: Lawrence Erlbaum Associates.

Amato, P., & Booth, A. (1997). *Generation at risk: Growing up in an era of family upheaval.* Cambridge, MA: Harvard University Press.

Ardelt, M. (2000). Still stable after all these years? Personality stability theory revisited. *Social Psychology Quarterly, 63,* 392–405.

Bengtson, V. L. (1989). The problem of generations: Age group contrasts, continuities, and social change. In V. L. Bengtson & K. W. Schaie (Eds.), *The course of later life: Research and reflections* (pp. 25–54). New York: Springer.

Brokaw, T. (1998). *The greatest generation.* New York: Random House.

Cohen, R. L., & Alwin, D. F. (1993). Bennington women of the 1930s: Political attitudes over the life course. In K. D. Hulbert & D. T. Schuster (Eds.), *Women's life through time: Educated American women of the twentieth century* (pp. 117–139). San Francisco, CA: Jossey-Bass.

Costa, P. T. Jr., & McCrae, R. R. (1994). Set like plaster? Evidence for the stability of adult personality. In T. F. Heatherton & J. L. Weinberger (Eds.), *Can personality change?* (pp. 21–40). Washington, DC: American Psychological Association.

Elder, G. H. Jr. (1974). *Children of the Great Depression.* Chicago, IL: University of Chicago Press.

Elder, G. H. Jr., Johnson, M. K., & Crosnoe, R. (2003). The emergence and development of life course theory. In J. T. Mortimer & M. J. Shanahan (Eds.), *Handbook of the life course* (pp. 3–19). New York: Kluwer Academic/Plenum Publishers.

Firebaugh, G. (1992). Where does social change come from? Estimating the relative contributions of individual change and population turnover. *Population Research and Policy Review, 11*, 1–20.

Glenn, N. D. (2003). Distinguishing age, period, and cohort effects. In J. T. Mortimer & M. J. Shanahan (Eds.), *Handbook of the life course* (pp. 465–476). New York: Kluwer Academic/Plenum Publishers.

Hagan, J. (2001). *Northern passage: American anti-Vietnam War resisters in Canada.* Cambridge, MA: Harvard University Press.

Heatherton, T. F., & Weinberger, J. L. (Eds.). (1994). *Can personality change?* Washington, DC: American Psychological Association.

Inkeles, A. (1983 [1955]). Social change and social character: The role of parental mediation. *Journal of Social Issues, 11*, 12–23. Reprinted, *Journal of Social Issues, 39*, 179–191.

Kertzer, D. I. (1983). Generation as a sociological problem. In R. H. Turner & J. F. Short Jr. (Eds.), *Annual review of sociology* (Vol. 9, pp. 125–149). Palo Alto, CA: Annual Reviews.

Mannheim, K. (1952 [1927]). The problem of generations. In P. Kecskemeti (Ed.), *Essays in the sociology of knowledge* (pp. 276–322). Boston, MA: Routledge & Kegan Paul.

McAdam, D. (1988). *Freedom summer.* New York: Oxford University Press.

McCluskey, K. A., & Reese, H. W. (1984). *Life-span developmental psychology: Historical and generational effects.* New York: Academic Press.

Modell, J. (1989). *Into one's own.* Berkeley, CA: University of California Press.

Newcomb, T. M. (1943). *Personality and social change: Attitude formation in a student community.* New York: Dryden Press.

Newcomb, T. M, Koenig, K. E., Flacks, R., & Warwick, D. P. (1967). *Persistence and change: Bennington College and its students after twenty-five years.* New York: Wiley.

Ortega y Gasset, J. (1933). *The modern theme.* New York: Norton.

Roscow, I. 1978. What is a cohort and why? *Human Development, 21*, 65–75.

Rosenberg, H. (1959). *The tradition of the new.* New York: Horizon Press.

Ryder, N. B. (1965). The cohort as a concept in the study of social change. *American Sociological Review, 30*, 843–861.

Settersten, R. A., Jr. (2006). Aging and the life course. In R. H. Binstock & L. K.

George (Eds.), *Handbook of aging and the social sciences* (6th ed., pp. 3–19). New York: Academic Press.

Sewell, W. H. Jr. (2005). *Logics of history.* Chicago, IL: University of Chicago Press.

White, H. (1992). Succession and generations: Looking back on chains of opportunity. In H. A. Becker (Ed.), *Dynamics of cohort and generations research* (pp. 31–51). Amsterdam: Thesis.

CHAPTER SEVEN

Toward Generational Intelligence

Linking Cohorts, Families, and Experience

Simon Biggs and Ariela Lowenstein

> Each age has its landscape, its atmosphere, its cities, its people . . .
> CHARLES GINNER (an English artist, 1878–1952,
> Camden Town Group)

Rarely have societies witnessed a "silent revolution" of such significance as population aging. Longer life spans and fewer births are transforming the age structure of societies from a triangle, with a few older adults at the top and an ever-larger number of younger people fanning out below them, into a rectangle with, until the very extreme of late life, roughly equal numbers of people in each part of the life course (Bengtson & Lowenstein, 2003). This transformation means that the proportions of children, young, middle-life, and older persons will be approximately the same. Such a change in age structure, affecting both the developed and the developing worlds (Aboderin et al., 2002) is historically unprecedented and may be expected to provoke challenges to existing norms of intergenerational behavior.

An implication of this transformation is that a new architecture for social relations may begin to emerge. Higher life expectancy is already creating new spaces for multigenerational interactions, as there are simply more family generations to interact with each other (Antonucci, Akiyama, & Merline, 2001). To this phenomenon can be added an increased complexity of extended family patterns arising from divorce, remarriage, and other forms of relationship (Bengtson, Lowenstein, Putney, & Gans, 2003). How then would an individual, a family, and a society cope with the above changes in their demographic maps and in changing norms and patterns of intergenerational relations?

Generations, Social Change, and Intergenerational Relationships

The goal of this essay is to examine the discourses regarding the concept of generation arising from the study of families and cohorts and to suggest a conceptual framework that may prove useful in engaging with novel and changing experiences of generational identity and intergenerational relations.

The rationale for addressing this conceptual problem is threefold. First, a number of social issues are emerging that have an intergenerational dimension. These include age discrimination in the workplace, elder abuse, and questions of generational equity around pensions and forms of care. Such issues have been recognized by the Second World Assembly on Ageing in Madrid, convened by the United Nations in 2002, which noted: "the need to strengthen solidarity between generations and intergenerational partnerships, keeping in mind the particular needs of both older and younger ones, and encourage mutually responsive relationships between generations" (United Nations, 2002, p. 4).

Second, there is a growing recognition that to study adult aging one has also to study intergenerational relationships (Antonucci, Jackson, & Biggs, 2007). Intergenerational relations provide the context within which individuals age, the way that they mark their own aging, and the relative value that is attached to that process.

Third, different disciplines are engaged with the concept of generation but rarely cross-communicate (Bengtson & Lowenstein, 2003). Each emphasizes a particular perspective but without delving into understanding how a multiplicity of different influences contribute to a singular experience that people use to navigate their social world. Generation is, then, a "packed social concept" (McDaniel, 2008), including a variety of social, familial, and personal associations, that may or may not explicitly influence personal identity. Taken together these factors point to a reexamination of the idea of generation, its constituent parts, and the way in which it is experienced by different age groups in families and in wider social contexts.

There are various meanings attached to the concept of generation in everyday experience. Bengtson (2001) distinguishes two levels of analysis, the micro and the macro. Here, the micro level pertains to relations between family members, for example, among children, parents, grandparents, and the extended family. The macro level refers to relationships between cohorts that are often defined in terms of specific national or global events. At a mezzo level, Biggs (2007) presents the inner-outer metaphor, which examines generational transformations in terms of the bidirectional movement between public and private self-location.

The concept of generation can be defined with regard to society or to family, to personal or to public events. At the level of the family, generation refers to position in the lineage. At the societal level, it refers to the aggregate of persons born in a limited period (i.e., a birth cohort, according to demographic parlance) who therefore experience historical events at similar ages and move up through the life course in unison. Sanchez and Diaz (2005, p. 397), based on a proposal by Donati (1999), present five meanings of the concept: (1) Cohort (generation in a demographic sense), a group of persons born in the same years or range of years; (2) age group (generation in a historic sense), a cohort of number of years which is considered as a social group; (3) generational unit (as proposed by Mannheim, 1952 [1928]), a subgroup that produces and guides social and cultural movements; (4) generation in a socio-anthropological sense, a group of persons who share a position regarding relationships of descendence, which are socially mediated; and (5) generation in a relational sense, a group of people sharing a relationship linked to their position in the family (son, parent) and a position in society depending on their social age (youth, adult). This last meaning combines historic-social age with family lineage and implies that one can look at generation as a concept that connects individuals and their capacities to make decisions with social structures over time (McDaniel, 2008).

In this essay we explore the notion of generation by using Bengtson's distinction between macro and micro structures while considering how the public and private spheres of generation interact, particularly as they relate to the iterative relationship between consciousness of family lineage and historical cohort.

Self-Awareness through Lineage

The familial approach to generations has been a powerful influence on mainstream social gerontology, arising from the discipline's roots in issues of health and social care. It is suggested that relationships among generations provide important security from external threats and that the maintenance of intergenerational relationships is therefore critical in providing a buffer against economic hardship, psychological isolation, and social anomie. Families, according to Bengtson and Putney (2006), are the "glue" that ensure social stability, personal security, and "continuity of the social order." Intergenerational solidarity provides a sense of identity and belonging and might increase family generational consciousness (Lowenstein, 2003).

Bengtson and colleagues (Bengtson & Roberts, 1991; Bengtson & Murray, 1993) developed an intergenerational solidarity-conflict paradigm, which has achieved predominance in the gerontological literature for the past 30 years and has been adopted in European as well as North American studies (Lowenstein, 2007). Intergenerational solidarity is manifested in six different dimensions that reflect relationships between older parents and adult children: structural solidarity, association, functional, emotional, normative, and consensus.

According to Bengtson & Putney, intergenerational solidarity within families answers the question: "How will the group deal with differences or conflicts that arise between generations and negotiate their resolution for the betterment of individuals, families and the social order?" (2006, p. 20). In a robust restatement of what is essentially the solidarity position, privileging family relations over social structures, these authors claim: "intergenerational relations at the micro-social level within multigenerational families have a profound but unrecognized influence on relations between age groups at the societal level. . . . The essence of multigenerational families is interdependence between generations and its members, and this will tend to mitigate schisms between age groups over scarce government resources" (2006, p. 28)

One of the main psycho-social approaches to the concept of generation is the life-course perspective, which encompasses the following premises. (1) The life course is a social phenomenon (Hagestad & Neugarten, 1985) that reflects the intersection of social, cultural, and historical factors with personal biography (Elder, 1985; Meyer, 1988). (2) The life-course perspective focuses on age-differentiated sequences of transitions (Rossi & Rossi, 1990), with transitions and trajectories as key concepts (Hagestad, 1990), and "cultural precepts underlying the life-course system define and locate the meaning of both the individual and the trajectory of the proper life" (Meyer, 1988, p. 62).

Perhaps the most widely known evidence of the relationship between family and historical and economic circumstances can be found in the work of Elder (1985, 1994), whose longitudinal study of life chances following the Great Depression and economic downturn in the North American Midwest has become a seminal point of reference. This life-course approach links the three metrics of individual lifetime, family time, and historical time. The life-time metric relates to chronological age and age stratification and to the meanings, behavioral expectations, and vulnerabilities associated with particular ages (Riley, Johnson, & Foner, 1972; Hagestad, 1990). The linkage between particular ages and family-event sequences assumes an underlying set of age norms. Lastly, historical circumstances and broad social changes such as migration, wars, or economic shifts mold and reshape mutual support within families (Bengtson et al., 2003; Hareven, 1996; Elder, 1985). Position in the family, age at which economic hardship is experienced, and gender were each found to mediate life chances and certain aspects of personality.

In France, Attias-Donfut (2003; Attias-Donfut & Wolff, 2005) has addressed generational interdependence in families as mitigating the effects of "discontinuity of social destinies." While identities partially flow from the vertical relations between generations within a family, they are also driven by the realities of social structure that commonly affect an age cohort. Attias-Donfut's work has focused on cultural transmission and generational memories and, as such, constitutes a powerful attempt to place the protective role of families within a social and historical context. The cohort one is born into, she states, shapes one's personal destiny through prevailing social conditions "at the time of entry into professional life, notably concerning the educational system and the labor market" (2003, p. 214). In the French postwar context, at least three socio-historical phases can be identified which have significantly affected the quality of family resilience. These she calls the generations of labor, of abundance, and of underprotection. Successive cohorts, therefore, do not have the same life chances. Family and kinship ties, which are themselves subject to multigenerational changes in fortune, can nevertheless protect family members through generational interdependence, mitigating the effects of this "discontinuity of social destinies "and offering an insight into the relationship between family lineage and class stratification. The memory of historical events is itself shaped by the role of family members in passing the experience of social events on to younger generations, as "each generation has one foot in the history which formed its predecessor and one in its own history and time" (Attias-Donfut & Wolff, 2005, p. 453).

The work of Elder, Attias-Donfut, and their associates demonstrates that the protective role of the family can be uneven and equivocal and does not perform a simple functionalist role of protecting families. An exclusively familist approach to the social order, however, can contribute to the maintenance of embedded social positions and the transfer of social and economic

life changes. It has been argued, for example, that a culturally specific emphasis on the family presupposes its positive value in some North American research (Marshall, 2002) and avoids problematizing family relations (Luescher
& Pillemer, 1998), the interrelationship between generational rivalry at work
and in families (Biggs, 2006), and the role of the family in maintaining social
inequality in wider society (Lorenz-Meyer, 2001). In an interesting twist regarding the effects of family solidarity on social structures, Attias-Donfut
(2003) points out that the transmission of generational memories can also
constitute an act of resistance to the social order insofar as these oral histories
can act as an alternative to dominant social messages promoted by powerful
groups in society at large.

Whatever the primacy of family or cohort on intergenerational interaction,
Hagestad (2003) has observed that families have functioned as critical mediators between individual experience and societies in flux, with Roos (2005)
adding that life's turning points are most often perceived as negative if they
arise from macro social change and positive if they are related to personal intergenerational events. Katz, Lowenstein, Phillips, and Daatland (2005,
p. 394) suggest that the typical sites for social gerontological discourse on generations in later life are "relations between older parents and their adult children when the parents are becoming frail". Changes that increase dependency
can highlight continuities and discontinuities in the balance between solidarity and conflict.

Much of Bengtson and his associates' work has concentrated on the family
as a place where the tensions of micro and macro meet. Here, intergenerational relations within families represent complex social bonds. Family members are linked by multiple types of solidarity that may be contradictory, and
conflict and ambivalent feelings may develop (Luescher & Pillemer, 1998; Pillemer et al., 2007). However, when a group like the family recognizes and be-
haves on the basis of a shared identity, it can act as an enfolding network that
distances within-group relationships from external threat, providing protection through care relations and reciprocity (Lowenstein, Katz, & Gur-Yaish,
2007). Attitudes between family members will determine how suited individuals are to roles and how effective social norms based on obligation or choice
will be (Finch, 1995).

Lineage and degrees of family solidarity have been put forward as important factors in the creation of generational identities. And while a number of
attempts have been made to identify the functions of family and transmission
between adult generations, the types of family interaction, and the effects of

different historical circumstances, there has been less attention devoted to the experience of generation as a source of personal identity and how this interacts with family structures. Family links private and public spheres and provokes expectations concerning intergenerational relations and responsibilities that may cause tension if these public expectations do not correspond to personal identifications and social attitudes.

Self-Awareness through Cohort

Adults use the term "generation" both to refer to their position in the micro sphere of lineage structures and also to identify certain large social groups who are growing older together. These groups would have been born at approximately the same time and been given a particular social and historical label. Examples in the United States would include the war generation; the baby boom generation, born after World War II between the late forties and the early sixties, a period characterized by a spike in the birth rate (Bengtson & Oyama, 2007); generation X, the age group born approximately between 1965 and 1976; generation Y, born from 1977 to 2002; and the "global generation, associated with the growth of global information technologies (Edmunds and Turner, 2005)." In India, the generation of the "zippies" ("Liberalization's Children"), born in the 1980s and 1990s, resides in new cities or suburbs and exhibits a sense of entitlement, coolness, self-confidence, and creativity (Lukose, 2008). In Singapore, generation M is the millennium generation, born in a time of economic prosperity and political stability and acculturated to the competitive Westernized culture (Koh, 2008). As such, birth cohorts that become identified as the carriers of social or historical meaning influence how members and nonmembers see themselves. They also may carry certain intergenerational attitudes that influence the way that one generation responds to another, which interact with familial forms (Biggs, Phillipson, Money, & Leach, 2007).

In the twentieth century, the social science of generation was underdeveloped when compared to other forms of social structuration, such as social class, gender, or race. Demographic transformations, global aging, and the ensuing political repercussions have increased contemporary interest in generations as birth cohorts. Here, generations are viewed as groups of individuals sharing similar histories and adapting together to a changing social climate.

Mannheim's (1997) pioneering work in this area first used the concept of a social generation in the seminal article "The problem of generations" (published first in 1928 and translated to English in 1952, with a renewed publication in 1997). Mannheim criticized previous assessments of generations for relying too heavily on the lineal and biological determinants of age categories. He drew attention to the role of generations in historical change, talking about "historical generation" and emphasizing the importance of forms of consciousness arising from these processes. His argument was that a generation represents a unique type of social location based on the dynamic interplay between being born in a particular year and the socio-political events that occur while that cohort emerges into adulthood. For him, generational location is a social fact similar to class position.

Mannheim (1952, 1997) also addressed the distinction between generational location, referring to individuals born in the same historical and cultural period, or *the birth cohort*; people exposed to the same concrete historical experiences, or *actual generation;* and individuals within the same generation who interpret their similar experiences in particular ways, or *generational units*. A key concept here was the degree to which a cohort developed "generational consciousness" (p. 311), which, similarly to Marxist visions of class consciousness, was contingent on surrounding social conditions. In certain historical circumstances a generation became conscious of itself and began to act as a politically self-conscious unit. Thus, in certain circumstances, generations may form close within-cohort identifications that will affect relations with other generations. At other times, when generational consciousness is less strongly formed, relations between generational groups would be more salient. Mannheim identified strong within-cohort consciousness with progressive social change and conflict with senior generations. Mannheim can be viewed as the first scholar who analyzed generational relations emerging between personal biography and social context as parameters relating to individual experiences of cultural and social change that form a particular social identity.

Following Mannheim, Bourdieu (1990, 1993) refined the concept of generational location as a generational "cultural field" characterized by the emergence of a changed relationship between past and present social spaces. He assumed that a generation is a social construction arising from the struggle for resources in a given field. Generational struggle, accordingly, is important in cultural transformation, with rate of change within the cultural space being a product of the intensity of the struggle for rare cultural resources between different generational groups. Generational style or consciousness is perceived by Bourdieu as generational "habitus," a collection of attitudes, lifestyles, and resources that generate and structure individual experience. This view, current within cultural gerontology, has also been used to imply that generational identities are becoming more fluid, suggesting that a set of new problems may emerge with few established norms for their resolution.

The shift from historically determined consciousness to generational habitus as a sort of social space that one can enter into frees generation from a fixed age group and allows it to be seen much more as a lifestyle choice. Gilleard (2004) has argued that generation can be thought of as a distinct, temporally located cultural field within which individuals from a potential variety of overlapping birth cohorts participate as generational agents. Gilleard further points out that generational styles of consciousness arising from a specific habitus, both generate and structure an individual's behavior and self-perception. Gilleard and Higgs (2002, 2005) discuss the blurring of generational differences and the creation of cohort-based "cultures of aging."

The association between particular cohorts and forms of consciousness has led to a number of reinterpretations of Mannheim's original position. Corsten (1999), for example, explores the concept of the "cultural circle" as formative of generational consciousness. Rather than being historical forces, generational identities are seen as something arising from interpersonal interactions: "People who spontaneously observe that other people use certain criteria for interpreting and articulating topics in a similar manner to themselves" (p. 262). Roos (2002), dealing with transition points, examines the intersections between birth cohorts and social experiences and posits that not all cohorts become generations. From his perspective, life transitions are not immediately relevant as generational experiences of the Mannheimian type. Mannheim assumed that a given experiential position with regard to important historical events and specific ages give rise to a generation, which could be called an "experience generation." However, according to Roos's (2002) data, important experiences are as likely to be private and personal events, so instead of an experience generation we actually witness event generations.

Cavalli (2004) and Pilcher (1994) argue that the formation of generational consciousness tends to occur in relation to events experienced in youth when people are coming of age. According to Vincent (2005), these elements of culture include both the formation of identity and lifestyle attributes, which are mainly formed in adolescence because experiences during that time influence the development of socio-interpretive maps and reactions to social phenomena that are used in adulthood. However, like Roos, Cavalli (2004) incorporates the concept of "crucial event" into the biography of individuals and considers that, while cohort effects are linked to self-identity, the concept of generation should be limited to definition of lineage relations and the private sphere.

Thus, the trend in exploring generational consciousness has gone from seeing it as a product of social structures that at some point appears as a self-conscious collective identity toward seeing it as an experience that is continually reshaped among individuals and depends largely on the personal interpretation of transitions and lifestyle choices. The flexibility that Bourdieu's habitus allows has led to its becoming a bridge between cohort and lineage and in this sense picking up on the work of Attias-Donfut outlined in the previous section. Here, lineage is always present in the background of generational consciousness, whereas the life chances of any one generation depend on the interaction between forms of familial identification and historical circumstances.

Bourdieu's (1996) perspective, when applied to the family, is based on the central themes of capital and habitus, focusing on intergenerational transmission of different types of capital. Bourdieu refers to three types of capital: economic, social, and cultural. Economic capital comprises income and inheritance. Social capital consists of the knowledge and specific identities of individuals and elite groups. Cultural capital is organized through habitus to legitimate preferences, practices, and behaviors based on past experiences within the family and shapes a person's future expectations. The family is a focus of accumulating capital, and there are family practices that promote inequality (Bourdieu, 1996). He therefore characterizes the family as both an objective and subjective social unit that organizes the way individual family members perceive social reality.

Eyerman and Turner (1998) define generation as "a cohort of persons passing through time that come to share a common habitus, hexis and culture, a function of which is to provide them with a collective memory that serves to integrate the cohort over a finite period of time" (p. 93). However, as Turner (1998), has pointed out, generational relations are not necessarily a source of cohort or familial cohesion. Each has a strategic temporal location relative to a set of resources, and access to these resources creates generational identity and solidarity that secures advantages against other generations. Rivalry therefore exists between generations, resulting in a "generational negotiation" for resources (Collard, 2001), with each generation activating power and social control (Dunham & Bengtson, 1986).

Edmunds and Turner (2005) stress the role of antagonistic social relations and processes in the formation of generational consciousness: "An age cohort comes to have social significance as a generation by creating a distinctive cultural or political identity. It is the interaction between historical resources, contingent circumstances and social formation that makes a 'generation' an interesting sociological category" (p. 561). They argue that in the twenty-first century this process has become global in nature, so that "globally experienced traumatic events may facilitate the development of global generations" (p. 564). Such generations are defined as being similar to the sixties or baby-boomer generations, who forged strong generational symbols and emotive connections through youth-driven social movements and the consumption of goods and services. Twenty-first-century generations are facilitated through developments in communications technology or an international crisis such as 9/11 (Turner, 2002; Edmunds & Turner, 2002b). They further note that technology has become salient in the formation of generational consciousness. However, such global generations are not homogeneous but vary according to national, regional, and local variation in technological access and interpretation of events.

When the studies of generations based on family, lineage, and social cohort are compared, one can see a move away from formal relations toward an understanding of generations based on personal or collective experience and self-conscious identities. If, as has been argued elsewhere, generation is a cross-roads phenomenon where a number of social influences intersect (Biggs, 2007), then it is not unreasonable to begin to explore the phenomenology of that experience and the processes that might make one factor more salient than others or make individuals more or less willing to use generation as a self-conscious form of identity.

Toward a Phenomenology of Generation

Arber and Attias-Donfut (2000) have observed that a feeling of generational belonging is created not just in a horizontal dimension of the birth cohort but also in a vertical dimension of familial lineage. Questions of generational awareness exist at the intersection of these axes. To this can be added the distinction that Biggs (1999) and Biggs et al. (2007) draw between depth and surface dimensions of the mature self, which creates a third context, that of the maturation of the personal consciousness. This third context is perhaps more difficult to explore empirically, yet it nevertheless exists tacitly in the life-course and generational consciousness models outlined above. The meeting point of birth cohort, familial lineage, and personal maturation creates a three-dimensional space in which the phenomenology of generational identity and its immediate experience exist. It is the quality and critical consciousness of this space, we would argue, that inform behavior in intergenerational settings and open the possibility of an holistic awareness of self as a generational entity. Taken together, these influences contribute to a specifically generational life world that influences thinking, emotions, and behavior. We would further argue that the experience of that space—the degree to which people are aware of it, how they react to it, and the effect it has on the sense of who they are and how they behave towards others—would form a bridge between familial and cohort-based understandings of generation.

By choosing a critical phenomenological form of inquiry, we recognize that while each dimension may be conceptually discrete, they are all experienced holistically, and it is their sum or balance which results in a particular experience of generation. Becoming conscious of one's own distinctive identity emerges as a force that both links and distinguishes particular generational groups insofar as it is not until one becomes conscious of generational distinctiveness that one can develop genuine relationships between generations (Faimberg, 2005).

The point here is not so much to rehearse the observation that adult demography consists of cohort, period, and lifespan effects as to suggest that generation is actually experienced as an amalgam of influences that give any one intergenerational decision its own phenomenal flavor. Consciousness of generation, in both micro and macro contexts, depends upon being able to recognize both one's generational identity and how that identity itself generates certain forms of relationship.

Toward Generational Intelligence

A phenomenological understanding, which we have called Generational Intelligence (GI), would raise some basic questions that have not been at the forefront of the debate on generational consciousness in families and societies. What does each individual bring into the intergenerational familial and societal exchange? How conscious are individuals of what they bring? How is generational consciousness performed and negotiated within the encounter? How does it impact the process and outcome of the encounter and the potential for connection, conflict, or ambivalence between generations? Does it lead to acquiring awareness and building capacity for understanding different generations and their needs?

Having reviewed current thinking on families and cohorts, we would argue that any definition of generation (See Alwin, Chapter 6) should be one that can answer the above questions and help examine the interrelationships among individual, familial, and societal levels of social consciousness. As such, Generational Intelligence would act as a bridging concept between the micro and macro spheres. This lies partly in the assumption that generation is experienced in immediate action as a phenomenological whole, even though it may arise from attitudes to life course, family, or cohort. As the relationship between cooperation, conflict, and ambivalence between generations is currently theoretically contested (Pillemer et al., 2007), we would argue that sustainable intergenerational relationships will need to rely on increased levels of generational insight, empathy, and mutually negotiated action. Intelligence of this sort facilitates the interplay among different levels of understanding associated with intergenerational exchanges. Ultimately, such deeper understanding should allow us to move beyond bipolar conceptual positions—such as family or cohort, macro or micro, obligation or choice—which can so often give credence to inflexible responses to related social issues. An intelligent approach to intergenerational relations would need to address the issue of how individuals become self-consciously aware of their generational status and how far this awareness influences their experience of and action toward others in the social world.

REFERENCES

Aboderin, I., Kalache, A., Ben-Shlomo, Y., Lynch, J. W., Yajnik, C. S., Kuh, D., & Yach, D. (2002). *Active aging*: A policy framework. Geneva: World Health Organization.

Antonucci, T. C., Akiyama, H., & Merline, A. (2001). Dynamics of social relationships in midlife. In M. E. Lachman (Ed.), *Handbook of midlife development*. Chichester, UK: Wiley.

Antonucci, T. C., Jackson, J., & Biggs, S. (2007). Intergenerational relations: Theory, research and policy. *Journal of Social Issues, 63*(4), 679–694.

Arber, S., & Attias-Donfut, C. (2000). *The myth of generational conflict*. London: Routledge.

Attias-Donfut, C. (2003). Family transfers and cultural transmissions between three generations in France. In V. L. Bengtson & A. Lowenstein (Eds.), *Global aging and challenges to families* (pp. 214–252). New York: Aldine de Gruyter.

Attias-Donfut, C., & Wolff, F.-C. (2005). Generational memory and family relationships. In M. L. Johnson (Ed.), *The Cambridge handbook of age and ageing* (pp. 443–454). Cambridge, UK: Cambridge University Press.

Bengtson, V. L. (2001). The Burgess award lecture: Beyond the nuclear family: The increasing importance of multigenerational bonds. *Journal of Marriage and the Family, 63*(1), 1–16.

Bengtson, V. L., & Lowenstein, A. (2003). *Global aging and challenges to families*. New York: Aldine de Gruyter.

Bengtson, V. L., Lowenstein, A., Putney, N. M., & Gans, D. (2003). Global aging and the challenges to families. In V. L. Bengtson & A. Lowenstein (Eds.), *Global aging and challenges to families* (pp. 1–26). New York: Aldine de Gruyter.

Bengtson, V. L., & Murray, T. M. (1993). Justice across generations (and cohorts): Sociological perspectives on the life course and reciprocities over time. In L. M. Cohen (Ed.), *Justice across generations: What does it mean?* (pp. 11–138). Washington, DC: AARP.

Bengtson, V. L., & Oyama, P. S. (2007). Intergenerational solidarity: Strengthening economic and social ties. In V. L. Bengtson & W. A. Achenbaum (Eds.), *The changing contract across generations* (pp. 3–23). New York: Aldine de Gruyter.

Bengtson, V. L., & Putney, N. M. (2006). Future conflicts across generations and cohorts? In J. A. Vincent, C. Phillipson, & M. Downs (Eds.), *The futures of old age*. London: Oxford University Press.

Bengtson, V. L., & Roberts, R. E. L. (1991). Intergenerational solidarity in aging families: An example of formal theory construction. *Journal of Marriage and the Family, 53*, 856–870.

Biggs, S. (1999). *The mature imagination*. Buckingham: Open University Press.

Biggs, S. (2006). Ageing selves and others: Distinctiveness and uniformity in the struggle for intergenerational solidarity. In J. A. Vincent, C. Phillipson, & M. Downs (Eds.), *The futures of old age* (p. 109–117). London: Oxford University Press.

Biggs, S. (2007) Thinking about generations: Conceptual positions and policy implications. *Journal of Social Issues 63*(4), 695–712.

Biggs, S., Phillipson, C., Money, A-M., & Leach, R. (2007). The mature imagination and consumption strategies: Age and generation in the development of baby boomer identity. *International Journal of Ageing & Later Life, 2*(2), 31–59.

Bourdieu, P. (1990). Youth is just a word. In *Sociology in question* (Chapter 12). London: Sage.

Bourdieu, P. (1993). *The field of cultural production: Essays on art and literature*. Cambridge, UK: Polity Press.

Bourdieu, P. (1996). On the family as a realized category. *Theory, Culture and Society, 13*(3), 19–26.

Cavalli, A. (2004). Generations and value orientations. *Social Compass, 51*(2), 155–168.

Collard, D. (2001). The generational bargain. *Intergenerational Journal of Social Welfare, 10*, 54–65.

Corsten, M. (1999). The time of generations. *Time and Society, 8*(2), 249–272.

Donati, P. (1999). Familia y generaciones. Desacatos. *Revista de Antropologia Social, 2*, 27–49.

Dunham, C. C., & Bengtson, V. L. (1986). Conceptual and theoretical perspectives on generational relations. In N. Datan, A. L. Greene, & H. W. Reese (Eds.), *Life span developmental psychology intergenerational relations* (pp. 2–27). Hillsdale, NJ: Lawrence Erlbaum Associates.

Edmunds, J., & Turner, B. S. (2002a). *Generations, culture and society.* Buckingham: Open University Press.

Edmunds, J., & Turner, B. S. (Eds.). (2002b). *Generational consciousness, narrative and politics.* Lanham: Rowman & Littlefield.

Edmunds, J., & Turner, B. S. (2005). Global generations: Social change in the twentieth century. *The British Journal of Sociology, 56*(4), 559–577.

Elder, G. H. Jr. (1985). Perspectives on the life course. In G. H. Elder (Ed.), *Life course dynamics: Trajectories and transitions, 1968–1980* (pp. 23–49). Ithaca, NY: Cornell University Press.

Elder, G. H. Jr. (1994). Time, human agency, and social change: Perspectives on the life course. *Social Psychology Quarterly, 57*(1), 4–15.

Eyerman, R., & Turner, B. S. (1998). Outline of a theory of generations. *European Journal of Social Theory, 1*(1), 91–106.

Faimberg, H. (2005). *The telescoping of generations: Listening to the narcissistic links between generations.* London: Routledge.

Finch, J. (1995). Responsibilities, obligations, and commitments. In I. Allen & E. Perkins (Eds.), *The future of family care for older people.* London: HMSO.

Gilleard, C. (2004). Cohorts and generations in the study of social change. *Social Theory and Health, 2*(1), 106–119.

Gilleard, C., & Higgs, P. (2002). The third age: Class cohort or generation? *Ageing & Society, 22*(3), 369–382.

Gilleard, C., & Higgs, P. (2005). *Contexts of ageing: Class cohort and community.* Cambridge, UK: Polity Press.

Hagestad, G. O. (1990). Social perspectives on the life course. In R. H. Binstock & L. K. George (Eds.), *Handbook of aging and the social sciences* (3rd ed., pp. 151–168). San Diego, CA: Academic Press.

Hagestad, G. (2003). Independent lives and relationships in changing times. In R. Stettersten (Ed.), *Invitation to the life course.* Amityville, NY: Baywood.

Hagestad, G. O., & Neugarten, B. L. (1985). Age and the life course. In R. H. Binstock & E. Shanas (Eds.), *Handbook of aging and the social sciences* (2nd ed., pp. 35–61). New York: Van Nostrand Reinhold.

Hareven, T. K. (1996). Introduction: Aging and generational relations over the life course. In *Aging and generational relations life-course and cross-cultural perspectives* (pp. ix–xxv). New York: Aldine de Gruyter.

Katz, R., Lowenstein, A., Phillips, J., & Daatland, S.-O. (2005) Solidarity, conflict and ambivalence in cross-national contexts. In V. L. Bengtson, A. C. Acock, K. R. Allen, P. Dilworth-Anderson, & D. M. Klein (Eds.), *Sourcebook of family theory and research.* Thousand Oaks, CA: Sage.

Koh, A. (2008). Disciplining Generation M: The paradox of creating a local national identity in an era of global flows. In N. Dolby & R. Fazal (Eds.), *Youth agency and globalization in India* (Chapter 11). New York: Routledge.

Lorenz-Meyer, D. (2001). *The politics of ambivalence.* New Working Paper Series 2, 1–24. Gender Institute. London: London School of Economics.

Lowenstein, A. (2003). Contemporary later-life family transitions: Revisiting theoretical perspectives on aging and the family—toward a family identity framework. In S. Biggs, A. Lowenstein, & J. Hendricks (Eds.), *The need for theory: Critical approaches to social gerontology* (pp. 105–126). Amityville, NY: Baywood Publishing.

Lowenstein, A. (2007). Solidarity-conflict and ambivalence: Testing two conceptual frameworks and their impact on quality of life for older family members. *Journal of Gerontology: Social Sciences, 62B,* S100–S107.

Lowenstein, A., Katz, R., & Gur-Yaish, N. (2007). Reciprocity in parent-child exchange and life satisfaction among the elderly: A cross-national perspective. *Journal of Social Issues 63*(4), 865–883.

Luescher, K., & Pillemer, K. (1998). Intergenerational ambivalence: A new approach to the study of parent-child relations in later life. *Journal of Marriage and the Family, 60,* 413–425.

Lukose, R. (2008). The children of liberalization. In N. Dolby & R. Fazal (Eds.), *Youth agency and globalization in India* (Chapter 8). New York: Routledge.

Mannheim, K. (1952). *Ideology and utopia: An introduction to the sociology of knowledge.* New York: Harcourt, Brace and Co.

Mannheim, K. (1997). The problem of generations. In *Collected works of Karl Mannheim.* London: Routledge.

Marshall, V. W. (2002). *Solidarity or ambivalence?* Paper presented to the annual general meeting of the Gerontological Society of America, Chicago.

McDaniel, S. (2008). The "growing legs" of generation as a policy construct: Reviving its family meaning. *Paper presented at Aging: Families and Households in Global Perspective.* Boston, MA.

Meyer, J. W. (1988). The life course as a cultural construction. In M. W. Riley (Ed.), *Social structures and human lives* (pp. 49–62). Newbury Park, CA: Sage.

Pilcher, J. (1994). Mannheim's sociology of generations: An undervalued legacy. *The British Journal of Sociology, 45*(3), 481–495.

Pillemer, K., Suitor, J., Mock, S., Sabir, M., Prado, T., & Sechrist, J. (2007). Capturing the complexity of intergenerational relations: Exploring ambivalence within later-life families. *Journal of Social Issues, 63*(4), 793–808.

Riley, M. W., Johnson, M., & Foner, A. (1972). *Aging and society* (Vol. 3): *A sociology of age stratification.* New York: Russell Sage.

Roos, J. P. (2002). The baby boomers, life's turning points and generational consciousness. *Paper prepared for the workshop on narrative, generational consciousness and politics, Faculty of Social and Political Sciences, University of Cambridge, Friday, June 30, 2000.*

Roos, J. P. (2005). *Life's turning points and generational consciousness.* Helsinki: University of Helsinki.

Rossi, A. S., & Rossi, P. H. (1990). *Of human bonding: Parent-child relations across the life course.* Hawthorne, NY: Aldine de Gruyter.

Sanchez, M., & Diaz, P. (2005). Cited in S. Newman & M. Sanchez (2007), *Intergenerational programmes: Concept, history and models.* In M. Sanchez et al., *Intergenerational programmes: Towards a society for all ages* (p. 37). Valencia: Obra Social.

Turner, B. S. (1998). Ageing and generational conflicts. *British Journal of Sociology,* *49*(2), 299–304.

Turner, B. S. (2002). The distaste of taste: Bourdieu, cultural capital and the Australian postwar elite. *Journal of Consumer Culture, 2*(2), *219–240.*

United Nations. (2002). *Madrid International Plan of Action on Ageing.* New York: United Nations.

Vincent, J. A. (2005). Understanding generations: Political economy and culture in an ageing society. *The British Journal of Sociology, 56*(4), 579–599.

CHAPTER EIGHT

Biography and Generation

Spirituality and Biographical Pain at the End of Life in Old Age

Malcolm Johnson

Families, generations, and relationships have been at the center of the study of aging as long as it has been as a recognized area of scientific study. Social scientists from a variety of disciplines have long been preoccupied with the connectedness of human beings from the primary social units called families through to those called communities and those called nation-states. They are the essential components of societies. Much of the attention was given to cross-sectional accounts that provided snapshots of life and relationships at a given point in time. There is value in such pictures, but that value is multiplied when the images are repeated over time, providing an understanding of the way social, economic, cultural, and personal factors interact over time. Such an approach is particularly apt if the object is to understand the processes of aging, which commence at birth and continue throughout the span of life. It is in the dynamics of living that human lives are shaped.

The search for understanding of the formative influences on identity and kinship; the modes of adaptation to economic and political changes; and the consequences of fresh conceptions of gender, race, and nationality have an established place in social gerontology. Driven largely by public policy concerns, the research has often been problem-focused, influenced by the need of governments to address pressing issues of the day. Retirement policies, the costs of pensions, illnesses in later life, inequalities between the genders, the quality of services to older people, and dementia are all perennial topics. The now well-known phrase describing this research is "data rich and theory poor" (Bengtson, Putney, & Johnson, 2005).

Despite its focus on the end of life, this chapter is firmly grounded in the life-span approach and the longitudinal studies of generations (see Alwin, Chapter 6) and intergenerational relations that Vern Bengtson has carried out over the past four decades. It considers the concept of biographical pain and the distinctive spiritualities of people living in the fourth age. This chapter's intellectual links to Bengtson's work are to be found in its parallel lines of development and common commitment to articulating theories of the life span that address the dynamics of human biographies. But here, as in other writings (Johnson, 2009), I am anxious to ensure that these theoretical discourses recognize that complex lives have endings and that death is treated as an integral feature of the life span, not simply a period at the end of the sentence. Biographies reach their conclusion as finitude translates into death, and in that last period of life, autobiographical reflection, dominated by intergenerational relations, is at its most intense.

Biography, Generations, and the New Demography of Death

The early years of the twenty-first century play host not only to the demographically oldest societies in human history but also to an unprecedented conjunction of old age and death. In Western Europe today, 80% of all deaths are of people over 65 years old and predominantly of men and women who are much older. The democratization of very old age has seen the average age of death move rapidly along the life path, extending the standard working-class period of lived retirement from around 3 years to 13. Among the expanding battalions of survivors in their tenth decade, men lose out to the extent that there are six women for every man. As a consequence, when we look for the oldest old in those places where one in three will find themselves—nursing homes or assisted living facilities—the average age is 90. Centenarians, so rare in the recent past, are almost commonplace. Residents of such establishments are overwhelmingly female.

Death has moved away from the newly born, mothers in childbirth, children with infectious illnesses, men involved in hazardous work, and adults with life-threatening illnesses into the province of old age. It has also become a correlate of late-life widowhood. This might be the major loss, but entry into these total-care facilities also means a marked deterioration of physical health, probably resulting in loss of mobility. Other correlates include loss of visual acuity, decline in hearing, and, for around half of the resident population, troubling memory loss or dementia. While many find that the supportive environment revives them and sponsors new friendships, others find their health profile and loss of independence deeply depressing. Although the topic is rarely mentioned, these individuals, with their long experience of adulthood, are well aware that this is "the last lap."

From a gerontological perspective, the changing character of death in old age accounts for the social geography of the general population's reactions to death. Public reactions to the premature death of a child, especially if the circumstances are mysterious or horrifying, are now inflated festivals of emotion and street symbolism. The public outpouring of emotion for strangers that is unleashed by the death of John Kennedy, Martin Luther King Jr., Diana, Princess of Wales, or even an appealing child brutally murdered has created new levels of ritual expression. Similar collective "grief" may also occur if a younger adult dies. Yet the assumed script for anyone over seventy is summed up by the phrases "she had a good run," "he is in a better place," "it must be a relief," and "that time comes for us all." These acceptable platitudes rarely carry the sense of loss that surviving relatives might be experiencing or the psychologically and financially gloomy future that many who are widowed will face.

Sociologically, we are observing a cultural lag as the mores of the times slowly develop an appreciation of the real and experienced deprivation that many endure but which is yet to become part of the body of knowledge. There are other factors in the current equation. Widowhood often impoverishes women who have outlived their resources. Yet their deaths will relieve family "carers" in their sixties of their responsibilities and release the assets tied up in a small house. For a very long time in public presentations on this topic I have used the phrase: "Where there's a will—there are families."

Here in the interstices of generational relationships, both macro and micro, there are unspoken fragments of social fabric which currently favor the middle-aged. Those in the last stages of their old age are seen as beneficiaries of the demographic revolution. Indeed, many are mindful of the life bonus they have unexpectedly gained and take pleasure in great-grandchildren, subsidized travel, the support of churches, and the experience of life at a slow pace. Others live in constant pain and have multiple pathologies that are treated by regular handfuls of polypharmacy. They experience the indignity of dependency, the uncertainties of memory loss and dementia, and the anxiety of life without a future.

This new group represents a succession of cohorts. Their lives began in the poverty and terror of the First World War, and their early adulthood was lived through the Great Depression and the Second World War. Most left school at 14 and experienced physical hardship in both their work and home lives. Born between 1900 and 1935, this group's members are markedly distinct from the baby boomers (born between1946 and 1964), whose lives have been characterized as economically and socially privileged (Achenbaum, 2005). Moreover, the differences in their life chances, their relative poverty of opportunity and money, and the nature of the society they lived in have, I assert, left them with considerably different spiritual concerns and moral frameworks.

Reflecting on the 25 years since the publication of his landmark text *Children of the Great Depression* (which provided a key foundation for life-span theories and longitudinal studies of aging), Glen Elder (1999) writes of the resilience of this cohort and the remarkable ways in which many turned their lives around. He draws attention to Michael Rutter's observation that "The quality of resilience resides in how people deal with life changes and what they do about their situations" (Rutter, 1985, p. 608). In reflecting on the findings of his Berkeley research contemporary Jean Macfarlane (1971), Elder gives approving support to her view that the most outstandingly mature adults from their study were those who confronted and overcame the great deprivations of their childhoods. Such interpretations were acknowledged as not being scientific observations, but she goes on to claim that "no one becomes mature without living through the pains and confusions of maturing experiences" (Macfarlane, 1971, p. 341).

As a non-American, I may be forgiven for seeing in these deductions a distinct structural optimism that reflects the powerful mythology of the American dream. This is not to cast doubt on the validity of views that overcoming adversity is maturational and character-building. But for the many who grew in emotional strength and prosperity, there is an equal number (there are no data to allow a less global approach to estimation) who were scarred for life by the ravages of their Depression childhoods and whose life chances were permanently inhibited by the loss of learning and the tarnished relationships that grew out of serious poverty. Arthur Miller's (1949) depiction of Willy Loman in *Death of a Salesman,* as the embodiment of the emptiness of the American dream, is just as authentic a presentation of the opportunity structure and so too is the context of failed aspiration, failing marriage, depression, and the loss of his success as a salesman, leading to attempts at suicide.

As life-span theorists have long known, history creates cohorts of individuals swept up within tides of events they can only respond to (Dannefer & Uhlenberg, 1999). Such societal (and now global) forces create cultural identities, which in retrospect become easily observable. Once the construct is voiced, these cohorts receive labels and typologies. In recent decades we have, for example, the baby boomers and generation X as clear demarcations. See Chapter 1 of Bengtson, Biblarz, and Roberts (2002) for explications. But just as diverse individuals live out their existence in these manufactured social vehicles, so too do they end their lives imbued with the beliefs, practices, rituals, and conventions of their lived experience.

Life-Span Theory Grounded in Longitudinal Research

What we have learned from Elder and his intellectual inheritors is that "social change has differential consequences for persons of unlike age, which suggests that age variations are related to variations in the meaning of a situation, in adaptive potential options, and thus linkages between the event and the lifecourse" (Elder, 1999, p. 8). Vern Bengtson was already engaged in his own analysis of the relationships between biography and generation before Elder's book was published. Indeed, the intellectual preoccupations this volume so rightly celebrates were clearly visible in his first book, *A Social Psychology of Aging* (1973), when the now legendary Longitudinal Study of Generations (LSOG) was already established and had carried out its first wave of data collection

Looking back on the core principles which underlay the LSOG studies, Bengtson (Bengtson, Biblarz, & Roberts, 2002) draws attention to three assumptions. "First is the assumption that human development is a *relational process*, profoundly shaping and shaped by our social connections to others. . . . The second . . . is that the microenvironmental context of individual development is linked to higher levels of social organization, a concept often referred to as *nested contexts*. . . . The third assumption guiding our analysis is that intergenerational transmission processes and outcomes unfold at the intersection of events occurring on two distinct timelines, *social history* and *individual biography*. From this perspective, individual development represents a biographical sequencing of critical periods that intersect with various macrolevel socioeconomic and cultural conditions existing in a particular historical epoch" (Bengtson, Biblarz, & Roberts, 2002, pp. 20–21).

More recently, Bengtson, Elder, and Putney (2005) wrote a joint chapter on the life-course perspective, in which they distilled the fusion of their separate but linked researches in this manner: The life course is conceptualized as a sequence of age-linked transitions that are embedded in social institutions and history. As a theoretical orientation, the life-course perspective sensitizes researchers to the fundamental importance of historical conditions and change for understanding individual development and family life. This complex of factors that bears upon cohorts and individual biographies as individuals progress along the life path sets expectations of "a good life" in the spiritual as well as the secular sense. Value frameworks emerge out of poverty and unemployment just as much as from prosperity and consumer boom.

Biography as the Key Source of Spirituality

As human beings we are the accumulation of our life experience. What we have lived, observed, thought, felt, and done are the essence of our personhood. Our journey along the life path is unique, even if it has been shared with others who have lived in the same places, lived in the same houses, been to the same schools, experienced the same world and local events, gone through the stages from childhood to the present, loved some people and disliked and been hurt by others, been sometimes lucky and also suffered hurtful losses. The distinctive nature of our journey is our personal biography. The story of our lives is a detailed narrative that we have constructed from millions of recollections to form an account of who we are. As we have gone through life we have been mentally writing this story, adding to it new features and editing others out.

Curiously, we very rarely get the opportunity to tell the whole life story. Many individuals will have heard fragments, episodes, and stories of special note. Some family members and close friends may have heard these noteworthy tales more times than they would have liked. But unless we have been in extended therapy, it is likely that even our closest kin have never heard the whole. There are two sides to this: lack of opportunity and an inbuilt restraint that makes us reluctant to expose the totality of ourselves to another person. We will come to the reluctance later. As for the opportunities, in a world of busyness and schedules, there are few people with whom we would feel comfortable enough to relate our story to, who would have the several hours it would take even to make a good start.

Being listened to, without constant interruption, by a nonjudgmental listener is a rare and special opportunity. Having your life recollections heard with engaged interest and your interpretations of what they mean to you taken seriously is a particular privilege. As a researcher, I have on innumerable occasions listened to an older person's life story, mindful of the trust invested in me and surprised at the extent of intimate revelation. Often, accounts of extramarital relations or of babies aborted or given up for adoption while husbands fought in a war, or revelations by women of sexual and physical abuse and dishonest practices, are told for the first time to what I describe to students as "a safe, interested stranger." All too often it becomes apparent that these are stories of deep guilt, protected over decades and made wholly unavailable to even the closest kin.

The converse of the rationing of significant biographical information is the frequent unwillingness of children to listen to the wishes of their elderly parents. "I want to talk to you about my funeral." "No, you don't want to talk that way. You will live for years yet." Children are frequently unable or unwilling to talk with their parents about issues of mortality and spiritual concern. So where do older people at the far end of life turn for a listener? Not for the first time, the insight of Maya Angelou (2008) captures the dilemma:

"Growing Older by Design"

When you see me
Sitting quietly like a sack
Left on a shelf
Don't think I need
Your chattering
I'm listening to myself.

This stanza written by the then-80-year-old writer and poet neatly reframes the aloneness of the older person. It highlights the continuing and ever-interesting inner reflection that all human beings have as a gift. Life review, reminiscence, or simply recalling a fragment of the past prompted by a random cue is the daily universal experience. But the nature of the experience is undoubtedly related to age. The older you are, the more you have to remember. The older you are, the closer you are to the end of your life, and the fewer opportunities you have to fulfill your dreams and deal with the failings, fissures, and hurts of the past. At the same time, those who live long are more alone. Aloneness in itself is not necessarily undesirable. But it does present unaccustomed unoccupied space for biographical reflection. This will provide pleasurable recall of the good times in every life. Maya Angelou's "Don't think I need your chattering; I'm listening to myself" seems to imply a satisfying inner life. It may also be the sponsor of depression (endemic among the very old, for clearly observable reasons), distress, and profound pain.

Remembering in Pain

Everyday experience of living or working with older people, particularly those who have lost their independence, reveals that the ones who maintain a positive hold on life are far outnumbered by the depressed and the disappointed. For a subset of this unhappy group, the sequence of losses they have experienced leads to a state of anguish that steals from them many if not all of the former pleasures of living.

In my own work I have interviewed many older people who have come under this unlifting shadow. These experiences have occurred throughout my professional life, but have recently reappeared through interviews with older people with severe visual impairment. Here the most prominent finding was of almost unrelieved isolation combined with a grieving for the losses that come with blindness and infirmity. For this group, which numbers almost 1 million across the United Kingdom (1 in 10 of the retired population), there is a disturbing paucity of services.

Inevitably, many of the most frail and dejected are to be found in residential (assisted living) and nursing homes. Entering reluctantly and distressed by the deprivation of their life's acquisitions and freedoms, such people are deeply unhappy despite the best possible care. Entry to a care home requires the individual to leave leaving the independent dwelling the regarded as home and transferring to a form of collective living, where much of each day is spent with unchosen strangers, both fellow residents and staff. Accompanying the multiple losses of personal space, familiar locality, personal domain, and personal and family history is the stark recognition that they have entered the "last lap" of life.

Religion and the support of faith communities can ease the path, especially for the current cohorts of elders, for whom religious values, beliefs, and practices were instilled early and transmitted across generations. Research conducted by Coleman and his colleagues (Coleman, 2004; Coleman, McKeirnan, Mills, & Speck, 2007) at Southampton on the spiritual beliefs of older people showed that those who had strong religious convictions were less likely to be depressed and more likely to be at ease with their personal past and the prospect of death. Moderate believers and those with little or no religious faith revealed lower estimates of personal worth and a proneness to depression. These results, added to the research-based estimates of declining levels of belief in later life, indicate two broad observations. Firstly, religious belief and spiritual capability are positive attributes in dealing with the decrements of old age. Secondly, there are indications of low levels of spirituality in old age even though today's old people have had much greater exposure to religious and spiritual experiences than have younger people.

In seeking a solid platform for a proposition to capture the all-too-common anguish found in life histories, I have turned again to the analysis of personal biographies. The distilled, refined, and polished but often flawed and jagged story we fabricate from the recollections of life lived, has been one of the tools I have used in attempting to explain the processes of ageing for over 30 years. (It was in 1976 that my paper "That Was Your Life: A Biographical Approach to Later Life" was first published). Through this work I have discovered, as did Kierkegaard, that life can best be understood backward, though it must be lived forward.

Biographical perspectives help to explain the new estimates of low late-life epidemiology of spirituality, even in contemporary societies which host obsessions with "discovering one's inner self," searching for holism in nature, alternative medicine, "talking therapies," and evangelical sects—let alone the largely spurious search for revelation through drugs.

Biographical Pain

The starting point for me was the claim of leading figures in the hospice movement, now received wisdom, that palliative medicine could deal with all kinds of physical pain, but there was also a neglected dimension of spiritual pain. This concept grew from the motivations and convictions of the pioneers of the modern hospice movement, notably Cicely Saunders. The hospice idea predates St. Christopher's Hospice by many centuries, but Dame Cicely's creation of that establishment marks the acknowledged commencement of the modern hospice movement and the serious beginnings of palliative medicine (du Boulay, 1984).

Soon spiritual pain became a portmanteau term to deal with pain which was not physical or demonstrably psychiatric. Because many people have little or no spiritual vocabulary, let alone experience of practice, I thought there was need for another category and another descriptor. Aware that the pain I have observed appears to grow in intensity as individuals get closer to death—either because of terminal illness or advanced old age—I created the term "biographical pain," which is defined as, "the irremediable anguish which results from profoundly painful recollection of experienced wrongs which can now never be righted. When finitude or impairment terminates the possibility of cherished self-promises to redress deeply regretted actions."

The presence of serious biographical pain is characterized by the surfacing of deeply buried fractures in the life biographies of individuals who always intended to "put things right" but have now run out of capability to bring about that resolution. They will no longer be able to apologize, seek or give forgiveness, deliver restitution, or deliver a good to balance out the bad for an evil act. The opportunity to redress wrongs has passed by, and the individual is left with an overwhelming sense of guilt.

It is the very slowness of late life which provides the opportunity for such life reviews to surface. During the busyness of independent living, we're able to submerge our worst worries and fears deep into our inner selves. Sometimes the repository becomes covered over; then the resurfacing of wiped-out recollections (of giving away a child born out of wedlock, cheating a relative or friend out of their business, or experiencing the breakup of a trusting relationship) is all the more painful .

Biographical pain is something we all experience in some degree. Sometimes we can "re-frame" the events and see them in a better light, or provide a personal accounting which balances them out. Those who have religious faith may seek forgiveness through a priest, by prayer, or via redemptive good works. But for the many who are spiritually unlearned, there are fewer options available.

Old people need spiritual care that embraces biographical pain without claiming it as a religious entity. We need to create new social rituals for this "putting right." When the churches and Christian communities in pre-industrial times provided asylum to those in desperate need, they offered more than food and shelter. Their Christian task was to help mend the broken spirit, through love and service and prayer. In our day this task is still needed, and the best old people's homes provide something that approximates it.

Secular society in Western Europe will not welcome a wholly religious formulation for addressing the spiritual needs and the biographical anguish of people coming to the close of their lives. But as we rethink the care of those who must live in grouped settings, ways of supporting residents with biographical disturbances (for which there are no drugs or potions) should be high on the agenda.

Fourth Age Spirituality

There has been extensive academic discourse about the meanings of the term "spirituality,"[1] seventeenth-century word that only gained currency in the nineteenth century and grew in usage in the twentieth. Broadly, we can identify two realms of meaning which seem to address the experience of fourth-agers, that is, those in the final stage of life, characterized by old age and dependency. (1) An individual's relationship with her God and how she stands in relationship to the mores, values, and practices of her religious denomination. (2) An individual's constant reappraisal of himself in relation to the values, standards, and practices which emanate from personal beliefs and convictions.

Definitions of spirituality conventionally begin with the spiritualities set within world religions, where the relationship with God and immersion in prayer generates a sense of otherness, which may become transcendent, and a deepening of selfhood. The religious spiritual life may include adherence to specified practices often repeated (such as the Protestant celebration of holy communion, the Islamic daily prayer schedule, or regular attendance at Mass and confession), where the rituals provide a devotional schedule of engagement with God, priest, and the community of the faithful.

Nonreligious models of spirituality are less easy to specify because there are so many and their form and purposes are extremely diverse. A recognized starting point is the work of Viktor Frankl, an Austrian psychiatrist who created the definition "the search for meaning." Frankl himself termed this as an existential rather than a spiritual search Nonetheless, many new and refurbished secular spiritualities are ready to shelter under this canopy definition, even if their practices, rituals, and orthodoxies are distinct.

Leading proponents of the search-for-meaning approach are to be found in the health professions, particularly nurses. In their paper on the links between spirituality and successful aging, Sadler and Biggs (2006), drawing on reviews of the nursing literature, report a series of elements in the nursing spiritual repertoire, which include transcendent belief in a higher power, experiencing a sense of connection, and drawing on inner resources, such as strength and peace. Other features, such as "meaning making" and "manifest expressions," are to be found in the literature. Rumbold (2000), writing from within the context of palliative care, provides some clarification by treating spirituality as a worldview, a way of looking at the meaning and purpose of life.

The debates about meaning will continue. If researchers and practitioners are trying to reveal, assess, measure, and interpret what we call the spiritual; further distillation will be required. Yet without this desired exactness there is more than sufficient evidence that human beings desire to understand themselves, the world they live in, and the forces which guide it. Their understandings provide them with a moral compass, an external source of reference, and a way of measuring themselves against higher standards than those of the society. This is clearly evident in the world religions and often in the revered writings which accompany other belief systems.

In an attempt to combine conceptualizing, empirical evidence, and practical application, Tornstam (2005) has developed a theory of *gerotranscendence*, which provides an explanatory framework for positive aging. His purposes have been to shift gerontological thinking from the despairing old age of Erikson (1982) and Cumming and Henry (1961) into a paradigm that sponsors old age as a period worth achieving because of its own true benefits. He questions the underlying assumptions of the concept of successful aging, "with the typical emphasis on activity, productivity, independence, efficiency, wealth, health and sociability" (Tornstam, 2005, p. 3). Having observed the normative expectation that good aging is the continuation of the midlife patterns indefinitely, Tornstam asserts that there is continuous development into old age. His theory of the gerotranscendent individual depicts him or her as someone who experiences a redefinition of the self and of relationships to others and a new understanding of fundamental, existential questions.

In this stage of transcendence (a term selected from the core lexicon of spirituality) the individual becomes less self-occupied and more selective about social activities, has a greater affinity with past generations, takes less interest in superfluous social interaction, exhibits a decreasing interest in material things, and develops a need for solitary meditation. After a thorough critique of the negative ascriptions made to old age by society and gerontologists alike and the false optimism of the "successful aging" movement, Tornstam takes his readers into a set of complex empirical analyses, which indicate the characteristics of gerotranscendence.

In addition to the substantive body of research it employs and the theoretical rigor of its argument, Tornstam's work marks a transition point in the gerontological discourse. He engages with both the theory and the knowledge base in order to reformulate received notions of aging. This radical redefinition places spiritual transformation in the central arena of late life. By challenging the functionalist assumptions not only of the early formulations but also of the life-course theorists, he marks out serious challenge to the existing paradigm and notions of the life span which has no end.

In the world of care for these very same individuals at the far end of life is another kind of discourse, which has its own powerful orthodoxies, incorporating entrenched presumptions about who should be the societal managers of dying, death, and bereavement. Palliative care and its sponsor, the hospice movement, has articulated its own rules about the appropriate ways to die and how pain should be palliated through a religio-medical model. Here concepts of spirituality and finitude are formulated in very specific ways and in line with the life-span theorists and the "successful aging" proponents; the focus is on "living to the end" while avoiding the distasteful reality of death and its aftermath.

Conclusions

For those cohorts born in the first three and a half decades of the twentieth century, the Christian religion was the dominant experience, both in terms of private and family practice and in terms of socially prescribed values.

What Carette and King in their book *Selling Spirituality: The Silent Takeover of Religion* (2005) call the corporate rebranding of spirituality (which has directly affected boomers) has left fourth-agers untouched. Their biographies are rooted in an earlier age, a different culture. Any attempt to understand and address their biographical pain must start from an understanding of a world we have largely lost—but which lives in them until the day they die.

NOTE

1. Some of this section draws from Johnson (2009).

REFERENCES

Achenbaum, A. (2005). *Older Americans, vital communities: A bold vision for societal aging.* Baltimore, MD: Johns Hopkins University Press.
Angelou, M. (2008). *Growing older by design.* Washington, DC : AARP. Available on AARP.org (posted September 22, 2008).
Bengtson, V. L. (1973). *The social psychology of aging.* Indianapolis, IN: Bobbs-Merrill.
Bengtson, V. L., Biblarz, T. J., & Roberts, R. E. L. (2002). *How families still matter: A longitudinal study of youth in two generations.* New York: Cambridge University Press.

Bengtson, V. L., Elder, G. H. Jr., & Putney, N. M. (2005). The lifecourse perspective on aging. In M. L. Johnson, V. L. Bengtson, P. G. Coleman, & T. B. L. Kirkwood (Eds.), *The Cambridge handbook of age and ageing* (pp. 493–501). Cambridge, UK: Cambridge University Press.

Bengtson, V. L., Putney, N. M., & Johnson, M. L. (2005). Are theories of aging necessary? In M. L. Johnson, V. L. Bengtson, P. G. Coleman, & T. Kirkwood (Eds.), *The Cambridge handbook of age and aging* (pp. 2–20). Cambridge, UK: Cambridge University Press.

Carrette, J., & King, R. (2005) *Selling spirituality: The silent takeover of religion.* London: Routledge.

Coleman, P. G. (2004). Is religion the friend of ageing? *Generations Review, 14*(4), 4–8.

Coleman, P. G., McKiernan, F., Mills, M., & Speck, P. (2007). In sure and uncertain faith: Belief and coping with loss of spouse in later life. *Ageing and Society 27*(6), 869–889.

Cumming, E., & Henry, W. (1961). *Growing old: The process of disengagement.* New York: Basic.

Dannefer, D., & Ullenberg, P. (1999). Paths of the lifecourse: A typology. In V. L. Bengtson & W. K. Schaie (Eds.), *Handbook of theories of aging* (pp 306–326). New York: Springer.

du Boulay, S. (1984). *Cicely Saunders: The founder of the modern hospice movement.* London: Hodder & Stoughton.

Elder, G. H. (1999) *Children of the Great Depression: Social change in life experience* (25th anniversary ed.). Boulder, CO: Westview Press.

Erikson, E. H. (1982). *The life cycle completed: A review.* New York: Norton.

Johnson, M. L. (1976). That was your life: A biographical approach to later life. In M. A. Munnichs & W. van den Heuvel (Eds.), *Dependency or interdependency in old age* (pp. 147–173). The Hague: Martinus Nijhoff.

Johnson, M. L. (2009). Spirituality, finitude and theories of the lifespan. In V. L. Bengtson, D. Gans, N. M. Putney, & M. Silverstein (Eds.), *Handbook of theories of aging* (2nd ed., pp. 659–674). New York: Springer.

Macfarlane, J. (1971). Perspectives on personality, consistency and change, from The Guidance Study. In M. C. Jones, N. Bayley, J. W. Macfarlane, & M. P. Honzik (Eds.), *The course of human development : Selected papers from the longitudinal studies, Institute of Human Development, The University of California, Berkeley* (pp. 410–415). Waltham, MA: Xerox College Publishing.

Miller, A. (1949). *Death of a salesman.*

Rumbold, B. (Ed.) (2000). *Spirituality and palliative care.* Melbourne: Oxford University Press.

Rutter, M. (1985). Resilience in the face of adversity: Protective factors and resistance to psychological disorder. *British Journal of Psychiatry, 147,* 598–611.

Sadler, E., & Biggs, S. (2006). Exploring the links between spirituality and "successful ageing." *Journal of Social Work Practice, 20*(3), 267–280.

Tornstam, L. (2005) *Gerotranscendence: A developmental theory of positive aging.* New York: Springer.

PART IV / Religion and Families

Contexts of Continuity, Change, and Conflict

Engaging the family solidarity paradigm, the authors in this section examine the role of religion in family and institutional settings and the intergenerational and social network processes embedded within these contexts. The two empirical studies in this section also reveal how religion often serves as the framework for understanding a family's or an individual's unique racial or ethnic identity and social connections.

Achenbaum takes a historical-institutional perspective with respect to the domains of religion, spirituality, and aging. He begins by considering the role that theory-building has played in Bengtson's treatment of religion, spirituality, and aging, especially as it relates to continuity and change in multigenerational families. Observing that baby boomers as religious consumers are more fluid in their spiritual choices than were their parents, the author concludes that not only do religious organizations have shallower institutional roots than in the past, they have not kept pace with the spiritual needs of a religiously pluralistic cohort of older adults.

Using both survey and interview data from the Longitudinal Study of Generations, Putney et al. explore the interconnections of ethnic and cultural heritage, religious identity or affiliation, and the transmission of a family's religious tradition across generations in eight racial and ethnic minority multi-generational families. They show that the quality of parent-child relations serves as the crucial mechanism for passing on a religious tradition to the next generation. In those families where there were clear patterns of religious continuity across generations, family members consciously linked their religious beliefs, family values, and racial and ethnic heritage. Ethnicity matters in their religious life because it is about their family.

Lincoln, Chatters, and Taylor bring the study of solidarity, conflict, and ambivalence into the realm of organizational culture by examining church congregations as a quasi-family form. They consider how involvement in both families and churches is important for receiving social support but can also be associated with negative social interactions. The authors show that because African Americans are historically well integrated within their religious institutions, they are often better able to tolerate negative interactions in church-based relations compared to Non-Hispanic White older adults. Demographic and church involvement characteristics affect the likelihood of experiencing negative interactions among religious congregants.

CHAPTER NINE

How Theory-Building Prompts Explanations about Generational Connections in the Domains of Religion, Spirituality, and Aging

W. Andrew Achenbaum

Few gerontologists have pursued theory-building with as much enthusiasm and insight as Vern Bengtson. Several generations of colleagues and students share his appreciation of the importance of taking theory-building seriously in advancing science. Researchers in aging understand the value of theories in identifying interesting questions and in setting boundaries. They recognize that a rigorous commitment to using the right lens to "see" the intellectual and methodological challenges at hand in a given project can enhance their investigations.

Theory-building has animated Bengtson's way of problem-solving as he has pursued multidisciplinary research in aging. The payoffs professionally for USC's AARP/University Professor of Gerontology Emeritus have been considerable. Vern Bengtson has won virtually every major prize in his field and served in most of the important elected offices in the American Sociological Association and the Gerontological Society of America, among other august professional groups.

Before I turn to the main thrust of this paper, I want to describe the ways that theory-building (broadly understood) has fired Vern Bengtson's gerontological imagination as it set boundaries for what he wanted to explore and explain empirically. I should admit at the outset that I will be illustrating my argument by focusing on what, frankly, has been a rather minor subject in Vern Bengtson's work. He did not write much about religion and spirituality in aging until late in his career, when he had refined his multidisciplinary approach to gerontological research.

I choose "religion and spirituality" because it is a domain where our interests intersect. It is a domain where theory-building is critical in order to conjoin hermeneutics with science. How does defining and solving problems in a multidisciplinary manner affect how gerontologists conceptualize and present their findings? Why might this approach afford advantages to researchers on aging who otherwise rely exclusively on discipline-based theories?

Commentaries on Theory-Building in the Writings of Vern Bengtson

Bengtson, Cara Rice, and Malcolm Johnson wrote (1999, p. 5) that theory is "the construction of explicit explanations in accounting for empirical findings." Because "theory" is a murky word, the trio distinguished theory from other facets of knowledge building. "Facts" and "empirical generalizations" clearly are part of the research enterprise, but the investigatory process entails more than the generation of measurable data interpreted statistically. "Models" resemble theories, but they do not provide explanations, the key word in the trio's definition of theory, "the *why* behind the *what* that is observed" (p. 6). Nor do all theories precipitate "paradigm shifts." Still, as Thomas Kuhn declaimed in *The Structure of Scientific Revolutions* (1962), the accumulation of anomalous theories for explaining natural phenomena sometimes forces the scientific community to question the accuracy of prevailing ways of seeing, causing them collectively to embrace (a) different (set of) theories and methods.

Theories, in Bengtson's view, serve several purposes. They help investigators to describe, integrate, and explain data. Good theories serve as filters, identifying those "facts" that are germane to the problem at hand and those (however intriguing) that should be excluded. Theories have predictive value. Finally, theories in basic sciences often have real-world applications (Bengtson, 1989; Bengtson & Schaie, 1999, p. 7; Hendricks & Achenbaum, 1999, p. 33).

Bengtson concedes that the quest for "grand theory" in aging has disenchanted gerontologists as well as researchers in other domains. As a graduate student he was privy to the internal politics at the University of Chicago's Committee on Human Development and professional reaction to the rise and fall of "disengagement theory" (Achenbaum & Bengtson, 1994). And Bengtson realizes that the demands and time pressures placed upon policy analysts and social practitioners to generate practical remedies to assist older people can be so great as to make theory-building seem to be a luxury. Nonetheless, he has consistently maintained that "applications in gerontology—whether in medicine, practice, or policy—demand good theory, since it is on the basis of *explanations* about problems that interventions should be made; if not, they seem doomed to failure. Without theory, the contributions of individual studies in aging are likely to have little impact" (Bengtson, Rice, & Johnson, 1999, p. 16).

Vern Bengtson throughout his career has championed the critical importance of theory-building in mapping the discourses and practices of scientific enterprises. He has been especially keen to advocate multidisciplinary theories in gerontology. Working with Bernice Neugarten, a polymath, at the University of Chicago in the mid-1960s instilled in Bengtson the value of integrating theories from several social sciences, notably sociology and psychology, to sharpen his own field of vision. The Committee on Human Development rightly prided itself as being one of those rare and rarefied centers of intellectual risk-taking. Its vitality owed much to the idiosyncrasies and brilliance of its instructors and students. Significantly, members of the committee individually and collectively realized that they were building on a tradition of cross-fertilizing ideas about aging in all its facets—biological, medical, behavioral, social, and applied.

Such a multidisciplinary approach had been launched by gifted scientists from more than a dozen disciplines, whose collective endeavors were published in E. V. Cowdry's handbook, *The Problems of Ageing* (1939). The handbook set high standards for gerontology as it emerged as a scientific field of inquiry (Achenbaum, 1995). As Lawrence Frank, a social scientist and program officer at the Josiah Macy Jr. Foundation who funded Cowdry's project and invested in gerontological research at Chicago, put it, "The problem is multidimensional and will require for its solution not only a multidisciplinary approach but also a synoptic correlation of diverse findings and viewpoints" (1942, p. viii).

Despite Frank's rhetoric and Macy's money, multidisciplinary theory-building proved easier to extol than to execute. Mechanisms of aging differ greatly at the cellular, molecular, organic, and environmental levels. Basic biological research often serves as the foundation for medical education, but it rarely informs how physicians and nurses care for their patients. University-based disciplines act like academic tribes (Becher, 2001). Rampant are intramural disagreements over the suitability of problems to be studied, the theories (if any) to be deployed, and the suitability of methods. While some eminent scholars emphasize "consilience" (Wilson, 1998) in the quest for knowledge, theirs is a minority position. Departments prefer to defend turfs, administratively and intellectually. Freestanding centers, which cannot typically grant tenure, rise and fall on the size of grants that they win. No wonder few rising scholars are inclined to take the risk of crossing academic boundaries in theory-building. Most senior scholars have too much invested in disciplinary mores that have guided how they go about their business to make radical changes. It is difficult enough to keep pace with developments within any single lively discipline, much less to gain expertise simultaneously in another field.

Vern Bengtson has been a risk taker, albeit a cautious one, in pursuing multidisciplinary approaches to doing gerontology. In his opinion, "major theoretical perspectives in social gerontology [emerged] according to the theoretical traditions in sociology" (Passuth & Bengtson, 1988, pp. 334–335). Vern was respectful of the intellectual traditions and the accomplishments of past masters of his tribe. Yet Bengtson felt that too much dependence on disciplinary-specific models would deter multidisciplinary theory-building in the aging enterprise. Thus he limited his focus to social gerontology. In so doing, Bengtson conceded that integrating biological approaches with behavioral and psychological orientations was too daunting a task. Bengtson nonetheless still had ample room to maneuver. Within the realm of social psychology, after all, there were incompatible camps. Some gerontologists had to overcome the dominance of structural functionalism. Others had to move beyond activity/disengagement theories about older people's life satisfaction (Passuth & Bengtson, 1988, p. 346).

With support from the National Institute of Mental Health and a private foundation, Bengtson launched what he figured would be a one-time survey of the "generation gap." The original 1970–1971 survey included 349 three-generation, White, working- and middle-class families (roughly 2,000 individuals) and was designed to investigate reciprocal linkages between individual development and intergenerational family relationships. The National Institute on Aging enabled the project to become a longitudinal survey in 1985; the renamed Longitudinal Study of Generations (LSOG) was subsequently expanded in 1988, 1991, 1994, 1997, 2001, 2003, and 2006. With the passage of time, assessments were broadened to enrich the original survey instrument. They recorded subjects' attitudes and values, mental and physical health, attainments at school and work, and relationships with kin. (Despite divorces and deaths over time, the sample pool now extends to four generations.) Bengtson and his team of researchers gathered macrolevel data along with microlevel assessments. They addressed and expanded the questions that informed the original project proposal (Bengtson, Biblarz, & Roberts, 2002, pp. 12, 169; USC, 2007).

Bengtson has had countless opportunities to showcase and defend his sample (and more critically, its intellectual underpinnings) in classrooms, professional gatherings, and grant proposals. In my opinion, Bengtson's most insightful presentation was delivered in his Burgess Award Lecture. (*Caveat lector:* The precise words Bengtson used in this address to describe theory-building differ sometimes from ones he deployed elsewhere, but they are consistent.) He began by paying special tribute to Ernest W. Burgess, who briefly served as one of his teachers, and to Matilda White Riley, surely one of his most important mentors (Bengtson & Achenbaum, 1993, pp. 261–264).

Vern Bengtson then elaborated "the theoretical construct of *intergenerational solidarity* as a means to characterize the behavioral and emotional dimensions of interaction, cohesion, sentiment, and support between parents and children, grandparents and grandchildren, over the course of long-term relationships" (Bengtson, 2001, p. 8). Consistent with earlier writings, he drew a distinction between macrostructural and microsocial continuities and changes in "the development and aging of each of the three and now four generations in our sample, as well as the sociohistorical context of family life as it has changed over the years of the study." Bengtson analyzed six dimensions of solidarity that he judged to be the basis of intergenerational relationships: affectual, associational, consensual, functional, normative, and structural (Bengtson, 2001; for the micro/macro distinction, see Bengtson, Biblarz, & Roberts, 2002, p. xviii; Bengtson & Achenbaum, 1993, pp. 5, 263; Bengtson & Schaie, 1999, pp. 27–28).

Modestly, Bengtson declared that "the intergenerational solidarity model represents only a start at understanding the processes and dynamics of multigenerational relationships over time" (Bengtson, 2001, p. 10). But we should not minimize Bengtson's intellectual achievement. The Longitudinal Study of Gerontology is not simply another collection of data. It was intended to activate a multidisciplinary theory of aging that examined and explained "the contextual features which surround the aging process. This includes historical, political, and economic features as well as the ongoing construction of every-day aging experiences" (Passuth & Bengtson, 1988, p. 349). Intergenerational solidarity is not grand theory in the tradition of Marx or Mannheim; it surveys a limited (albeit important) gerontological domain. And while Bengtson's training in social psychology and human development at the University of Chicago is evident in the LSOG's formulation, it is also clear that his theoretical field of vision widened as he matured. He was open to new ideas and criticism even when they stung. Bengtson mentored many, including those who did not intend to replicate or emulate his studies.

Consider the range of dissertations (hardly exhaustive) that Bengtson supervised between 1971 and 1988 in which students used the LSOG dataset in the course of identifying fruitful gerontological problems. William Martin, one of his first students, studied alienation and age across three generations in 1971. Five years later, James Dowd defended his thesis on "Age-stratum consciousness in an older sample: The effects of status inconsistency," and David Haber elaborated "Creativity over the career course: An adult socialization perspective." Steven McConnell's "Bureaucrats and old clients: Dependence, stigma, and negative sentiment in the service relationship," in 1977, helped to prepare him for a distinguished career as a Senate aide, advocate for older Americans, and senior foundation officer. In 1984, Carolyn Paul, relying on the Retirement History Study instead of the Longitudinal Study on Generations, gauged "The calculus of deferred retirement." Linda Burton analyzed "Early and on-time grandmotherhood in multi-generation families." At least 18 other Bengtson students based their dissertations on the LSOG (USC, 2007); most put findings into an historical context that supported a life-course perspective. Bengtson's multidisciplinary theory not only served his research agenda but also gave others considerable latitude in pursing ideas, without being diffuse.

Examining Bengtson's grant record offers another aperçu into how multidisciplinary approaches to research on aging open vistas and (hopefully) avert sinkholes. Initially focusing on mental health, Bengtson's proposals later clustered around generational themes: aging parents, new roles for the aged, generational differences, intergenerational solidarity (as it affected mental health and aging parents), and sociocultural contexts of aging. Having identified areas of interest and created a construct suitable to generate questions and explain findings, Bengtson could build on past accomplishments. Occasional setbacks did not deter him for long. Expositions on theory-building matured his scholarship, opening new possibilities.

This observation leads us, at last, to core of the paper: What role has theory-building played in Bengtson's treatment of religion, spirituality, and aging? Neither religious experiences in his formative years nor stints as a chorister in maturity predisposed Bengtson to pursue the topic of religiosity as a major strand of his research. Bengtson only occasionally wrote about the importance to the mental well-being of older Americans of forging intergenerational connections in religious settings (Bengtson & Achenbaum, 1993, pp. xi, 6; Bengtson & Harootyan, 1994, pp. 81–82, 215)

An invitation from the John Templeton Foundation to submit a proposal to study "the transmission of religion across generations" spurred Bengtson's interest in religion. The foundation gave Bengtson and his team $840,000 from July 2006 through June 2008 to conduct a pilot study. In January 2006, Bengtson invited roughly two dozen scholars, mainly sociologists of religion, to the University of Southern California to discuss theories of generational transmission in faith-based contexts. The participants were to identify questions and issues for a new survey that would be added to previous survey panels of the Longitudinal Study of Generations. Some guests questioned the feasibility of the proposed project on methodological grounds. They noted (and Bengtson freely acknowledged) that there were flaws in the LSOG sample: it was not, among other things, representative of the United States or other countries in terms of ethnic and racial diversity or income.

Yet no one challenged the sample's longitudinal design, developmental thrust, or multigenerational scope—its linking of families and individuals, its psychosocial focus, or its usefulness in putting trends into broader historical context. The sociologists of religion who were present, leaders in a subfield of a major discipline, were satisfied that an age-based multidisciplinary theory originally crafted to probe the "generation gap" of the late 1960s and early 1970s was sturdy enough to address and explain a very different set of issues: How do religious beliefs converge and diverge across generations? How great was the variance within generations and cohorts? How much did new religious currents affect people's religiosity and cause them to adapt their behavior?

Well-constructed datasets like the LSOG, in other words, often help discerning researchers to engage in theory-building to address problems for which surveys originally had not been intended. Bengtson could widen his field of vision by refining the questions that he asked respondents across generations. But, as he would be the first to acknowledge, there are other ways of seeing.

Another Way of Building Theories about Aging, Religion, and Spirituality

Like Vern Bengtson, I have maintained dual allegiances with my "home" discipline (in my case, history) while identifying as a gerontologist. Like Bengtson, I take pleasure in thinking critically about the place of theories in advancing gerontology as an intellectual enterprise. I agree with Vern that multidisciplinary approaches to problem solving are more effective than any single discipline or profession has yet to provide. Some of his mentors (especially Bernice Neugarten, Jim Birren, and the Rileys) greatly affected the way I think about gerontology.

But there is a major difference between us: Most academic historians are not trained to be theoreticians. I critique theories; I rarely test hypotheses or deploy theoretical constructs to shape an inquiry. Insofar as historians like me build theories in to our work, we typically borrow metaphors from the humanities or bench sciences, constructs from the social and behavioral sciences, or conceptual frameworks generated by scholars in interdisciplinary programs in African American studies, women's studies, or gay/lesbian/bisexual/transgender studies.

Historians tell stories and write narratives. Clio's heirs embed the theories that they utilize into their texts. It is important not to overstate the differences, however, between historians and sociologists interested in building theories in gerontology. Bengtson declares that "there may be other ways to describe" [theory-building], "such as 'telling a story' about empirical findings, or 'developing a narrative accounting' about observations" (Bengtson, Rice, & Johnson, 1999, p. 5). Bengtson's concept of theory-building privileges function over form. By that criterion, he invites historians to contribute to theory-building in accordance with their tribal customs, on the condition that they appreciate how scholars in other disciplines use theories. It is not a difficult hurdle.

Having been trained to rely on verifiable facts, students of the past require enough statistical training to be able to assess the quality of quantitative data. Historical descriptions and explanations of phenomena at the individual, community, national, and global levels must meet disciplinary-specific standards to be accepted by peers. The standards are sufficiently stringent to assure their usefulness to gerontologists. Good history is more than a sequence of facts strung together. Historians ground their contingent, ironic, paradoxical findings in an appropriately framed context.

So how would I go about studying the transmission of religion across generations? Unlike Bengtson, who inductively contextualized information from respondents in his LSOG data set, I generally proceed deductively. I need a sense of the big picture. Whereas Bengtson seeks explanations that make connections among individuals, families, communities, and the state, I ask questions about changes and continuities at the institutional level and then move to micro and macro levels of analysis, keeping track of continuities and changes over time.

I cannot overemphasize the importance that I place on studying institutions. They provide me links to individual- and global-based data. Institutions have a life of their own, trajectories typically independent of individual life courses or broad societal developments. Some fade or disappear after their founders or charismatic leaders leave the scene. Others implode when they no longer serve a purpose or turn a profit. Religious institutions have long played a central role in bringing Americans together. They too have changed over time, though not always in keeping with the times.

"The religious atmosphere of the country was the first thing that struck me on arrival in the United States," declared Alexis de Tocqueville in *Democracy in America* (1969 [1836–1840], p. 295). "In France I had seen the spirits of religion and freedom almost always marching in opposite directions. In America, I found them intimately linked together in joint reign over the same land." The America of de Tocqueville was a Protestant republic.

According to surveys, the United States remains faith-based. There has been some flight lately from the pews, however. In 2001, 81% of all Americans claimed affiliation with a religious community, down 9% from 1990 (Kosmin, Mayer, & Keysar, 2001, p. 10). Mainstream Protestant denominations lost the most ground. Schism and property suits threaten the Episcopal Church, which is embroiled in a controversy over homosexuality, itself a result of an unresolved conflict that split liberals and conservatives over the ordination of women in the mid-1970s. Sexual scandals and cover-ups may be part of the reason why roughly 30% of all Roman Catholics do not belong to a parish and only 5% of those under 30 attend Mass (Leege & Trozzolo, n.d., pp. 4–5).

These data indicate that baby boomers are less inclined to seek sustenance from the institutions that nurtured their forbears. Other facts bolster the plausibility this generalization. That a third of all Episcopalians are over the age of 65 might signal institutional stagnancy. But there may be other factors at play. Boomers prefer folk songs to Victorian hymns. The stately but sexist language of *The Book of Common Prayer* is off-putting. Others respond to different cultural forces. Some boomers and their families who have left the church are uncomfortable with embracing "inclusivity," just as they chafe at attitudes supporting the empowerment of women and racial, ethnic, and sexual minorities. Those who remain in the fold often feel marginal: Older Episcopalians on average receive less pastoral care and participate less frequently in parish life than they did when they were younger. Clergy, with an eye on numbers, are most interested in reaching and retaining couples with children.

Yet if we cast a wider net, a different picture of religious life in America emerges. With globalization has come an infusion of believers and congregations representing all the world religions (Tirrito & Cascio, 2003, pp. 32–35). First-generation Catholic immigrants are less likely to participate in congregations than members of the third generation; the reverse trend obtains among Protestant immigrants. Furthermore, both within and outside our borders, evangelical groups have flourished since the 1990s; more than a quarter of all Spanish-speaking residents claim to be born again. Nondenominational churches grew dramatically during the same period (Cramer, 2003; Stern, 2003). Nearly two-thirds of all Americans who have access to a computer use the Internet for religious purposes; that has prompted mainstream churches to stay wired to congregants (Pew Foundation, 2004).

Meanwhile, the baby boomers shop around, taking cues from family members to determine if and when they transfer in and out of parishes. Some return to their denomination of origin after their children are grown or join their significant others in a place where they feel comfortable. Others pursue options their parents were unlikely to consider. Celtic, Franciscan, and Benedictine inspirations vie with Wicca and Druids for their souls (Fairgrove, 2004). New Agers are likely claim to be "spiritual," not "religious"; they seek guides that blend healing and self-help. Still others take advantage of unprecedented access to world religions. Not only have White boomers incorporated Eastern sources into their religious lives, but Buddhist practices appeal to African Americans and Latinos/as (Arthur, 2004). So does Islam, which is predicted to become the second-largest religion (after Christianity) in the United States by 2015. Some Blacks join to affirm their pan-African identity; the urban poor often join mosques in response to charitable giving by Islamic social-service agencies (Haddad, 1991).

There certainly are other data points worth adding into any consideration of the transmission of religion from the great generation to the baby boom generation in the United States (for transmission of religion, see Putney et al., Chapter 10). I have, for instance, overlooked the growth of faith-based social services, which results from holes in the safety net as well as federal financial initiatives. Nor have I addressed the role of ideology—Liberation Theology especially—in mobilizing poor immigrants to advocate for social justice and to assist comrades in need. Still, I have gathered enough information with which to schematize a theory-driven narrative that would complement Vern Bengtson's account.

Like Bengtson, I am struck by the continuities I encountered in my analysis of the transmission of religion across generations. Some continuities are surprising; others set important parameters for evaluating the magnitude of change that has occurred since World War II. Let me cite three American traits affecting baby boomers that have existed since de Tocqueville chronicled *Democracy in America* 180 years ago:

1. A majority of Americans remain drawn to religious institutions. "In the United States associations are established to promote the public safety, commerce, industry, morality, and religion," observed de Tocqueville (1940 [1836–1840], Vol. 1, p. 198). A distinctive institutional arrangement, voluntary associations (including religious communities) attract individuals to participate in collective activities as long as they are useful and meaningful. Such institutions dissolve when no longer useful to their constituencies (de Tocqueville, 1940 [1836–1840], Vol. 1, p. 299).

2. While we tend to focus on a select group of Christian and Jewish faith-based communities and social-service agencies, the United States has long been a refuge for those persecuted for their beliefs. Religion in America is very pluralistic. "From time to time strange sects arise which strive to open extraordinary roads to eternal happiness" (de Tocqueville, 1969 [1836–1840], p. 535). Choices abound for baby boomers.

3. Americans are constantly seeking new ways to satisfy needs—whether religious yearnings or bellicose ambitions. This is consistent with their self-reliant, inward commitment (the French nobleman called it *individualisme*) to put their self-interest above concern for others. The quest can be frenzied. "The restlessness of the heart is the same, the taste for enjoyment is insatiable, the ambition of success as great; the means of gratifying it alone are different" (de Tocqueville, 1969[1836–1840], pp. 281–282). Boomers are fickle consumers in matters of faith.

Thus, while most parents have historically chosen to expose their offspring to the realm of religion, it is not enough for analysts to focus on the act of transmission itself. The form of religious institutions and the content of their teachings are ever in flux. As we shall see, many baby boomers received a particular cluster of messages that they then edited, modified, and even transmogrified to serve their own restless yearnings.

What has been occurring at the macro-societal level that might account for diverse transformations of the transgenerational transmission? Let me propose three factors:

1. Globalization has made the United States less parochial. Long accustomed to receiving immigrants, America has become at least temporarily home to markedly increased numbers of peoples from the subcontinent, Oceania, the Middle East, and Latin America. They bring with them their indigenous faiths and practices. As a result, traditional U.S. pluralism has given way to eclectic religious cosmopolitanism.

2. Fundamentalism has become a predominant strain in virtually every faith tradition, here and abroad. Certain in their beliefs, groups of fundamentalists expect others to read their sacred texts as they do. To do violence to the Truth justifies in many minds the right to do violence to others. Fundamentalism has polarized peoples within and across faith traditions, politically and socially (Marty, 1994).

3. Unlike their parents, baby boomers do not have to travel to remote places in order to witness the myriad ways that humans individually and collectively give thanks to an Ultimate Reality or celebrate life. They can stay at home and learn about other faith traditions via the media and the Internet. Hence, Americans' access to eclectic religious cosmopolitanism is greater than ever before.

Two microsocial changes merit note. On the one hand, the diminishing engagement in religious institutions—such as less regular weekly attendance at services—noted among baby boomers may become a lasting trend. The pattern is noticeable among that cohort's children and grandchildren. To varying degrees, it obtains across racial and ethnic lines. On the other hand, the rising interest in spirituality, particularly forms outside of prescribed institutional practices, may be yet another indication that the varieties of religious experiences in America among baby boomers have become less denominational. Spirituality, usually defined as an inwardly driven dialog with the Ineffable, takes many other forms. Neighbors, kindred souls, and strangers gather together in spiritually based voluntary associations of their own making.

Amid these constellations of continuities and changes are structural lags (Riley, Kahn, & Foner, 1994). Religious institutions have not kept pace with societal aging. As noted earlier, most clergy and lay leaders appeal to younger parishioners while they marginalize their older ones. This is counterproductive on two counts.

First, every faith tradition acknowledges its responsibility to care for widows and orphans, but not to empower them. Longtime members are not fed spiritually by a network of health-care and social-service delivery for elders— a safety net that only large, affluent congregations usually can provide anyway. In any case, focusing only on needs ignores the fact that many older Americans have much to contribute, liturgically and pedagogically, to the faith-based community. Having accepted a variety of changes over their lifetimes, most are still willing to make adjustments. Their voices of experience can help younger congregants to identify those lively traditions worth saving (Pelikan, 1986). Will baby boomers—now well into the third quarter of life—accept a roleless role in faith communities, or will they act out?

Second, most religious institutions rigidly compartmentalize the stages of life. Sunday school is age based. Most congregations have youth ministers, but their adult education programs are uneven in quality because organizers must appeal to a broad age span. Boomers are diverse, facing distinctive challenges and opportunities along their life journeys. (Perhaps this is one reason for marginalizing the aged; it reduces one age group from the pool of participants.) Faith-based communities should do more to promote intergenerational activities in outreach and in educational settings. They should provide opportunities for newcomers of all ages to find an appropriate niche regardless of their date of birth. They should not homogenize programs for baby boomers.

In addition to structural lags, let me underline two very different cultural lags (Ogburn, 1922). Religious institutions by and large have ignored or underestimated the powers of ideas that in recent decades have transformed how many people perceive human relations. First, they resist theologians who have recovered the power of the Feminine Divine and of documenting the historical and current role of women in faith-based communities. The make-over of Mary Magdalene (Dan Brown notwithstanding) and the creation of Magdalene communities (Adam, 2006) represent a profoundly significant effort to extirpate stereotypes about gender roles and sexuality. Eco-feminist theologies provide the intellectual girding to return women, especially of the baby boom cohort, to leadership roles they once held in many religious traditions. At the same time, strong theological arguments have been advanced to encourage the laity to take charge of many religious functions. Some propose that properly trained laypersons assume ecclesiastical ministries, defying to centuries-old beliefs that clergy undergo an ontological transformation upon ordination. The theological lag in both instances has unsettling implications: Does authority convey authenticity? If male/female, clergy/lay distinctions are obsolescent, why continue to perpetuate rigid boundaries, especially when we need to tap potential resources, notably among baby boomers?

I would not tell the story of the boomers' religious pathways the way I have just organized it. Actually, I have written parts of this narrative elsewhere, with greater emphasis on the impact of religion and spirituality on health and well-being than on the transmission of religion across generations (Achenbaum, 2005, pp. 103–128). But I hope that outlining the theoretical structure informing this vignette shows that Bengtson and I rely on many of the same theorists (including several contributors to this volume). Our modus operandi in building theories emphasizes historical context, microsocial and macrosocietal levels of analysis, and attention to cultural and structural lags. We both seek to describe, explain, and interpret data, differences in our themes and styles notwithstanding.

And so I end where I began. Vern Bengtson is right: Gerontologists have done much to promote multidisciplinary approaches to theory-building. To say this is not to minimize the importance of disciplinary-specific theories in aging to those within specific tribes or to the confederation of scholars worldwide. The great virtue of multidisciplinary theories is adaptability. With so many facets to aging, which manifest themselves on so many different planes in a dynamic fashion, we need a set of reliable lenses that can adjust from one essential puzzle to another while keeping track of the peripheral elements that might unlock some of the keys to the mysteries of aging.

REFERENCES

Achenbaum, W. A. (1995). *Crossing frontiers: Gerontology emerges as a science.* New York: Cambridge University Press.
Achenbaum, W. A. (2005). *Older Americans, vital communities: A bold vision for societal aging.* Baltimore, MD: The Johns Hopkins University Press.
Achenbaum, W. A., & Bengtson, V. L. (1994). Re-engaging the disengagement theory

of aging: On the history and assessment of theory development in gerontology. *The Gerontologist, 34,* 756–763.

Adam, B. (2006). *The Magdalene mystique: Living the spirit of Mary Magdalene.* New York: Morehouse Publishing.

Arthur, C. (2004). A revolution in religious consciousness. *Religious Pluralism, 6,* 19–41.

Becher, T. (2001). *Academic tribes and territories.* Buckingham, UK: Open University Press.

Bengtson, V. L. (1989). The problem of generations: Age group contrasts, continuities and social change. In V. L. Bengtson & K. W. Schaie (Eds.), *The course of later life* (pp. 25–54). New York: Springer.

Bengtson, V. L. (2001). The Burgess Award Lecture. *Journal of Marriage and Family, 63,* 1–16.

Bengtson, V. L., & Achenbaum, W. A. (Eds.). (1993). *The changing contract across generations.* New York: Aldine de Gruyter.

Bengtson, V. L., Biblarz, T. J., & Roberts, R. E. L. (2002). *How families still matter: A longitudinal study of youth in two generations.* New York: Cambridge University Press.

Bengtson, V. L., & Harootyan, R. A. (Eds.). (1994). *Intergenerational linkages: Hidden connections in American society.* New York: Springer.

Bengtson, V. L., Rice, C. J., & Johnson, M. L. (1999). Are theories important? Models and explanations in gerontology at the turn of the century. In V. L. Bengtson & K. W. Schaie (Eds), *Handbook of theories of aging* (pp. 3–20). New York: Springer.

Bengtson, V. L., & Schaie, K. W. (Eds.). (1999). *Handbook of the theories of aging.* New York: Springer.

Cowdry, E. V. (Ed.). (1939). *Problems of ageing.* Baltimore, MD: Wilkins & Williams.

Cramer, M. L. (2003). Mainline churches again filling pews. www.thetimesherald. com/news/stories/20030525/localnews/365206.html

de Tocqueville, A. (1969 [1836–1840]). *Democracy in America.* J. P. Mayer (Ed.). Garden City, NY: Doubleday & Co.

de Tocqueville, A (1945 [1836–1840]). *Democracy in America* (2 vols.). P. Bradley (Ed.). New York: Vintage Books.

Fairgrove, R. (2004). Links to multifaith and religious sites. (www.conjure.com/religion .htm).

Frank, L. (1942). Foreword. In E. V. Cowdry, *Problems of Ageing* (2nd ed., pp. v–ix). Baltimore, MD: Wilkins & Williams.

Haddad, Y. Y. (1991). *The Muslims in America.* New York: Oxford University Press.

Hendricks, J., & Achenbaum, W. A. (1999). Historical development of theories of aging. In V. L. Bengtson & K. W. Schaie (Eds), *Handbook of theories of aging* (pp. 21–39). New York: Springer.

Kosmin, B. A., Mayer, E., & Keysar, A. (2001). *American religious identification survey, 2001.* New York: Graduate Center of the City of New York.

Kuhn, T. (1962). *The structure of scientific revolutions.* Chicago, IL: University of Chicago Press.

Leege, D. C., & Trozzolo, T. A. (n.d.). *Participation in Catholic parish life: Religious rites and parish activities in the 1980s.* Report #3. University of Notre Dame: Notre Dame Study of Catholic Parish Life.

Marty, M. (1994). *Accounting for fundamentalism: The dynamic character of movements.* Chicago, IL: University of Chicago Press.

Ogburn, William F. (1922). *Social change: With respect to culture and original nature.* New York: Heubsch.

Passuth, P. M., & Bengtson, V. L. (1988). Sociological theories in aging: Current perspectives and future directions. In J. E. Birren & V. L. Bengtson (Eds.), *Emergent theories of aging* (pp. 333–355). New York: Springer.

Pelikan, J. (1986). *The vindication of tradition: The 1983 Jefferson lecture in the humanities.* New Haven, CT: Yale University Press.

Pew Foundation (2004). Internet and American life. (www.pewinternet.org/reports/toc/asp?Report=106).

Riley, M. W., Kahn, R. L. & Foner, A. (Eds.). (1994). *Age and structural lag: Society's failure to provide meaningful opportunities in work, family, and leisure.* New York: Wiley Interscience.

Stern, G. (2003). Mainstream Protestants reeling. *JournalNews.com.*

Tirrito, T., & Cascio, T. (Eds.). (2003). *Religious organizations in community services.* New York: Springer.

USC (2007). Longitudinal study of generations. Retrieved September 7, 2007 (http://www.usc.edu/dept/gero/research/4gen/history.htm).

Wilson, E. B. (1998). *Consilience.* New York: Vintage.

The Transmission of Religion across Generations

How Ethnicity Matters

Norella M. Putney, Joy Y. Lam, Frances Nedjat-Haiem, Thien-Huong Ninh, Petrice S. Oyama, and Susan C. Harris

How does racial, ethnic, or cultural heritage relate to the continuity of a religious tradition in multigenerational families? Have religious transmission patterns changed over time and between generations in ethnic families, particularly between today's youth and their elders? The long-term processes of assimilation and acculturation in the United States suggest that the passing on of a religious tradition from great-grandparents or earlier generations to younger generations is unlikely or perhaps has disappeared altogether. But is this the case? As the immigrant experience has grown more distant, are third- and fourth-generation ethnic families less interested in transmitting their religious tradition to younger generations?

Religion often serves as the framework for understanding a family's or an individual's unique ethnic identity. Many studies have observed the close linkage between ethnic and religious identities among immigrant families, how religion helps to ease and sustain an ethnic group's adjustment or even survival in a new cultural and political environment, and how a religious tradition and its institutions serve as a vehicle for sustaining ethnic identity (Cadge & Ecklund, 2007; Ebaugh, 2003; Herberg, 1960; Min & Kim, 2005; Warner, 2005).

A racial or ethnic heritage may be nearly coextensive with or defined by a particular religious identity and its practices. The historical relationship between Hispanics and Catholicism is an example. While this close connection between religion and ethnic heritage is enduring in many multigenerational families, in others the connection has become attenuated or altogether severed for younger generations. When members of an ethnic family reject their religious heritage, convert to another faith, or marry someone of a different faith or of no religious faith at all, consciousness of their ethnic background may be weakened as well. Family dysfunctions may similarly intrude on the traditional linkage between religion and ethnic identity.

In this chapter we focus on the interconnections of ethnic and cultural heritage, religious identity or affiliation, and the transmission of a family's religious tradition across generations in eight multigenerational families from different racial or ethnic backgrounds: Hispanic, African American, Jewish American, Asian American, and Italian American. These families are three and four generations removed from their immigrant experience, with the exception of the African American families. Using data from the 38-year Longitudinal Study of Generations and in-depth interviews with a subsample of four-generation families of diverse ethnic and religious backgrounds, we explore how a family's racial, ethnic, and cultural heritage matters in the reproduction of a religious tradition across generations. Despite the extraordinary social and cultural changes of the past several decades, we suggest that in many ethnic families their religious tradition has been sustained or even revitalized as a central feature of everyday life.

Background of the Study

In exploring the intergenerational transmission of religious tradition in ethnically diverse families, we first discuss religious socialization in families, the central role of intergenerational relationship quality for religious transmission, and how these processes can vary by ethnicity. We then discuss the linkages between religious and ethnic identities as they relate to the immigrant experience in the United States. Massive immigration over the past four decades has greatly increased the ethnic and religious diversity of American families and communities. The effects of this surge of immigration are revealed in recent ethnic population figures and the changing religious profiles of ethnic groups, factors arguing for the relevance of ethnicity for understand-

ing religious transmission. Researchers have noticed a shift from ethnic assimilation to cultural and ethnic pluralism as the desired immigration goal.
We comment on the implications of this change for religious continuity across
generations.

Religion and Families

In the United States there has long been a synergistic connection between
religious institutions and the family, which work together to ensure the maintenance and reproduction of beliefs and values in society through moral and
religious socialization of the young. The influence of religion pervades almost
every aspect of social life, including demographic patterns of marriage and
fertility as well as education and occupational pursuits (Edgell, 2006; King &
Elder, 1999; Roof, 1999). Religious beliefs and rituals enacted within the family have a definable impact on individual choices and trajectories across the
life course.

Central to this interrelationship is the passing on of the family's religious
heritage to younger generations, which has implications for the continuity of
the religious tradition itself (Roof, 1999). Yet we know too little about how religious values and practices are transmitted from parents to children, or from
grandparents to grandchildren (Myers, 1996), or how these processes may
have been altered as a consequence of the rapid social and technological
changes of recent years. It is also unclear how religious transmission, or its
lack, varies by a family's racial, ethnic, or cultural background.

Religious Socialization in Families

While often thought of as attributes of an individual, religious identity and
commitment are also social phenomena resulting from childhood religious
socialization occurring primarily in nuclear and extended families. The family and religious institutions are closely related to one another because of the
cultural emphasis on the value of children's religious socialization in the family (Dillon & Wink, 2007). Studies have shown that parents make a lasting
imprint on the religious belief orientations and commitments of their children
(Glass, Bengtson, & Dunham, 1986; Myers, 1996; Sherkat, 1998; Smith & Denton, 2005). Parents make sure their children participate in Sunday school and
other religious schools in committed ways to ensure the religious socialization
process continues. Pearce and Thornton (2007) found that the religious beliefs
and practices learned early in life from mothers are related to young adults'

family ideologies well into their thirties, supporting a family religious social-ization model. Individuals raised in a particular religious tradition were more likely to remain religiously active through young adulthood or return to that tradition when they start their own families than those who were raised with-out a religious identity (Stolzenberg, Blair-Loy, & Waite, 1995).

Intergenerational Relationships and Religious Socialization

The quality of intergenerational relations and the closeness of the parent-child relationship is perhaps the strongest predictor of religious continuity across generations (Bengtson, Biblarz, & Roberts, 2002; Myers, 1996; Sherkat, 1998; Smith & Denton, 2005). Myers found that although the recent experi-ences of adult offspring—such as attending college or the influence of peers—did affect their religiosity, these experiences did not reduce the influence of parents and family context. Myers concludes that "parental influences have considerable staying power even as offspring move out of the home and form independent households" (1996, p. 864). In the area of religiosity, there seems to be an enduring effect of childhood socialization. In their investigation of Jewish group identity, Dashefsky, Lazerwitz, and Tabory (2003) found that family socialization and social interaction with significant others were pri-mary sources of Jewish identity but that sustaining that identity also depends on being structurally integrated into the larger Jewish community as adults, such as synagogue involvement.

How families transmit religious beliefs and practices can take on various configurations depending on race and ethnicity, or cultural background, as well as gender, and socioeconomic position. For example, ethnic groups differ in family structures and patterns of interaction, which in turn can affect reli-gious socialization. Compared to Whites, Hispanic families remain larger, multigenerational coresidence is more likely, and members live closer to one another (Gonzales, 2007; Landale & Oropesa, 2007; McAdoo, Martinez, & Hughes, 2005). Among Mexican American families compared to European American families, ethnicity is regarded as a crucial link to family integration (Sarkisian, Gerena, & Gerstel, 2007). Dowd & Bengtson (1978) found that Mexican American respondents reported more frequent contact and interac-tion among extended family members than did White respondents. Blacks showed slightly higher rates of contact with extended kin and fictive kin than Whites. Asian American families are on average larger than White or Black families, and 15% of Asian American households contain three or more gen-erations (Park & Ecklund, 2007). Interracial and intercultural marriages are contributing to an even greater array of ethnic family patterns (McAdoo, Martinez, & Hughes, 2005).

Religion, Ethnicity, and the Immigrant Experience

Religion in America has deep roots in the immigrant experience. Researchers have observed that when members of these ethnic groups immigrated to religiously pluralistic urban areas, their traditional, family-centered religious faiths allowed them to retain, or even strengthen, their ethnic identities (Ebaugh, 2003; Herberg, 1960; Wittberg, 1999). From his mid-twentieth century vantage point, Herberg (1960) traced how religion affected the different generations of immigrants in the United States. He suggested that after the first generation, the children of immigrants tended to abandon their ethnic traditions as well as their native languages, but they retained their religion, as was more likely in a religiously pluralistic society. As religion was transmitted to the third and later generations, it became a central source or carrier of the family's ethnic identity, the vehicle for American acculturation.

Religion remains a major factor shaping ethnic adaptation and assimilation of new immigrants (Ebaugh, 2003; Warner, 2005). Cadge and Ecklund (2007) suggest that religious identities have become more salient for immigrants in the United States than in their nations of origin because of the role religion has in maintaining ethnic identity for the next generation. However, a religious tradition does not always enable the transmission of cultural identity across generations. Min and Kim (2005) found that Korean immigrants were able to transfer their Protestant religion, but not their Korean cultural traditions, which were not incorporated into their new congregations' worship services and activities. Nonetheless, for generations of immigrants, religion has served to integrate individuals and families into American society, and in the process contributed to family and cultural continuity.

Ethnic and Religious Diversity Trends

Recent trends in U.S. immigration highlight the relevance of studying religious transmission in ethnically diverse families. Massive immigration over the past four decades (since the passage of the Immigration and Naturalization Act of 1965) is altering the ethnic and religious landscape of the United States. Warner (2005) points out that the extent of the new religious and racial diversity in the United States is unprecedented, surpassing that of the late nineteenth and early twentieth centuries. While the new waves of immigrants are primarily from Latin American and eastern Asian countries, Christianity retains its predominance among these groups (Warner, 2005).

By 2050, Hispanics will almost double their share of the population (from 12.6% to 24.4%). Immigration as well as higher birth rates will account for this increase. Blacks will increase from 13% in 2000 to almost 15% in 2050. Asians will increase from 4% in 2000 to 8% in 2050. The Non-Hispanic White population will represent only half of the United States population by 2050 (U.S. Census, 2004).

Ethnic Group Differences in Religious Identities

There are major differences in the religious identities and commitments of various racial and ethnic groups. For example, today more than three-quarters of Blacks (78%) are Protestant, compared with just over half of Whites (53%) and about a quarter of Asians (27%) and Latinos (23%). The ethnic composition of religious institutions also varies by age. While almost half of all Catholics under age 30 are Hispanic, most Catholics over 70 are White (PEW Forum, 2008).

Religion has always been of great importance to African Americans. They have a high frequency of church attendance and church membership and a high prevalence of prayer in daily life (Lincoln & Mamiya, 1990; Pattillo-McCoy, 1998). Compared to other racial and ethnic groups, African Americans are the most likely to report a formal religious affiliation (Pew Forum, 2008). Beyond that, Black churches are the center of activity in the African American community.

Hispanics remain predominantly Catholic (68%) although a sizable proportion have switch to evangelical Protestant or other churches over the past four decades (Pew Forum, 2007). The proportion of native-born Hispanics who leave the Catholic Church has been offset by immigrants in the last few decades. Very few older Mexican-born Hispanics are converts, and most are members of families that have been Catholic for generations (Hill, Angel, Ellison, & Angel, 2005).

Among Asians in the United States, 17% are Catholic, an equal number are evangelical Christians, and 14% are Hindu. Asians are the most likely to be unaffiliated (23%) compared to other racial categories (Pew Forum, 2008). Jewish Americans constitute about 2% of the U.S. population. While affirming a Jewish heritage, many consider themselves to be culturally rather than religiously Jewish (Cadge & Davidman, 2006).

From Assimilation to Cultural Pluralism

For third- and fourth-generation immigrant families, it is likely that over time acculturation pressures weakened the transmission of religion to younger generations. However, a change in American cultural attitudes toward immigrant and minority groups has emerged in the past few decades, one that values diversity and cultural pluralism rather than assimilation (Garces-Foley, 2008; Warner, 2005). Garces-Foley observes that beginning in the early 1980s, the Catholic Church changed its stance toward immigrant groups, departing from its traditional role as an agent of assimilation and embracing the norm of cultural pluralism. Its new aim was to help immigrant groups retain their distinctive religious and cultural traditions. African American Catholics also benefited from this ethic of cultural pluralism, garnering additional resources from the Catholic Church for their local Black parishes. Warner (2005) observes a related change in ethnic churches: a move toward religious particularism, which celebrates in-group uniqueness but absent out-group enmity. He cites as an example how Jewish services, even in Reform synagogues, now emphasize the use of Hebrew and the wearing of yarmulkes to a greater degree than they did just two decades ago. More recently, the notion of multiculturalism has emerged, particularly as it applies to the desirability of multicultural congregations (Marti, 2006).

Intergenerational transmission processes and outcomes are not static; they occur in a continuously changing historical context. Nevertheless, we suggest there is religious continuity across generations in many families, and this may be especially the case for ethnic families. Because religion and ethnicity have been and continue to be so closely linked—as reflected in lives of generations of African Americans and American immigrants—examining intergenerational transmission of religion in racial and ethnic minority families can deepen our understanding of these processes.

Method
Sample

This analysis draws from the Longitudinal Study of Generations (LSOG), a study of over 3,000 respondents, ages 16–91, from 350 three- and four-generation families (for more details, see Bengtson et al., 2002). Individuals eligible for sample inclusion were generated from the families of grandparents randomly selected in 1970 from the membership of a large (840,000-member) health maintenance organization in the Los Angeles area. The sample pool was generally representative of White, economically stable, and middle and working class families. Self-administered questionnaires were mailed to the grandparents and their spouses (G1s), their adult children (G2s), and their grandchildren aged 16 or older (G3s). In 1985, 1,331 of the original sample were surveyed again, and since then data have been collected at three-year intervals through 2005. The response rate between 1971 and 1985 was 65% and has averaged 74% between waves since then. Additions to the eligible sample have included new spouses (mostly G3s), and, since 1991, great-grandchildren (G4s) who reached 16 years of age. The G3s in our sample are members of the baby boom generation while the G2s are their parents and the G1s their grandparents. The G4s in our sample are otherwise known as generation X and the millennial generation.

Relevant to the present inquiry, family members have been surveyed about their religious affiliation, practices, and beliefs over eight time waves, providing a picture of individuals' religious stability or change across the course of their lives and of families' similarities or differences in religiosity over time.

To explore in more depth the complexities of religious transmission in multigenerational families, we selected a subsample of 25 four-generation families from the LSOG panel and conducted in-depth interviews with 156 members of these families. A purposive sample, the families were chosen to represent a diversity of racial and ethnic groups, religious affiliations, levels of religious involvement, and variations in family cohesion or conflict. Our aim was to interview as many of the G1 great-grandparents as possible. The racial/ethnic minority composition of this subsample of families is 32%. The interviews focused on family relationships and traditions and the ways in which parents and grandparents pass on values (religious and nonreligious) from one generation to the next. The interviews ranged from 30 minutes (primarily with the older, more frail members of the sample) to more than three hours in length.

The transcribed interviews were coded using several strategies. Initially, we used a "grounded" approach, using the qualitative data analysis software Atlas.ti to code line by line the transcripts from several families. Our collective review of these coded transcripts resulted in the identification of many themes that emerged repeatedly in centrally important ways related to the transmission of religious identities and values within families, such as the significance of culture, race, and ethnicity, the impact of marriage, divorce, and remarriage, and the role of "rebels" and "zealots" in families. Once these themes were identified, we shifted our analysis from the individual to the family level, examining the interviews for material related to each of the themes we identified in our initial analysis.

We employed a mixed-methods analytic approach in examining religious transmission in our subsample of 25 families. In addition to the interview data, we examined the original LSOG surveys for each family, including those from family members who were not interviewed. This expanded the number of family members we were able to include in the analysis. Analyzed together, the survey and interview data helped us to develop a detailed, thematic case study for each family. While we quickly learned that religious affiliation is a particularly unstable and slippery characteristic of individuals and especially families, we nevertheless can describe the current affiliation of this purposive qualitative sample as approximately 16% evangelical Protestant, 18% mainline Protestant, 12% Catholic, 15% Mormon, 13% Jewish, 22% no affiliation, and 2% other.

For the present study we selected from the subsample eight minority families: the Sanchez and Garcia families (Hispanic), the Johnson and Walker families (African American), the Goldman and Lieberman families (Jewish American), the Yamamoto family (Asian American), and the Sabelli family (Italian American). Seven individuals from these families are first- or second-generation immigrants, but most are three or more generations removed. For this analysis we used both interview and survey data collected from 44 family members and survey data only from an additional 37 family members. Thus the total number of subjects is 81, for an average of 8 per family. To tap directly into the family members' own perspectives on the significance of race and ethnicity for their family traditions, especially their religious traditions, we conducted follow-up interviews with 15 of these individuals.

To understand the transmission processes of religion within racial and ethnic families, we focused on the interconnections of four elements: (1) racial, ethnic, and cultural background; (2) the family's religious experience; (3) individual religious involvement and choice; and (4) intergenerational relationships (see figure 10.1). The quality of parent-child relations serves as the crucial mechanism for passing on a religious tradition to the next generation. One of the advantages of this model is that as we analyzed the narratives and other data, it provided a useful framework for linking and understanding the complexities involved in the transmission of religion within multigenerational families of different racial, ethnic, and cultural backgrounds.

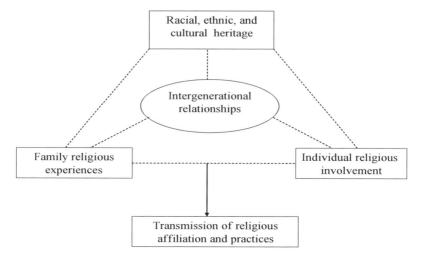

Figure 10.1. Conceptual model of the transmission of religion across generations.

Religious Transmission

Our central outcome of interest is the transmission of religion across generations. Here we are looking at religion as an identity or affiliation (how do subjects identify themselves when asked "what is/was your religion?"). We are also concerned with religious practices (how do subjects describe their religious activities now or in the past). Beyond this, we examine how subjects describe the role of religion in their lives and the meanings of religion and spirituality.

Racial, Ethnic, or Cultural Background

We examined four subthemes related to a family's racial, ethnic, or cultural background and how these experiences are described by subjects across generations. These subthemes reflect (1) immigrant experience, (2) racism or ethnic persecution, (3) the presence or absence of an ethnic community, and (4) intended assimilation. In order to examine how these subthemes play out at the family level, we looked at how each individual talked about his or her own experience. Thus at the individual level, we looked at: (1) how individuals identify themselves racially or ethnically or culturally and (2) how they talk about (or do not talk about) their connection to older generations' experience of immigration, racism or ethnic persecution, or assimilation. We traced how historical events or trends discussed in ethnic family stories as they related to specific racial or ethnic experience played a significant role in shaping how religion is being narrated and "passed on" within ethnic families.

Family Religious Experiences

We also coded for collective family religious experiences—how religion was experienced with family members and subjects' perceptions of these experiences. These include (but are not limited to) (1) a family history closely linked to a particular religion or church; (2) religious practices that are viewed as family tradition or tied to family history (e.g., the celebration of religious holidays as a family); and (3) childhood religious schooling experience (e.g., putting children in Sunday school, or teaching in Sunday school). Further, racial, ethnic, and cultural background or heritage can interact with a family's religious experience to affect ethnic and religious identities.

Individual Religious Involvements

While racial and ethnic history interacts with a family's religious experience to promote religious transmission to the next generations, this is not the whole story. Individual religious choices and involvement can reinforce or alter this process. We consider the effect of individual choice or circumstances (such as the experience of going to college) on religious identity and commitment and how this may have affected religious transmission.

Intergenerational Relationships

Closely linked to family religious experiences, the quality of intergenerational relations represents the central mechanism for religious transmission in our conceptual model. Collective religious experiences within the family are closely related to the quality of the parent-child relationship and its effect on the religious socialization of youth. Close grandchild-grandparent relations can also promote transmission. Parental marital stability or divorce can play a pivotal role in the degree of religious socialization that occurs between parents and children (as we observe in several of our family cases). A close grandparent-grandchild relationship may foster religious transmission when relations with a mother or father are not close or when their religious influence is compromised by divorce.

Results

Our cross-family analysis revealed four important themes related to religious transmission in these ethnically diverse families: (1) religious education and parenting; (2) the role of marriage (interfaith marriage, marital stability, or divorce); (3) intergenerational relationship quality; and (4) racial, ethnic, and cultural community and historical experiences of persecution. These themes exemplify ways in which racial, ethnic and cultural identities interact with processes of religious identities and the passing on of a religious tradition. While there are certainly other themes we could explore, we chose to organize our findings around these particular themes, recognizing of course that there is considerable interplay among the themes and complexities of influence on religious transmission across generations. In those families where we observed clear patterns of continuity in religious identity across generations, we also find that the family members consciously link their religious beliefs, family values, and racial and ethnic heritage together. Ethnicity matters in their religious life because it is about their family.

Religious Education and Parenting

In many of these families we found significant efforts by parents to provide their children with religious education programs organized within their ethnic communities and institutions (e.g., Sunday school, Hebrew school, catechism classes, or church youth education programs). Family narratives suggest this had a direct impact on parents' ability to pass on their religious affiliation to their children. However, providing children with formal religious training does not necessarily ensure the passing on of a religious tradition (Dillon & Wink, 2007; Hout & Fischer, 2002). The degree of parents' religious commitment and involvement in their children's religious education is also an important factor.

The two Jewish families in our study illustrate that parents' efforts to provide religious education for their children did not in itself guarantee the transmission of Judaism as a *religious* identity. The Lieberman family emphasized the importance of having their children attend Hebrew school. However, the great-grandparents in this family, while Jewish, were not religious. They thought of themselves as secular Jews with no religious commitment. Defining themselves as atheists, they were political activists. Their maintenance of a strong *cultural* Jewish identity, however, translated into providing a Jewish education for their children, grandchildren, and great-grandchildren.

For the second-generation son, a religious education in his youth was not necessarily determinative of religious commitment in adulthood. He became more religious than his parents by marrying an Orthodox Jewish woman. He indicated that he "became involved with the Jewish religious practices through [his] wife." The high value of having a Jewish education and transmitting a Jewish identity is evident among the third- and fourth-generation family members who had a bar or bat mitzvah. The Jewish subjects we interviewed affirmed that being Jewish is understood more as a cultural and ethnic identity than a religious identity; Judaism in this sense was successfully transmitted. As one G4 granddaughter indicates:

> Like I dropped off of my religious stuff, and so did my parents . . . they don't belong to synagogue anymore. My religious practices probably dropped off, not like permanently . . . as my daughter gets older . . . I want to kind of get back into [it], as she gets like old enough to kind of understand things.

A similar pattern can be found for the Goldman family, in which parents initiated religious schooling not to promote continuation of the Jewish religion across generations but to foster a cultural Jewish identity. There are nuances. In her interview, the G2 grandmother deliberately emphasized a value of having religious choice, a value her children absorbed. In consequence, her children halted their religious participation right after they were bar or bat mitzvah'd. Although her G3 son and his wife continued the practice of engaging their children in religious schooling, what was transmitted was not a religious Jewish identity but a cultural practice of Judaism in the family. As their G4 son says, "I see that I'm Jewish, and I see my parents are Jewish, my grandparents are Jewish . . . this is the way I'm supposed to do it." However, the religious aspect of being Jewish is not involved. While religious socialization is strong in these families, it is in the service of promoting a cultural Jewish identity.

The Walker family (African American) also demonstrates a strong tradition of religious schooling, but theirs is totally integrated in their Episcopalian church and family life. As such, religious education for youth contributes significantly to the transmission of religious affiliation across the generations in the family. There is a strong tradition of having children participate in Sunday school and attending church together as a family. The G2 grandmother was actively involved in attending church together with her G3 children. Two of her daughters in turn continued being involved in their church and teaching Sunday school, which their own children attended. A G4 son explains:

We were the ones that would go to church every week. We went as a family and as a church member I became, like, very active or I would do things in the church like an acolyte, which is the one who assist the priest, and then beyond that also, like, I became more and more . . . I helped out with the youth group, the Sunday school.

Across the generations, parents' consistent religious involvement in the same church in combination with close parent-child relationships explains the successful transmission of their religious identity.

In the Walker family, there is also a tradition of sending children to religious schools rather than public schools. The G2 grandmother attended a grade school sponsored by an evangelical church. Her G3 daughters attended Catholic high schools, and all her G4 grandchildren attended a high school sponsored by their Episcopal church. Two G4 grandchildren also attended Catholic colleges. The G4 grandson explains that the reason his parents put him into religious schools is not only because of their good academic record but also because

they looked at the people who, kind of, ran it and it was the same people that we would see at church. So it was, kind of, like, they knew, kind of, what they were getting before they got it and definitely just the quality of education. . . . So it's, kind of, word of mouth passed through the family that there's something that they're doing differently at these schools that do have this religious affiliation that is tangible in the success of the children.

This family strongly values educational achievement, and it associates a high quality of education with schools operated by churches.

The Sanchez family, a very large Hispanic family with a Catholic heritage, presents a different religious education scenario, one that reveals the crucial role of parent-child relationships for fostering or inhibiting religious transmission. With the exception of the G1 great-grandfather, commitment to the Catholic tradition has been more or less taken for granted. Aside from having their children attend catechism classes in preparation for First Communions, the second-generation parents' efforts to socialize their children into their Catholic faith have been minimal.

The great-grandparents and earlier generations all attended Catholic schools and married other Catholics. The great-grandfather attended church weekly and made sure his children attended. His G1 wife remembered, "My husband always make them go to church. He was always after the kids." When asked if she went with them, she said, "No, I used to go alone." His daughter, Julia, noted that her father's strict parenting "backfired," with negative consequences for his children's later religious commitment. All stopped going to church when they married in their teens. Julia and her five siblings attended public schools, not Catholic schools, as did their G3 children. While most continue to identify with the Catholic tradition, church attendance is infrequent for the third and fourth generations. As Julia said, "I don't know what it means . . . we just go." Religion was not talked about in the home. Julia's G3 son indicated, "I don't re-member going to church with my parents." He adds, "I don't think that my mom really knew what the baptism meant. But it was just a thing to do as a Catholic." Julia's G3 daughter, Connie, observed:

> My grandfather was Catholic, and my mother was raised Catholic. But I don't remember my mother . . . she didn't take us to church very often. I made my First Communion, I didn't go on with that, I didn't go to the Catholic Church. My mom always spoke about being Catholic, but in reality it was really some-thing we did every Sunday or Saturday or any other day.

In adulthood, Connie experienced growing disillusionment with the Catholic Church and switched to an evangelical Protestant church.

The Role of Marriage (Interfaith Marriage, Marital Stability, and Divorce)

The Garcia family is a very large and close Hispanic family with a strong Catholic tradition. Marriage within their Catholic faith is extraordinarily im-portant, a wellspring for expanding and revitalizing their Catholic religious practices and beliefs. Divorce is rare, as is marriage to a non-Catholic. In their interviews, the G2 grandmother, her G3 adult children, and her G4 adult grand-children all emphasized the importance of integrating religious activities into family life, such as celebrating religious holidays and attending church. Within-faith marriage reinforces this alignment of religion and family. A G3 son and his wife talked about how their common Catholic faith strengthens their marriage. Together they teach classes for confirmation and marriage at their church. Their G4 son and his spouse have continued this tradition, teach-ing catechism and marriage classes in their own church.

This pattern of within-faith marriage has expanded religious life in the family by integrating Spanish culture. Having married into the Garcia family, a G3 spouse, Maria, with the support of her husband, introduced the tradition of *curanderos* to the family. Thus, in this line of the Garcia family there is a parallel quasi-religious tradition. Maria finds her traditional healing practices to be compatible with her Catholic beliefs. She wants to transmit this Mexican healing tradition to her children and grandchildren, as she inherited it from her mother, grandmother, and great-grandmother before her. Her G4 son said that he believes in this healing practice although he is also a strong Catholic believer. His wife introduced her own family of origin's Spanish customs into her nuclear family's religious life, such as *Las Posadas* on Christmas and *cascarones* on Easter. Her G3 mother-in-law, Maria, reported that she likes these practices because they bring the family together.

The interviews of these ethnic family members reveal how important marrying someone of the same religious faith is for religious transmission. In both the Lieberman and Goldman families, the G1s emphasized the importance of marrying someone Jewish, which was passed down to the G2s in these families as they also married Jewish spouses. In both of these Jewish families, marrying within their faith led to the transmission of Jewish identity.

While the G1 parents in the Lieberman family were atheists, both G2 sons married Jewish women who were very religious. For one G2 brother, marrying a Jewish woman fostered the transmission of their Jewish identity and customs to their G3 children and G4 grandchildren. An exception occurred with the son of the other G2 brother in the Lieberman family. This G3, Stan, married an evangelical Protestant. His parents boycotted the wedding because "You don't marry outside of religion." Stan divorced and remarried twice after that. In his third marriage, Stan converted to his wife's mainline Protestant religion. Stan's G4 children from his first wife became confused about their religion, at times being pushed by their grandparents to unlearn what they had learned from their mother. Conflict over their religious identity arose for the G4 children because of the interfaith marriage and subsequent divorce of their parents.

In the Goldman family there are no interfaith marriages. Across the generations, all married within the Jewish faith. As relayed by a second-generation daughter, "My parents used to drum into [the children] that they're Jewish, they're Jewish, they're Jewish." The G1s were strict with their children about being Jewish, marrying within the Jewish faith, and staying within the Jewish community. For a G2 daughter, this exhortation was accompanied by a prejudice against those who were not Jewish. Talking about her parents, she says, "[They] were narrow-minded. . . . If somebody was different than us, they weren't any good." A G3 daughter said that being Jewish "was very important to [her] grandparents." Several family members talked about the importance of having a Jewish wedding and how doing so demonstrated being active or participating in an important Jewish tradition within the larger, extended family as well as the Jewish community.

In the Catholic Sanchez family, religious continuity and individual religious commitment diverge among the G3 siblings and cousins. A major reason for these different religious pathways is divorce and marrying someone of a different religious tradition. For two G3 members of the Sanchez extended family, their own or their parents' divorce seems to have played a role in their switching from the Catholic faith of their youth to another religious affiliation. G3 Connie's divorce prompted her to leave Catholicism and join a nondenominational Christian church. She talks about being born again and being touched by the Holy Spirit. In a certain way, she was primed for this shift. Connie's first husband, the father of her four children, is an evangelical Christian. Interviews suggest he may have influenced his ex-wife's and children's religious orientation, an influence manifested long after the marriage ended. While Connie identified as Catholic during the period of her marriage, her experience as a single person following divorce and the "emptiness" she felt caused her to question her Catholic faith. She came to see her parents' Catholicism as hypocritical and ineffective at curbing what she saw as the bad behaviors (using foul language and drinking) of her father, grandfather, and other family members. She transmitted her evangelical Christian religion to her four G4 children. Her second marriage to a Catholic ended in divorce several years later.

The religious pathway for her G3 brother, Jim, is different. In adulthood, his Catholic faith was revitalized through his marriage to a devout Catholic woman who remained committed to their marriage despite his previous difficulties. She had a strong Catholic upbringing and attended Catholic schools. She made sure their G4 children attended Catholic schools. While previously passive in his religious commitment, Jim had no problem with his wife's religious education of their children. Through his wife's influence, he became much stronger in his Catholic faith. Jim's Catholic wife transmitted her strong faith to their G4 children.

Intergenerational Relationship Quality

Whether involvement in a religious faith translates into religious transmission is very much affected by the quality of relations between parents and children and between grandparents and grandchildren. This dynamic in turn is linked to a family's racial and ethnic background.

In the Garcia family, there is high intergenerational solidarity. Across generations, their Catholic faith helped to sustain intergenerational relationships in the nuclear and extended family. In their interviews, family members emphasized the importance of Catholic religious practices and involvements because these activities cultivate family togetherness and cohesion. The older generations expressed the importance of transmitting their Catholic beliefs and practices to younger generations. Members see attending church together as a family tradition they would like to see continued with the younger generation.

Mothers play an important role in transmitting the importance of attending Mass to younger generations. A G2 daughter remembered that her mother always reminded her to go to church. In the next generation, her G3 son, who became a priest, said that his mother's "faith and belief in the Lord" instilled in him that the church "cannot be second to anything." Taken as a whole, this family's story indicates that the reinforcement of familism through religious practices rooted in family tradition was an important factor in the high transmission of their Catholic faith across four generations.

The quality of relations between the generations of the Johnson family (African American) is closely linked to their family's relationship with their church and religious continuity. Over the generations, family members have shared religious experiences at this church, including church attendance, baptisms, and catechism classes. The G1 grandfather played a significant role as both a religious leader and family figure, cofounding the first Black Catholic church in the city. Multigenerational family life revolved around this church. As G3 Joan indicates,

> I can honestly say that my mother's children and my aunt's children were more like sisters and brothers than cousins. We were many times in the same house . . .because my grandparents were very much involved in what was going on with the kids. We went to the same church. All the children were baptized in the same place.

Yet for a time, relations between Joan and her G2 mother were estranged, largely because of the G2 parental divorce. The divorce caused Joan to forge an even closer relationship with her grandparents, who were highly involved in the religious lives of their grandchildren. This strong skipped-generation influence may have contributed to the family's continued participation in its Black Catholic church. The family's connection to the same church across generations is strengthened by the high relevance of their racial background to religious transmission. Their racial and religious identities are interconnected.

In adulthood Joan has an extremely close relationship with her G4 daughters. Both daughters see their mother as the person who most influenced and shaped their values. However, the religious commitment of the G4 sisters diverges. In adulthood, the older sister and her mother attend church together, whereas the younger sister does not attend church at all. The younger sister says she is not interested in religion. "As far as religion is concerned . . . I don't go to church, so I know my mama's upset about that. I'm not really into Catholicism, or any other religion, at this point." Her mother, Joan, indicates this is probably a phase her daughter is going through, just as Joan did at that age. Despite this divergence, there has been high transmission of religious affiliation across four generations in this African American family.

In the Italian American Sabelli family, we found differences in the religious transmission pathways and outcomes of two sibling lineages, all of whom share the same ethnic heritage. Theirs is a complicated story of how religious affiliation may or may not be transmitted across generations and how the quality of intergenerational relationships over time is centrally involved in these processes. The Sabelli family history reveals the diminishing relevance of their Italian ethnic identity over generations. For the Go immigrant generation and their G1 children, their Italian and Catholic identities were tightly intertwined. When interviewed in 1986, the G1s expressed pride in being Italian and described the distinctiveness of their ethnic identity amid the dominant American culture. They also viewed attending the Catholic Church together as a family tradition. Growing up in an ethnic neighborhood and multigenerational household, the G2s witnessed their grandparents' immigrant experience firsthand. This experience instilled in them an Italian-Catholic identity rooted in family tradition. However, with the G2s, the tight connection between the family's ethnic heritage and its Catholic faith begins to unravel. To the extent that ethnic and religious identities remain relevant, their linkage is tenuous, although this varies by sibling line.

In G2 Bill's line of the family, there is relatively high transmission of their Catholic religious identity across generations. In G2 Betty's line of the family, there is low transmission of religious identity with little religious meaning remaining for the youngest generation. In both lines, there is decreasing appreciation or awareness of the family's Italian heritage. And in both lines, the quality of intergenerational relationships is significant for individual members' experiences with religion, with consequences for the transmission of the family's Catholic heritage down the generational ladders.

In G2 Betty's line, we observed that initially Catholicism and the family were mutually important, but the family's Italian heritage, though relevant for Betty earlier in her life, became less and less relevant for Betty's children and grandchildren. Betty's immigrant heritage shaped her values regarding the paramount importance of both family and her Italian-Catholic identity. This close association between religious and ethnic identities changes in the next generation because of Betty's divorce and its negative effect on Betty's relationship with her G3 daughter, Susan. Susan talks about the contradiction between her mother's professed family values and her relationship with her children. This intergenerational conflict diminishes the importance of the family's Italian heritage for the G3 Susan and her G4 children. Interestingly, G3 Susan maintained a close relationship with her G1 grandfather, and their shared experience of Catholic church activities encouraged her "sense of faith in God," which provided a source of comfort during her "crazy childhood" (the divorce of her G2 parents). Later in adulthood, following her own divorce and remarriage, Susan left the Catholic Church and adopted her second husband's evangelical Protestant religion. Although Susan was no longer a Catholic, the importance of religiousness that was transmitted from grandfather to granddaughter persisted.

Turning to the second line, G2 Bill's Italian ethnic identity remained strong during his early adult years but became less relevant over time. Bill's Catholic identity also faded when he was divorced during his daughter's growing-up years (he later remarried to a non-Catholic woman). Nevertheless, the family's Italian-Catholic identity was inherited by his G3 daughter, Amelia—not from her father but from her G1 grandfather, with whom she had a close relationship. Describing herself as "of Italian descent, a devout Catholic," Amelia links religious traditions and ethnicity together. Being Italian and Catholic go hand in hand, and family is important. "We're pretty Italian . . . The most important thing . . . is family. And at the center of that is the church." She goes on, "family and the church are pretty much tied together if you're Italian; they're just part of the same thing." The G1 grandfather exerted a similar long-term influence on the religiosity of Amelia's G3 cousin, Susan.

Over time, G3 Amelia's relationship with her nearly estranged G2 father, Bill, became very close. E-mail contact with her father gave him an opportunity to share old photos and stories of his youth and family, an expression of their Italian ethnic identity. In this case, we can see how parent-child relationship quality across the life course can be influenced by the sharing of ethnic family history.

Moving on to the next generation, identification with the family's religious heritage is maintained by Amelia's G4 daughter, Brooke. Influenced by her G2 grandfather Bill, Brooke identifies as Italian, but the close link between Catholicism and her family's Italian identity is broken. Brooke's relationship with her mother, Amelia, has its share of conflict, stemming from their different views on religion and politics, but both feel close to each other because they share their Catholic faith.

Racial/Ethnic Community and the Historical Experience of Persecution

As reflected in these family stories, maintaining a strong connection with a racial or ethnic community seems to promote religious identity and transmission across generations. We observe that the African American and Jewish families in this study have strong ethnic identities, in part because of their tight connection to their ethnic communities but also because of their historical experience as minority groups. Their sense of community is reinforced by their family religious experiences of going to their church or synagogue and sharing a strong religious, cultural, and racial or ethnic group consciousness. In the African American Johnson family, the G2 grandmother recalls how her parents went to "a Black church and most of our family was there, and everybody knew us and everything. Everybody knew us, because they were [there] at the beginning."

For the Jewish families in the study, maintaining a connection to the community is more about maintaining a cultural identity across generations. Jewish identity and a history of being Jewish across generations are a part of a "way of life" for many in these families. Describing his cultural background, a G2 Jewish man says, "I identified as being a cultural Jew . . .a person who has a Jewish perspective on life and the concept of paternity with people." He attributes his connection with cultural Judaism to his parents, who were connected to a Jewish community: "their best friends were all Jewish. They all spoke Yiddish."

A recurring theme that emerged from the interviews was the family's experience or deeply embedded memory of persecution, such as slavery and subsequent discrimination and exclusion, the Holocaust, the Japanese internment during World War II, and difficulties surrounding immigration and employment discrimination that continue to this day.

In the Lieberman and Goldman families, these events were personally experienced by the G1s and G2s because of their direct exposure to anti-Semitism or to the deaths of family members in the Holocaust. However, the

G3s and G4s in these families learned more about persecution and the Holocaust through family stories, from friends, and in school. A G3 woman in the Lieberman family said that being Jewish:

> was very important to [her] grandparents . . . [and] one of the reasons is because they lived, you know, and my mother, too actually—they lived through the wars . . .during a time where . . . [there was] a lot more anti-Semitism.

A G4 grandson comments on the way in which persecution influenced his family:

> They were alive during the Holocaust . . .[which] played a big role in shaping them . . .[which] ultimately rubs . . . shapes us in a way.

When a G2 in the African American Walker family married and moved to a different state, her racial experience in a church of the same denomination in which she grew up caused her to change her religious affiliation.

> When I went back East, the church was White, and they were all prejudiced Southerners, and so—even though I was living in New England, anybody from the Church of Christ is going to come from Texas or one of the southern states—they were very nice, there was not a problem; but I didn't feel about them the way I felt about the church. And so it was okay but it wasn't something I wanted to get up for on a Sunday morning.

She switched to the Protestant religion of her husband and mother-in-law, which she passed on to the next generations. This G2 grandmother's narrative illustrates the high relevance of racial background in the religious experience of members in this family, even as she changed to a church more welcoming to African Americans. Her change to what she described as a mixed-race congregation defined the trajectory of her children, grandchildren, and great-grandchildren. However, for the younger generations, the relevance of racial background relative to their religious experience became less direct than it was for the older generations. While most remained affiliated with the G2 grandmother's church, what has been passed on is the strong sense of family religious experience, reflected in frequent family rituals and celebrations during religious holidays.

Members of the African American Johnson family also spoke about their experiences of racism, saying that common involvement in their church provided both a buffer and a resource for coping with a difficult social environment. For some members, the significance of the family church has been strengthened because of their racial experience. A G3 daughter explains why her mother is so attached to their Black church. "It was one of the first churches where African Americans were accepted . . . so she has an attachment to that church because she grew up in that church."

The ethnic background of the Japanese American Yamamoto family was highly relevant for the G1 great-grandfather and his G2 son because of their experience in a Japanese internment camp during World War II. However, this experience of ethnic persecution later influenced the great-grandfather's strong encouragement of his son's American acculturation, which he saw as necessary in view of the anti-Japanese sentiment during World War II. The family lived in an area where there were very few Japanese, and Japanese cultural traditions were not encouraged in the absence of a Japanese American community. Because of the sociohistorical context, Japanese cultural identity was not relevant for the G2 son, and as a result he did not encourage an interest in Japanese culture among his G3 children and G4 grandchildren.

The Yamamoto family's experience of persecution is also linked to religion. In this case, being Protestant, the dominant religion in American culture, was perceived by the G1 great-grandfather as a means for his family members to earn respect as American citizens. Encouraged by his father, the G2 son attended a variety of Protestant churches with his friends during his adolescence. The lack of choice and opportunity that the G2 felt in his childhood because of his family's internment experience may have encouraged him to give his own G3 children much greater choice in their religious identity.

The older generations' need to assimilate to American culture through religious training—"being good citizens and just good people"—is not relevant to the G3 children and G4 grandchildren. They are removed from the G2's and G1's internment experience and no longer feel the same acculturation pressure to participate in institutionalized religious activity. The Japanese ethnic identity of the Yamamoto family has lost its relevance for the younger generations.

In the very close Garcia family, ethnic identity has become more important for the younger generations. A G4 grandson spoke about wanting to pass on to his children his values of cultural diversity, rooted in his racialized experiences and awareness of discrimination and prejudice. He wants his children to "view people beyond just the Black kid, the Chinese kid, the White kid." He said that he has learned from his experiences as a Hispanic male the value of not "[making] assumptions about people based on their appearance alone." He elaborated on these experiences of being judged based on his "brown skin pigmentation." Though a college graduate, he says,

> I'm still seen as a Hispanic male, first and foremost . . .all of which are tied to illegal immigration . . .not knowing how to speak English, and being janitors.

He hopes his children will be

> not [just] bilingual, but maybe even speak three languages . . .because it [would give] them more of an appreciation for the [Hispanic] culture.

This value is rooted in knowing that racism and discrimination had caused his parents to lose their Spanish language, and thus they were unable to pass the language on to him. He said that as a Hispanic, he internalized a certain mindset in terms of a work ethic and achievement, believing that he had to prove himself "more than anybody whose last name is Smith or Jones [in order] to be considered as equal." He identified himself as Mexican American, but "first and foremost" he is an American; he was born in the United States and has more emotional ties to the United States than to Mexico. However, he clarified that he and his family are certainly "not vanilla" because they are culturally a "big mix."

Discussion and Conclusion

For many of the families in this study, ethnic and religious identities have retained a certain affinity and interconnectedness across generations such that they jointly foster the intergenerational transmission of a religious tradition.

While all the families in the study are ethnic minorities (African American, Hispanic, Jewish American, Asian American, and Italian American), they differ in the degree to which their racial or ethnic identities remain relevant down the generations and over time, and in the ways these identities intersect with and find expression in family religious beliefs and practices. For the African American, Hispanic, and Jewish families, their racial and ethnic identities have not only been retained but have become more relevant for the younger G4 generation (for Hispanic ethnic groups, see Markides, Angel, and Peek, Chapter 15). The stories of the African American Walker and Johnson families in this study are similar in that their family histories are so intertwined with Black churches in their communities.

For the Lieberman and Goldman families, their ethnic identity also retains its relevance across generations, although in a different way. In these two Jewish families, ethnic and religious identities are so closely intertwined as to be almost indistinguishable (except for the few Orthodox Jews in our study). In both families, the religious Jewish experience evolves over the generations. In the Goldman family (but not in the Lieberman family), the older generations identify closely with Judaism as a religion, but for the younger generations Judaism is a cultural identity.

Our analysis confirms the significance of formal religious education in the process of transmitting religious affiliation. We also found important nuances in the religious socialization process, especially regarding parents' individual religious involvement, or its lack, and the quality of their relationships with their children. Intergenerational relationships and the quality of parent-child relations are essential conduits for the transmission of a religious tradition.

There is no single religious transmission pathway or pattern. For the Sabelli and Yamamoto families, tracing the racial ethnic and cultural influences of the oldest generations down the family lineages is complicated as these influences intersect and influence family religious values and practices. The Yamamoto family displays low religious continuity across generations and provides an example of changing religious practice as a product of changing sociohistorical experiences. Acculturation pressures experienced in the anti-Japanese climate of World War II prompted the first and second generations' practice of Protestantism, but this faded away for later generations. The family's Japanese American identity weakens as younger generations intermarry and divorce occurs. Nevertheless, family memory of their ethnic heritage has not been lost; the first and second generations' internment story was passed down to the third and fourth generations.

The picture is more complex with the Sabelli family. As with many immigrant groups, their Catholicism was almost synonymous with being Italian. But across time, this tight ethnic-religious coupling weakens, buffeted by societal changes, such as high rates of divorce and remarriage and an ethic of expressive individualism urging parents to allow their children to chose their own religion, if any. In the G2 grandparents' generation, both the Sabelli and Yamamoto families experienced marital instability and divorce as well as increasing interethnic and interfaith marriage.

Not surprisingly, we found religious switching in this study of ethnic families (although to a lesser degree than what we have observed in the White families in our larger study). Religious switching seems to be precipitated by religious disillusionment; a crisis or turning point, often divorce; and "lousy" parent-child relationships. More likely than not, a family's strong sense of ethnic identity will favor continuity of a religious tradition across generations.

The divergent religious transmission pathways of siblings are significant. We see this in the Sabelli family, where one sibling line retains its strong traditional allegiance to the Catholic faith even as the other sibling line has weak religious allegiance. Although the sibling lines stem from the same ethnic background, the relevance of ethnicity for religious affiliation transmission also varies. We know too little about the religious transmission patterns of these lateral relationship lineages in multigenerational families. New research directions should focus on examining sibling differences in religious transmission. What are the precipitating conditions? Does childhood sibling rivalry or parental favoritism play a role?

Religious transmission across generations is complex. In this research we sought not to generalize about the transmission of religion across generations in ethnic minority families but to discover some of the ways ethnicity might matter for religious transmission over time and to reveal some of the nuances and meanings of transmission patterns. What we observed suggests that the study of religion and ethnicity in multigenerational families offers promising opportunities for expanding our knowledge of religious influence across generations.

ACKNOWLEDGMENTS

The authors are indebted to the leadership and guidance of Vern L. Bengtson, who served as the principal investigator of the Longitudinal Study of Generations as well as the Transmission of Religion across Generations study on which this research is based. They also wish to express their gratitude to The Templeton Foundation for its generous support of the Transmission of Religion across Generations study.

REFERENCES

Bengtson, V. L., Biblarz, T. J., & Roberts, R. E. L. (2002). *How families still matter: A longitudinal study of youth in two generations.* New York: Cambridge University Press.

Cadge, W., & Davidman, L. (2006). Ascription, choice, and the construction of religious identities in the contemporary United States. *Journal for the Scientific Study of Religion, 45,* 23–38.

Cadge, W., & Ecklund, E. H. (2007). Immigration and religion. *The Annual Review of Sociology, 33*, 17.1–17.21.

Dashefsky, A., Lazerwitz, B., & Tabory, E. (2003). The journeys of the "straight way" or the "roundabout path": Jewish identity in the U.S. and Israel. In M. Dillon (Ed.), *Handbook of the sociology of religion* (pp. 240–260). New York: Cambridge University Press

Dillon, M., & Wink, P. (2007). *In the course of a lifetime: Tracing religious beliefs, practice, and change.* Berkeley, CA: University of California Press.

Dowd, J., & Bengtson, V. L. (1978). Aging in minority populations: An examination of the double jeopardy hypothesis. *Journal of Gerontology, 33*, 427–436.

Ebaugh, H. R. (2003). Religion and the new immigrants. In M. Dillon (Ed.), *Handbook of the sociology of religion* (pp. 225–239). New York: Cambridge University Press

Edgell, P. (2006). *Religion and family in a changing society.* Princeton, NJ: Princeton University Press.

Garces-Foley, K. (2008). Comparing Catholic and evangelical integration efforts. *Journal for the Scientific Study of Religion, 47*, 17–22.

Glass, J., Bengtson, V. L., & Dunham, C. (1986). Attitude similarity in three-generation families: Socialization, status inheritance or reciprocal influence? *American Sociological Review, 51*, 685–698.

Gonzales, A. M. (2007). Determinants of parent-child coresidence among older Mexican parents: The salience of cultural values. *Sociological Perspectives, 50*, 561–570.

Herberg, W. (1960). *Protestant, Catholic, Jew: An essay in American religious sociology* (2nd ed.). Garden City, NY: Doubleday.

Hill, T. D., Angel, J. L., Ellison, C. G., & Angel, R. J. (2005). Religious attendance and mortality: An eight-year follow-up of older Mexican Americans. *Journal of Gerontology: Social Sciences, 60B*, S201–S109.

Hout, M., & Fischer, C. S. (2002). Why more Americans have no religious preference: Politics and generations. *American Sociological Review, 65*, 165–190.

King, V., & Elder, G. H. Jr. (1999). Are religious grandparents more involved grandparents? *Journal of Gerontology: Social Sciences, 54*, S317–S328

Landale, N. S., & Oropesa, R. S. (2007). Hispanic families: Stability and change. *American Review of Sociology, 33*, 18.1–18.25.

Lincoln, C. R., & Mamiya, L. (1990). *The Black church in the African American experience.* Durham, NC: Duke University Press.

Marti, G. (2006). Fluid ethnicity and ethnic transcendence in multiracial churches. *Journal for the Scientific Study of Religion, 47*, 11–16.

McAdoo, H. P., Martinez, E. A., & Hughes, H. (2005). Ecological changes in ethnic families of color. In V. L. Bengtson, A. Acock, K. Allen, P. Dilworth-Anderson, & D. Klein (Eds.), *Sourcebook of family theory & research* (pp. 191–212). Thousand Oaks, CA: Sage.

Min, P. G., & Kim, D. Y. (2005). Intergenerational transmission of religion and culture: Korean Protestants in the U.S. *Sociology of Religion, 66*, 263–282.

Myers, S. M. (1996). An interactive model of religiosity inheritance: The importance of family context. *American Sociological Review, 61,* 858–866.

Park, J. Z., & Ecklund, E. H. (2007). Negotiating continuity: Family and religious socialization for second-generation Asian Americans. *The Sociological Quarterly, 48,* 93–118.

Pattillo-McCoy, M. (1998). Church culture as a strategy of action in the Black community. *American Sociological Review, 63,* 757–784.

Pearce, L. D., & Thornton, A. (2007). Religious identity and family ideologies in the transition to adulthood. *Journal of Marriage and the Family, 69,* 1227–1243.

Pew Forum on Religion & Public Life. (2007). *Changing faiths: Latinos and the transformation of American religion.* Retrieved October 28, 2008 (http://pewforum.org/surveys/hispanic).

Pew Forum on Religion & Public Life. (2008). *U.S. religion landscape survey.* Retrieved February 25, 2008 (http://pewforum.org/reports).

Roof, W. C. (1999). *Spiritual marketplace: Baby boomers and the remaking of American religion.* Princeton, NJ: Princeton University Press.

Sarkisian, N., Gerena, M., & Gerstel, N. (2007). Extended family integration among Euro and Mexican Americans: Ethnicity, gender and class. *Journal of Marriage and the Family, 69,* 40–54.

Sherkat, D. E. (1998). Counterculture or continuity? Competing influences on baby boomers' religious orientations and participation. *Social Forces, 76,* 1087–1114.

Smith, C., & Denton, M. (2005). *Soul searching: The religious and spiritual lives of American teenagers.* New York: Oxford University Press.

Stolzenberg, R., Blair-Loy, M., & Waite, L. J. (1995). Religious participation in early adulthood: Age and family life cycle effects on church membership. *American Sociological Review, 60,* 84–103.

U.S. Bureau of the Census. (2004). Census bureau projects tripling of Hispanic and Asian populations in 50 years; Non-Hispanic Whites may drop to half of total population. March 18. CB04-44. Retrieved September 7, 2009 (http://www.census.gov/Press-Release/www/releases/archives/population/001720.html).

Warner, R. S. (2005). *A church of our own. Disestablishment and diversity in American religion.* New Brunswick, NJ: Rutgers University Press.

Wittberg, P. (1999). Families and religions. In M. B. Sussman, S. K. Steinmetz, & G. W. Peterson (Eds.), *Handbook of marriage and the family* (2nd ed., pp. 503–523). New York: Plenum Press.

CHAPTER ELEVEN

Church-Based Negative Interactions among Older African Americans, Caribbean Blacks, and Non-Hispanic Whites

Karen D. Lincoln, Linda M. Chatters, and
Robert Joseph Taylor

There is a long history of research and scholarship on the importance of family and religion in the lives of African Americans (Billingsley, 1992, 1999; Hill, 1999; Taylor, Chatters, & Levin, 2004; Taylor, Jackson, & Chatters, 1997), and an emerging literature has begun to investigate the intersection of religion and family (Chatters & Taylor, 2006). One major intersection between religion and family is found in research examining family and church-based informal social support networks (Chatters, Taylor, Lincoln, & Schroepfer, 2002; Krause, 2002; Taylor, Lincoln, & Chatters, 2005). This work indicates that church members are an integral component of the social support networks of many older African Americans. However, increased interaction with any social group has both positive and negative consequences. Involvement in both families and churches is important for receiving social support, but it can also be associated with negative social interactions involving criticism, gossip, and other types of interpersonal conflict. This particular type of conflict is especially important because it involves interactions with members of an individual's social support network and has been shown to have adverse effects on health and well-being in late life (Lincoln, 2007; Mavandadi, Rook, & Newsom, 2007; Newsom, Nishishiba, Morgan, & Rook,

2003; Newsom, Rook, Nishishiba, Sorkin, & Mahan, 2005; Sorkin & Rook, 2006).

Although there is a fairly developed literature on negative interactions with family members, there is very little information on negative interaction with church members. Further, very limited attention has been paid to negative interactions involving social networks among racial and ethnic minority older adults. Accordingly, the goal of the present study is to examine the relationships among demographic factors, church involvement, and church-based negative interaction among a nationally representative sample of African American, Caribbean Black, and Non-Hispanic White older adults.

Race, Ethnicity, and Religious Participation

Religion plays an important role in the lives of Americans, particularly older adults and African Americans. These two groups have high rates of religious involvement across a variety of indicators including religious service attendance, church membership, and prayer. Recent investigations of religious participation have examined differences and similarities in religious participation for older African Americans, Black Caribbeans, and Non-Hispanic Whites. Both older Black Caribbeans and African Americans have high rates of religious involvement and report higher levels of religious involvement compared to older Non-Hispanic Whites (Taylor, Chatters, & Jackson, 2007a). These initial comparisons suggest that race is more important than ethnicity in patterning religious participation among older adults. That is to say, older African Americans and Caribbean Blacks were similar to one another in their religious involvement profiles, and both groups were different from Non-Hispanic Whites. However, a number of interesting differences distinguish African American and Black Caribbean older adults with respect to religious participation. Although older Black Caribbeans display levels of attendance, nonorganizational religious activity (e.g., prayer, reading religious materials), and subjective religiosity (e.g., perceived importance of religiosity) that are comparable to African Americans, they are less likely to be official members of a church, to ask others to pray for them, and to have distinctive denominational profiles (i.e., Caribbean Blacks are more likely to identify as Episcopalian, Pentecostal, and Catholic) (Taylor, Chatters, & Jackson, 2007a,b).

Negative Interaction in Church-Based Networks

Due to the high levels of religious service attendance among older adults, especially African Americans, church members are an important aspect of their social support networks (Chatters, Taylor, Lincoln, & Schroepfer, 2002; Krause, 2002; Taylor & Chatters, 1986, 1988). An emerging body of research indicates that church members provide both emotional support and tangible assistance (such as running errands or providing transportation) to older adults. Church members may be a particularly important source of assistance for older individuals without family members in close proximity (Chatters, Taylor, Lincoln, & Schroepfer, 2002). While church-based support may contribute to positive health outcomes, Ellison and Levin (1998) note that involvement in church-based networks may also be associated with negative social interactions that adversely impact health and well-being (see Krause, Ellison, & Wulff, 1998; Krause & Wulff, 2005). For example, church networks may make excessive demands on members' time, resources, and energy. Continued unequal or unreciprocated support exchanges may lead members to perceive that they are being taken advantage of and are unappreciated. Further, participation in church networks may expose members to judgment, criticism, and negative sanctions directed at personal behaviors, actions, and life circumstances that are deemed to be at odds with religious teachings and doctrines. Possible adverse consequences of negative social interactions include low psychological well-being (Krause, Ellison, & Wulff, 1998), anxiety, and mood disorder episodes (Bertera, 2005; Zlotnick, Kohn, Keitner, & Grotta, 2000).

An emerging body of research provides a detailed examination of the nature of negative interactions in church settings and between church members. In a focus group study of older White and Black adults, Krause and colleagues (Krause, Morgan, Chatters, & Meltzer, 2000) identified three major areas of interpersonal conflict among church members: (1) conflict over religious doctrine, policy, or religious teachings, (2) conflict between church members and their pastors, and (3) conflict between fellow congregants. Conflict over religious doctrine typically involved major issues in contemporary religion such as abortion, the role of women in the family, and the role of gays and lesbians in churches. General conflict involving church members included problematic interpersonal behaviors and social interactions such as gossiping and the development of cliques and church factions. Taylor, Chatters, and Levin (2004,

Chapter 7) conducted a focus group study of African American adults which investigated negative interaction among church members. Focus group participants noted the presence of a number of problematic interactions among church members, including interpersonal conflict, jealousy, and envy. However, they also stated that these kinds of problems should be expected in any social organization or group. For instance, two participants noted:

- "Well, I think with churches, with family, you are always going to have conflict. I think, in our church, some of the things we've seen are probably not unnatural."
- "They talk about people and they get into other people's business. They do what human people do, you know, and it's normal" (Taylor, Chatters, & Levin, 2004, p. 174).

Probably the most frequently mentioned form of negative interaction was gossip. Focus group participants noted that gossip caused a tremendous amount of strife in churches and made it difficult for people to grow and rebound from mistakes they had made in the past. Many of the focus group members noted that they actively tried to avoid gossip. Several African American participants noted how they tried not to engage in gossip (p. 176):

- "I don't want to—I really don't like to take in a lot of negative things, and I stay away from people that feed a lot of negative stuff, because, you know, that stuff, it gets into your spirit."
- "I came here to praise and worship God. I didn't come for—to know who's pregnant or who's doing this and doing that."
- "I don't want to know. I don't want to know who did this and who done that and why they did what they did. I tell my wife the same thing all the time, you know. Why you want to hear something if it ain't going to benefit you, me, our family, it's not going to do anything for us?"

In addition to gossip, focus group members mentioned several other types of conflict involving issues of power and authority, seniority within the church, responsibilities, and duties. These problematic interactions include disputes during church board meetings, conflicts between recent and long-term members of the church, and conflict during special church programs and events such as Women's Day. Several focus group participants discussed issues of church climate and instances in which church members were aloof and made them feel unwelcome. In particular, focus group participants noted that people were made to feel unwelcome in churches because of their clothing, hair styles, and class or lifestyle differences.

Negative interactions like gossip and conflict are important because research has proven that negative interactions are associated with lower levels of life satisfaction, happiness, self-esteem, and other indicators of psychological well-being (Lincoln, 2007; Lincoln, Chatters, & Taylor, 2005; Lincoln, Chatters, Taylor, & Jackson, 2007). Negative interactions are also associated with physical health problems such as higher rates of heart disease (Krause, 2005), heightened physiological reactivity (King, Atienza, Castro, & Collins, 2002), susceptibility to infectious disease (Cohen, Doyle, Skoner, Rabin, & Gwaltney, 1997), declines in physical functioning (Seeman & Chen, 2002), and mortality (Tanne, Goldbourt, & Medalie, 2004). In fact, because they are unexpected, negative interactions have a stronger impact on outcomes than do positive, supportive interactions (Rook & Pietromonaco, 1987). Although the vast majority of this research on negative interaction focuses on family and friends, an emerging body of work examines the damaging effects of negative interaction with church members on mental health. For instance, Krause, Ellison, & Wulff (1998) found that negative interaction from church members decreases psychological well-being. Overall, findings from these studies confirm that involvement in church networks is associated with both positive and negative social interactions (Krause, Morgan, Chatters, & Meltzer, 2000), and negative interactions, in turn, have consequences for health and well-being outcomes (Krause, Ellison, & Wulff, 1998; Krause & Wulff, 2005).

Theoretical Perspectives on Social Interactions in Churches

Prior work on church-based networks has been informed by conceptual frameworks and research on social networks and social support (Chatters, 2000; Idler & George, 1998). However, particular features of religious institutions deserve special attention when investigating social interactions in these settings. First, as alluded to earlier, because they are explicitly religious settings, social interactions within churches carry particular import as representing idealized norms and expectations for interpersonal behaviors (e.g., the golden rule, prohibitions against idle gossip), and social relationships relate to a number of different social roles (e.g., fellow congregant, coworker, neighbor, spouse). Furthermore, African American churches possess a group or collectivist orientation (Krause, 2003; Lincoln & Mamiya, 1990) which emphasizes concern for the common welfare of the congregation and strong norms for providing assistance to others. Given high expectations for appropriate codes of conduct, departures from expected norms for interpersonal behaviors (i.e., negative social interactions) may be particularly disconcerting and harmful to the individual. Second, as a social setting, churches in general and African American churches in particular share many functional similarities to families (Chatters & Taylor, 2006). Identification and involvement with one's church is often couched in terms of a family's history with the church as founding or pivotal members of the congregation. Consequently, involvement with religious institutions can span the life course of the individual and encompass several generations within a family. As such, churches often constitute what has been termed a "support convoy" (Kahn & Antonucci, 1981) that accompanies individuals as they face both major and minor life experiences and transitions (e.g., marriage, births, illness, death). Given the noted similarities between families and churches, this study of negative social interactions within religious communities uses relevant theoretical and conceptual models from research on family and intergenerational relations (Taylor, Lincoln, & Chatters, 2005).

Family Solidarity

The first framework considered here is the family solidarity model (Landecker, 1951; Nye & Rushing, 1969), or the intergenerational solidarity paradigm (Bengtson, Giarrusso, Mabry, & Silverstein, 2002). The family solidarity model is characterized by six core constructs of family relations—affectual, consensual, functional, associational, structural, and normative solidarity— each of which reflects a dialectic of family function, structure, and process (Bengtson, Giarrusso, Mabry, & Silverstein, 2002). The six solidarity constructs allow for an assessment of family behaviors and attitudes with respect to closeness to or distance from one another (affectual), dependency vs. autonomy (functional), integration vs. isolation (associational), agreement vs. dissent (consensual), opportunities vs. barriers (structural), and familism vs. individualism (normative).

Several of these core dimensions of the family solidarity model (e.g., affectual, functional, associational, and normative solidarity) are similarly reflected in the processes and structure of African American religious congregations and have been examined in relation to Black churches (Taylor, Lincoln, & Chatters, 2005). For example, similar to findings from studies on Black family networks, perceptions of closeness to church members and degree of interaction with church members were related to one another (i.e., perceived closeness is positively associated with level of interaction), and both closeness and interaction were independently associated with increased support from church members (Taylor, Lincoln, & Chatters, 2005). Overall, church-based networks embodied several core constructs of the family solidarity model, including high levels of emotional closeness (affectual solidarity), frequent interaction (associational solidarity), and significant amounts of received church support (functional solidarity). Similar to relationships observed in family networks, higher levels of integration (affectual and associational solidarity) in church-based support networks were positively associated with receiving assistance (functional solidarity) from these networks.

Family Ambivalence

The ambivalence perspective (Connidis & McMullin, 2002) focuses explicit attention on issues of difference and conflict in family relations. The basic tenets of the ambivalence perspective are that (1) conflict is inherent in all social relations, (2) family relationships are characterized by ambivalence, (3) ambivalence is associated with structured social relationships in which specific groups are privileged, and (4) individuals are active participants in negotiating and resolving ambivalence. Like other social organizations, religious institutions embody structured social relationships in which particular groups are privileged, which, in turn, gives rise to ambivalent relationships and conflict (Krause, Ellison, & Wulff, 1998; Krause, Morgan, Chatters, & Meltzer, 2000). Interpersonal conflicts with church members can involve the structured social relationships and privileged positions associated with differences in gender, socioeconomic status, and church seniority (Krause, Morgan, Chatters, & Meltzer, 2000).

In sum, constructs from both the family solidarity paradigm and the intergenerational ambivalence perspective inform the present study. African American churches closely identify with and incorporate distinctive family structures, functions, and processes that embody and reproduce the roles, relationships, and statuses that are characteristic of family. The intergenerational solidarity paradigm's focus on various dimensions of family relations (e.g., affectual, functional, associational, and normative solidarity) is well suited as a framework for exploring the character of interpersonal interactions and relations among church members. Similarly, the intergenerational ambivalence perspective's particular focus on structured social relations as a source of difference and conflict is an apt framework for capturing noted status differences (e.g., seniority, social class, and gender) that exist within African

American churches and appear to underlie instances of negative social interactions.

Purpose of the Study

The present study examines negative interactions with church members within a sample of older African Americans, Caribbean Blacks, and Non-Hispanic Whites. This investigation uses constructs from both the intergenerational solidarity paradigm and the ambivalence perspective to examine church-based negative interaction. Our purpose is to examine church-based negative interactions within and across these three groups of respondents and empirically identify subpopulations of individuals that are homogeneous for a given set of demographic and religious involvement characteristics. Several independent factors that characterize religious participation (i.e., attendance) and church relationships (i.e., emotional closeness, support, and contact) are examined while controlling for the effects of demographic factors that have known associations with religious involvement (e.g., age, education, poverty status, gender, marital status, and region). Our specific focus is on how relational aspects of church-based networks—specifically, select constructs identified in the family solidarity paradigm (i.e., reported closeness, support, and contact)—are associated with church-based negative interactions within and across the three race-ethnicity groupings.

Methods
Sample

This analysis utilizes the National Survey of American Life (NSAL) dataset to identify profiles of church-based negative interaction among older adults. The present analyses are based on complete data for 1,095 African American, Caribbean Black, and Non-Hispanic White respondents (55+ years). The average age is 66.67 years, and approximately 60% of the respondents are women. Approximately 44% of respondents are African American (e.g., U.S.-born Blacks of non-Caribbean descent), 2.8% are Caribbean Black, and 53% are Non-Hispanic White adults. Approximately 60% of respondents live in the South, 51.4% are married, the average number of years of education is 12.25 years, and 14.3% of respondents have incomes below poverty (these figures are based on weighted frequency distributions).

The National Survey of American Life: Coping with Stress in the 21st Century was collected by the Program for Research on Black Americans at the University of Michigan's Institute for Social Research. The field work for the study was completed by the Institute for Social Research's Survey Research Center in cooperation with the Program for Research on Black Americans. The NSAL includes the first major probability sample of Caribbean Blacks ever conducted. For the purposes of this study, Caribbean Blacks are defined as persons who trace their ethnic heritage to a Caribbean country but now reside in the United States, who are racially classified as Black, and who are English-speaking (but may also speak another language).

The NSAL sample has a national multistage probability design. The interviews were face-to-face and conducted within respondents' homes. Respondents were compensated for their time. The data collection was conducted from 2001 to 2003. A total of 6,082 interviews were conducted with persons aged 18 and older, including 3,570 African Americans, 1,621 Blacks of Caribbean descent ("Caribbean Blacks"), and 891 Non-Hispanic Whites. The overall response rate was 72.3%; 70.7% for African Americans, 77.7% for Caribbean Blacks, and 69.7% for Non-Hispanic Whites. This response rate is excellent when considering that African Americans (especially lower-income African Americans) and Black Caribbeans are more likely to reside in major urban areas which are more difficult and much more expensive for conducting interviews. Final response rates for the NSAL two-phase sample designs were computed using the American Association of Public Opinion Research guidelines (AAPOR, 2006).

The Black Caribbean sample was selected from two area probability sampling frames: the core NSAL sample and an area probability sample of housing units from geographic areas with a relatively high density of persons of Caribbean descent (more than 10% of the population). Of the total Black Caribbean respondents (n = 1,621), 265 respondents were selected from the households in the core sample and 1,356 were selected from housing units from high-density Caribbean areas (see Heeringa et al., 2004, and Jackson et al., 2004, for a more detailed discussion of the NSAL sample). Caribbean Blacks reported over 25 different countries of origin, which were characterized as Spanish-speaking Caribbean countries (e.g., Puerto Rico, Dominican Republic, or Cuba), English-speaking Caribbean countries (e.g., Jamaica, Barbados, or Trinidad & Tobago), and Haiti.

In both the African American and Black Caribbean samples, it was necessary for respondents to self-identify their race as Black. Those self-identifying as Black were included in the Black Caribbean sample if (1) they answered affirmatively when asked if they were of West Indian or Caribbean descent, (2) they said they were from a country included on a list of Caribbean area countries presented by the interviewer, or (3) they indicated that their parents or grandparents were born in a Caribbean area country. All study procedures were approved by the Institutional Review Board of the University of Michigan.

Measures

Church-based negative interaction was assessed by respondents' perceived frequency of negative interactions with their fellow church members. Church-based negative interaction is measured by an index of three items. Respondents were asked: (1) "How often do the people in your church make too many demands on you?" (2) "How often do the people in your church criticize you and the things you do?" and (3) "How often do the people in your church try to take advantage of you?" The response categories for these questions were "very often," "fairly often," "not too often," and "never." Higher values on this index indicate more frequent negative interaction with church members. Cronbach's alpha for this three-item index is 0.72 for African Americans, 0.65 for Caribbean Blacks, and 0.66 for Non-Hispanic Whites.

Church attendance was assessed by asking respondents, "How often do you usually attend religious services?" The response categories for this question were "very often," "fairly often," "not too often," and "never." Higher values on this variable indicate more frequent church attendance. *Subjective closeness* to church members was measured by asking respondents "How close are you to the people in your church? Would you say very close, fairly close, not too close or not close at all?" Higher values on this item indicate higher levels of closeness to church members. *Size of helper network* assessed the number of church members whom respondents indicate as potential providers of social support. Respondents were asked, "How many people in your church (place of worship) would help you out if you needed help?" The response category for this question was continuous and ranged from 0 to 97 people. Response categories were recoded into an ordinal variable ranging from zero to four, with higher values indicating a larger helper network. *Contact with church members* assessed the frequency of interactions that respondents had with church members. Respondents were asked, "How often do you see, write, or talk on the telephone with members of your church (place of worship)? Would you say nearly every day, at least once a week, a few times a month, at least once a month, a few times a year, hardly ever or never?" Higher values on this item indicate more frequent contact with church members.

Finally, several demographic factors are included in this analysis including race (African American is the referent), age and education (measured continuously), poverty status (<100% is the referent), gender (0 = male; 1 = female), marital status (married is the referent), and region (0 = South; 1 = non-South).

Analysis Strategy

Descriptive analyses were conducted to examine the distribution of demographic and church involvement variables in the total sample. Table 11.1 presents the characteristics of the sample for the current investigation. We then conducted latent class analysis to classify the nature of church-based interaction in the sample. All analyses were weighted to account for unequal probabilities of selection, nonresponse, and post-stratification such that respondents are weighted in accordance with their numbers and proportions in the full population. In addition, all analyses accounted for the complex, multistage clustered design of the NSAL sample (i.e., clustering and stratification) when computing standard errors.

Latent Class Analysis

This study uses latent class analysis (LCA) to identify the nature of unobserved religious participation and church relationships among respondents. The LCA was accomplished using Mplus version 5.1. LCA characterizes the independent action of multiple church involvement features from a single respondent. Unlike variable-centered approaches (e.g., regression or factor analysis) that independently model church involvement variables across all respondents, LCA is a "person-centered" approach designed to divide the population under study into a set of latent subpopulations that share a distinct, interpretable pattern of relationships among the indicators (Meiser & Ohrt, 1996). Because membership in the subpopulation is generally unknown to the researcher, a latent categorical variable (composed of "classes") is assumed to exist and inferred from the data. These classes represent subgroups of individuals who are similar to each other on the variables entered into the analysis and different from individuals in the other subgroups. LCA identifies the fewest number of mutually exclusive, homogeneous classes of persons based on the pattern of individual characteristics (McCutcheon, 1987).

We performed LCA to identify classes of individuals based on their demographic profiles, religious participation, and characterization of church involvement. This technique capitalizes on the associations between the variables entered in the model, allowing researchers to see how they operate together

Table 11.1. Characteristics of the sample (n = 1,512)[1]

Variable	African American (n = 837)		Caribbean Black (n = 304)		Non-Hispanic White (n = 298)	
	Frequency	%	Frequency	%	Frequency	%
Sex						
Male	300	40.4	133	53.0	110	47.2
Female	537	59.6	171	47.0	188	52.8
Age						
55–64 years	384	46.3	153	47.2	132	47.0
65–74 years	301	36.9	98	36.1	101	31.6
75+ years	152	16.8	53	16.7	65	21.5
Poverty status						
Poor (<100%)	227	24.7	49	19.1	32	6.8
Near poor (100–199%)	249	26.6	74	24.5	80	22.3
Non-poor (200–399%)	213	26.7	98	26.2	103	36.8
Non-poor (400% or more)	146	21.8	83	30.2	82	34.0
Education						
Less than high school (<12 years)	360	31.7	91	29.7	70	34.3
High school (12 years)	254	38.2	96	34.7	110	24.6
Some college (13–15 years)	108	14.6	44	10.2	61	20.6
College or more (16+ years)	115	15.5	73	25.4	57	20.4
Marital status						
Married	252	39.5	134	55.0	113	50.4
Previously married	517	53.3	141	39.8	160	42.4
Never married	60	6.1	29	5.2	23	6.7
Region						
South	525	44.4	97	65.1	198	42.7
Non-south	312	55.6	207	34.9	100	57.3
Church attendance						
Very often	427	49.9	169	56.1	138	41.3
Fairly often	197	22.9	48	15.9	38	13.0
Never/not too often	213	27.2	87	28.0	122	45.7

to create classes. This is in contrast to variable-based models that use predictive approaches in which shared variance among the predictors allow only some to appear to be associated with the outcome, although in actuality they all may be. Multinomial logistic regression models were used to examine the associations between covariates and the latent classes. Finally, to examine the overall differences in characteristics among the classes, we used analysis of variance (ANOVA) for continuous variables and χ^2 tests for categorical variables. All tests of difference were performed in SPSS 15.0.

Variable	African American (n = 837)		Caribbean Black (n = 304)		Non-Hispanic White (n = 298)	
	Frequency	%	Frequency	%	Frequency	%
Contact						
Nearly every day	212	26.7	60	26.1	51	21.2
At least once a week	208	29.1	69	29.9	61	23.8
A few times a month	104	14.5	45	16.6	33	14.3
At least once a month	68	9.3	17	6.9	16	7.7
A few times a year	71	10.5	36	11.7	33	18.1
Never	68	9.9	30	8.7	29	14.9
Size of helper network						
None	36	5.0	13	3.4	15	10.3
1–5 people	202	30.0	102	34.2	36	20.3
6–10 people	156	22.3	49	20.7	40	17.0
11–20 people	117	17.1	28	26.2	33	15.4
21 people or more	167	25.7	33	15.4	81	37.0
Subjective closeness						
Very close	382	51.0	104	48.5	79	27.0
Fairly close	233	32.9	108	32.0	81	41.3
Not too close	74	10.5	37	17.1	36	17.9
Not close at all	40	5.5	10	2.4	27	13.7
Negative interaction						
Very often	17	2.1	4	2.3	1	0.4
Fairly often	73	10.2	28	9.5	11	5.8
Not too often	302	43.4	118	49.5	92	41.1
Never	337	44.3	109	38.6	119	52.8

[1] Weighted percentages

Results

Descriptive information (table 11A.1) indicates that African Americans, Caribbean Blacks, and Non-Hispanic Whites reported fairly low levels of church-based negative interaction. Approximately 44% of African Americans, 39% of Caribbean Blacks, and 53% of Non-Hispanic Whites indicated that they "never" experienced negative interaction with their church members, whereas 2.1% of African Americans, 2.3% of Caribbean Blacks, and 0.4% of Non-Hispanic Whites indicated experiencing negative interaction "very often."

Means of church-based behaviors are shown by race in figure 11.1. Caribbean Blacks and African Americans reported a significantly higher mean number of negative interactions than Non-Hispanic Whites. There were significant dif-

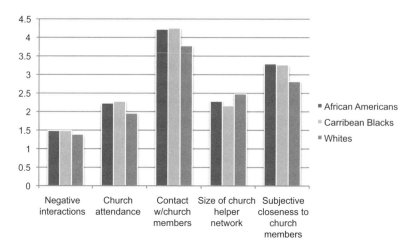

Figure 11.1. Mean church-based behaviors by race.

ferences in reported levels of subjective closeness to church members, size of helper network, contact with church members, and church attendance. African Americans and Caribbean Blacks reported stronger feelings of subjective closeness to church members, higher levels of contact with church members, and greater church attendance compared to their Non-Hispanic White counterparts. However, Non-Hispanic Whites reported having more church members who would provide social support compared to African Americans and Caribbean Blacks.

Model testing began with identifying the number of subpopulations (or "classes") needed to describe the data. The model was specified such that means and variances among the covariates were estimated within each class while the correlations between covariates were not estimated, thus specifying a latent class model. The number of latent classes is determined iteratively. An initial model with one class was specified, and then an increasing number of classes were added while examining the goodness-of-fit indices, interpretability of the results, and meaningfulness of the classes. The Bayesian Information Criterion, or BIC, values (Kass & Raftery, 1995; McLachlan & Peel, 2000) were used to determine the optimal number of classes for the best representation of the data, with smaller BIC values indicating improvement over the previous model with one less class. For the present study, the overall model selection is guided not only by BIC values but also by entropy indices, class sizes, and the interpretability of the classes, since the BIC criterion tends to favor models with fewer classes (Wiesner & Windle, 2004). Model selection was also guided by examining the reliability of the classifications via the estimated posterior probabilities of class membership for each individual (Muthén & Muthén, 2000). The precision of the classification can be assessed by how well respondents are classified into each class. A reliable classification will require the respondent to have posterior probabilities that are very high for belonging to a single class and very low for belonging to all other classes. Finally, the overall interpretability of the model based on class counts and substantive theory for model selection were considered.

Latent Class Enumeration and Class Differentiation

The three-class solution was determined to be optimal based on improvements in model fit and the ability of the three-class solution to identify well-differentiated classes and capture theoretically meaningful structures of church-based negative interaction. Estimated population-average probabilities of class membership for the three classes were derived from the model-based probabilities for all respondents to be in each class (each respondent has a probability of membership for each of the three classes that sums to 1.00). The average across-class probabilities were 0.930 for class one, 0.919 for class two, and 0.899 for class three, suggesting good definition of class membership. Accordingly, individuals in the sample have, on average, a relatively high probability of being a member of the class to which they were assigned. While there are no specific guidelines regarding acceptable probability levels for determining class membership, some have suggested that each class should differ from others with respect to at least one model parameter (Greenbaum, Del Boca, Darkes, Wang, & Goldman, 2005). The results from the present analysis meet these criteria. Overall, the probabilities associated with class assignment indicted that the classes were well differentiated.

The three derived latent classes were *low church involvement/low negative interaction* (n = 741), *high church involvement/high negative interaction* (n = 262), and *low church involvement/high negative interaction* (n = 92). As shown in figure 11.2, the low/low class is characterized by respondents who reported the least frequent experiences of church-based negative interaction and the lowest level of contact with church members compared to the other two latent classes. The high/high class is characterized by respondents with the highest level of church attendance, the highest level of contact with church members, and the highest level of subjective closeness to church members compared to their counterparts in the other two classes. Members of this class also had

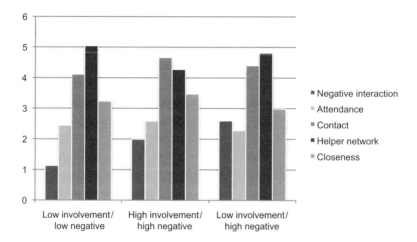

Figure 11.2. Latent class profile by church-based behaviors. *Note:* Size of helper network divided by four for scalability. Multiple group differences are statistically significant except size of helper network.

higher-than-average negative interaction. The low/high class is characterized by respondents who reported the most frequent experiences of church-based negative interaction compared to the other two latent classes. Members of this class also reported the lowest level of church attendance and the lowest level of subjective closeness to church members compared to their counterparts in the other two latent classes. (Socio-demographic differences across the classes are shown in table 11A.2 at the end of the chapter.)

Association with Latent Class Membership

Multinomial logistic regression analysis was performed to compare the latent classes with the set of covariates examined in the study, using the low church involvement/low negative interaction class as the reference group. These results (shown in table 11A.3) indicate that race, gender, poverty status, marital status, and region significantly differentiated the high/high and the low/high classes from the low/low class. The associations between race and latent class membership (independent of age, gender, education, poverty status, marital status, and living in the South) are shown as odds ratios in figure 11.3. Whites were more than two and a half times more likely than African Americans to be in the low/high class characterized by low levels of church involvement and more frequent negative church-based interaction, and they were less than half as likely as African Americans to be in the high/high group characterized by high involvement

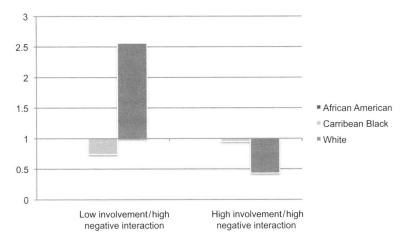

Figure 11.3. Odds ratios predicting latent class membership by race (low involvement/low negative interaction class is reference group).

and more negative interaction. Caribbean Blacks did not differ significantly from African Americans in their class membership.

Members of the low/high class were also more likely to be male, never married, under the poverty line, to reside in non-Southern regions of the United States, and less likely to be previously married. Members of the high/high class were more likely to be married than be previously married or never married.

Discussion

Research on social support typically focuses on social networks and support relations involving family, friends, and coworkers; comparatively few studies investigate church-based networks and interactions with church members. This is also true with regard to research on negative interaction: except for research by Krause (e.g., 2002, 2005), there is very little work on this topic. This analysis provided an in-depth examination of negative interaction within church settings among a national sample of older African Americans, Caribbean Blacks and Non-Hispanic Whites. Prior work in this area is based on a "variable-centered" approach in which independent variables are examined for their discrete relationships to a dependent factor. In contrast, the specific strength of latent class analysis is that it utilizes a "person-centered" approach whereby the population in question is divided into a set of latent subpopulations that share a distinct, interpretable pattern of relationships among the indicators (Meiser & Ohrt, 1996). LCA revealed several interesting relationships involving church-based negative interaction and church involvement that enhance our understanding of how these factors are related.

The analysis distinguished three distinct latent classes of church involvement and negative interaction. Study findings were largely consistent with prior research by Taylor, Chatters, and Jackson (2007a) on the demographic correlates of religious participation that identifies specific groups of respondents who display extensive (e.g., African Americans, women, Southern residents, married) vs. more limited (e.g., Whites, men, non-South resident, not married) involvement in religious networks. Present findings verified the presence of race effects on church-based behavior. Higher proportions of African Americans and Caribbean Blacks were represented in the latent class reflecting high involvement and high church-based conflict, suggesting a degree of social integration within a church context that is reminiscent of involuntary kinship relations. This suggests a tolerance of negative aspects of church participation, echoing work by Pargament and colleagues (1983) regarding racial differences in church climate and interaction.

Non-Hispanic Whites demonstrated lower intensity (of simultaneously positive *and* negative) religious involvement than African Americans, a pattern consistent with prior findings for race differences in religious involvement (Taylor, Chatters, & Jackson, 2007a) and specifically research on church networks (Krause, 2002) and congregational climate (Pargament et al., 1983). Notably, African Americans and Caribbean Blacks were no different from one another, indicating that race differences were more important than ethnicity with regard to latent class membership (Taylor, Chatters, & Jackson, 2007a).

Findings for marital status were somewhat mixed. Prior research indicates that married African Americans display higher levels of church involvement (Taylor, Chatters, & Levin, 2004), suggesting that because marriage is formally endorsed by the church, being married is a privileged status that provides a link to networks within religious settings. Persons who are divorced, on the other hand, generally have lower levels of participation in church networks, potentially due to stigma associated with being divorced. Further, among divorced persons, involvement in religious networks may be accompanied by negative interactions such as gossip and social isolation (Taylor, Chatters, & Levin, 2004; Taylor, Chatters, & Jackson, 2007a). The present findings indicated that a high proportion of married individuals were represented in the low/high profile, partially supporting prior work stressing the integrative functions of marriage; the high proportion of never-marrieds in the low/low class (and the low proportion of marrieds) may suggest that never-marrieds are tenuously connected to church networks and consequently have a low risk for negative interactions.

However, the relatively high proportion of marrieds in the low/high group suggests that because married persons have a spousal relationship that constitutes a source of social support and contact, they may choose to moderate their involvement in problematic church networks and thus have low levels of church involvement. This is reminiscent of depictions of churches as greedy and intrusive institutions which, while providing significant resources, make substantial demands of time and effort, encroach on members' privacy, and often censure attitudes and behaviors that are deemed unacceptable (Ellison & Levin, 1998; Taylor, Chatters, & Levin, 2004).

Interpreting study findings from a substantive perspective requires us to think about what the derived classes of religious involvement and negative interaction potentially mean in relation to respondents' status characteristics as well as the nature of their associations within church settings. Latent class analysis provided specific patterns of demographic factors, religious participation, and characterizations of church involvement, allowing us to understand how the variables operate together to form distinct classes within this sample of older adults. The findings were largely consistent with prior research using traditional, variable-centered analysis approaches in indicating that groups that are unique in their religious experiences (e.g., high levels of religious involvement) were more likely to be associated with classes that embodied that distinctiveness. Using prior information about religious involvement and church-based negative interaction, we can offer several speculations about what these latent classes might mean in terms of the "natural history" of involvement with church networks.

The classes may represent differing levels of church involvement or "investments" (i.e., attendance, closeness, contact, helper network size) as well as related disadvantages or "costs" (i.e., demands, criticisms, being taken advantage of) that are associated with involvement in church networks. The high/high class may indicate that both high investments and high costs are part and parcel of being associated with these church networks for a particular subpopulation of older adults. For example, African American church networks have been characterized as providing extensive forms of emotional and instrumental support to members as well as having a warm, congenial and expressive congregational climate. As such, they embody high support environments with close interdependent relations, but these relations could encroach on privacy and become a source of conflict. In contrast, church networks characterized by more tenuous attachments and investments may result in fewer problematic interactions. Finally, lower levels of commitment and investment may be either the cause or consequence of experiences of negative interactions (e.g., too many demands, being taken advantage of, or criticism) within church networks. This may be the case with never-married persons who anticipate lower levels of connections to these networks and preemptively limit their investments in church networks (e.g., fewer people in helper network, lower subjective closeness), which results in negative interactions. Alternatively, never-marrieds may voluntarily curtail their involvement in church networks (e.g., reduce attendance and contact with members) after having experienced negative interactions.

Finally, this study of relational aspects of church-based networks and negative interactions within and across the three race-ethnicity groupings indicated that core constructs of the family solidarity paradigm (e.g., affectual, associational, functional) were important for differentiating distinct classes of church involvement and negative interaction that coupled significant investments in religious pursuits and identities (e.g., contact, closeness, available helpers) with apparent costs in terms of interpersonal relations (e.g., criticism, being taken advantage of, too many demands). As such, respondents in this class may be involved in church networks that most closely approximate the nature of interpersonal relationships in families. Curiously, no class emerged with a profile of high involvement and low conflict, suggesting that negative interactions may be unavoidable when investment in church activities is high and raising the intriguing possibility that conflict may serve an integrative purpose in church life.

Conclusion

The majority of older adults are involved in social networks in religious settings, although to varying degrees. The findings from this study generated heterogeneous groups of individuals in the population based on patterns of religious involvement. Three unique subpopulations have demonstrated that there are differences in average involvement, or patterns within the older adult population. The use of a latent variable approach identified two high-negative-interaction classes that are quite distinct demographically and with respect to their levels of church involvement. This variation would suggest that even low levels of church involvement may be associated with negative outcomes.

Findings from the current study illuminate the merits of investigating a wide range of church involvement indicators to identify whether some types of activities for particular subpopulations of older adults are more beneficial or detrimental to their social relationships within church settings compared to other types. Findings also empirically highlight heterogeneity among the older adult population as represented by the various compositions of the latent classes. This heterogeneity is important to consider when investigating the influence of religious involvement on the social relationships of older adults and how these relationships might impact health and well-being.

APPENDIX

Table 11A.1. Comparison of mean characteristics by race

	African American (n = 616)	Caribbean Black (n = 41)	Non-Hispanic White (n = 855)	ANOVA test for overall difference	
	Mean	Mean	Mean	F-statistic	P value
Negative interaction	1.4887	1.4906	1.3907	18.228	0.000
Education	11.55	12.03	12.52	17.550	0.000
Age	66.63	65.89	66.82	0.285	0.752
Church attendance	2.2271	2.2813	1.9567	17.336	0.000
Contact	4.2254	4.2547	3.7757	10.276	0.000
Size of helper network	2.2854	2.1604	2.4838	3.325	0.036
Subjective closeness	3.2939	3.2658	2.8174	38.943	0.000
	Proportion %	Proportion %	Proportion %	χ^2 test for overall difference χ^2	P value
Marital status					
Married	39.9	56.1	50.6		
Previously married	53.9	39.0	42.6		
Never married	6.2	4.9	6.7	20.020	0.001
Gender					
Male	40.4	53.7	47.2		
Female	59.6	46.3	52.8	8.031	0.018
Region					
South	55.6	34.1	57.3		
Non-south	44.4	65.9	42.7	8.580	0.014
Poverty status					
Poor (<100%)	24.8	19.0	6.8		
Near poor (100–199%)	26.7	23.8	22.3		
Non-poor (200–399%)	26.7	26.2	36.9		
Non-poor (400%+)	21.8	31.0	34.0	113.560	0.000

Table 11A.2. Comparison of characteristics between classes weighted by class probabilities (means)

	Low/low (n = 741)	High/high (n = 262)	Low/high (n = 92)	ANOVA test for overall difference	
	Mean	Mean	Mean	F-statistic	P value
Negative interaction	1.134	1.994	2.598	1,339.865	0.000
Age	66.833	66.729	65.457	1.088	0.337
Education	11.756	11.760	12.600	2.807	0.061
Church attendance	2.443	2.588	2.283	6.683	0.001
Contact	4.115	4.664	4.402	11.569	0.000
Size of helper network	20.173	17.111	19.250	1.526	0.218
Subjective closeness	3.239	3.477	2.989	13.586	0.000

				χ^2 test for overall difference	
	Proportion %	Proportion %	Proportion %	χ^2	P value
Race					
African American	60.1	69.1	47.8	41.728	0.000
Caribbean Black	19.7	24.0	17.4		
Non-Hispanic White	20.2	6.9	34.8		
Marital status					
Married	33.1	37.4	54.3	58.986	0.000
Previously married	59.1	61.8	27.2		
Never married	7.8	0.8	7.0		
Gender					
Male	32.9	31.3	53.3	16.355	0.000
Female	67.1	68.7	46.7		
Region					
South	59.8	60.7	58.7	0.127	0.938
Non-south	40.2	39.3	41.3		
Poverty status					
Poor (<100%)	22.5	22.9	12.0	8.122	0.229
Near poor (100–199%)	27.8	27.5	29.3		
Non-poor (200–399%)	28.9	25.2	31.5		
Non-poor (400%+)	20.8	24.4	27.2		

Table 11A.3. Adjusted odds of latent class membership using *low/low* class as referent

Variable	Adjusted odds ratio (95% confidence interval)			
	Low/high		High/high	
Race *(ref = African American)*				
Caribbean Black	0.74	(0.27, 2.03)	0.95	(0.37, 2.46)
White	2.56	(1.94, 3.39)	0.43	(0.35, 0.52)
Age	0.98	(0.86, 1.13)	0.99	(0.87, 1.13)
Gender *(ref = male)*				
Female	0.56	(0.47, 0.66)	0.97	(0.85, 1.10)
Education	1.17	(0.51, 2.70)	1.08	(0.59, 1.97)
Poverty status *(ref = poor <100%)*				
Near poor (100–199%)	1.39	(0.82, 2.37)	0.82	(0.57, 1.18)
Non-poor (200–399%)	0.62	(0.41, 0.92)	0.85	(0.60, 1.19)
Non-poor (400%+)	0.52	(0.39, 0.69)	0.88	(0.72, 1.08)
Marital status *(ref = married)*				
Previously married	0.14	(0.12, 0.16)	0.74	(0.65, 0.85)
Never married	1.68	(1.42, 1.98)	0.20	(0.18, 0.23)
Region *(ref = South)*				
Non-south	2.09	(1.77, 2.47)	1.02	(0.89, 1.16)
Church attendance	0.55	(0.24, 1.27)	1.11	(0.61, 2.02)
Contact	1.49	(0.46, 4.83)	1.12	(0.56, 2.25)
Size of helper network	1.00	(0.59, 1.69)	0.99	(0.69, 1.41)
Subjective closeness	0.76	(0.51, 1.13)	1.30	(0.93, 1.82)

REFERENCES

American Association of Public Opinion Research (AAPOR). (2006). *Standard definitions: Final dispositions of case codes and outcome rates for surveys* (4th ed.). Lenexa, KS: AAPOR.

Bengtson, V. L., Giarrusso, R., Mabry, J. B., & Silverstein, M. (2002). Solidarity, conflict, and ambivalence: Complementary or competing perspectives on intergenerational relationships? *Journal of Marriage and the Family, 64*, 568–576.

Bertera, E. M. (2005). Mental health in U.S. adults: The role of positive social support and social negativity in personal relationships. *Journal of Social and Personal Relationships, 22*(1), 33–48.

Billingsley, A. (1992). *Climbing Jacob's Ladder: Enduring legacy of African American families.* New York: Simon & Schuster.

Billingsley, A. (1999). *Mighty like a river: The Black church and social reform.* New York: Oxford University Press.

Chatters, L. M. (2000). Religion and health: Public health research and practice. *Annual Review of Public Health, 21*, 335–367.

Chatters, L. M., & Taylor, R. J. (2006). Religion and families. In V. L. Bengtson, A. C. Acock, K. R. Allen, P. Dilworth-Anderson, & D. M. Klein (Eds.), *Sourcebook of Family Theory and Research* (pp. 517–522). Thousand Oaks, CA: Sage.

Chatters, L. M., Taylor, R. J., Lincoln, K. D., & Schroepfer, T. (2002). Patterns of informal support from family and church members among African Americans. *Journal of Black Studies, 33*, 66–85.

Cohen, S., Doyle, W. J., Skoner, D. P., Rabin, B. S., & Gwaltney, J. M. (1997). Social ties and susceptibility to the common cold. *Journal of the American Medical Association, 277*, 1940–1944.

Connidis, I. A., & McMullin, J. A. (2002). Ambivalence, family ties, and doing sociology. *Journal of Marriage and the Family, 64*, 595–601.

Ellison, C. G., & Levin, J. S. (1998). The religion-health connection: Evidence, theory, and future directions. *Health Education & Behavior, 25*, 700–720.

Greenbaum, P. E., Del Boca, F. K., Darkes, J., Wang, C.-P., & Goldman, M. S. (2005). Variation in the drinking trajectories of freshmen college students. *Journal of Consulting and Clinical Psychology, 73*, 229–238.

Heeringa, S. G., Wagner, J., Torres, M., Duan, N., Adams, T., & Berglund, P. (2004). Sample designs and sampling methods for the Collaborative Psychiatric Epidemiology Studies (CPES). *International Journal of Methods in Psychiatric Research, 13*, 221–240.

Hill, R. B. (1999). *The strengths of African American families: Twenty-five years later* (2nd ed.). Thousand Oaks, CA: Sage.

Idler, E. L., & George, L. K. (1998). What sociology can help us understand about religion and mental health. In H. Koenig (Ed.), *Handbook of Religion and Mental Health* (pp. 51–62). New York: Academic Press.

Jackson, J. S., Torres, M., Caldwell, C. H., Neighbors, H. W., Nesse, R. M., Taylor, R. J., Trierweiler, S. J., & Williams, D. R. (2004). The National Survey of American Life: A study of racial, ethnic and cultural influences on mental disorders and mental health. *International Journal of Methods in Psychiatric Research, 13*, 196–207.

Kahn, R. L., & Antonucci, T. C. (1981). Convoys of social support: A life course approach. In S. B. Kiesler, J. N. Morgan, & V. K. Oppenheimer (Eds.), *Aging: Social change* (pp. 383–405). New York: Academic Press.

Kass, R. E., & Raftery, A. E. (1995). Bayes factors. *Journal of the American Statistical Association, 90*, 773–795.

King, A. C., Atienza, A., Castro, C., & Collins, R. (2002). Physiological and affective responses to family caregiving in the natural setting in wives versus daughters. *International Journal of Behavioral Medicine, 9*, 176–194.

Krause, N. (2002). Church-based social support and health in old age: Exploring variations by race. *Journal of Gerontology: Social Sciences, 57*(6), S332–S347.

Krause, N. (2003). Religious meaning and subjective well-being in late life. *Journal of Gerontology: Social Sciences, 58B*, S160–S170.

Krause, N. (2005). Negative interaction and heart disease in late life: Exploring variations by socioeconomic status. *Journal of Aging and Health, 17*, 28–55.

Krause, N., Ellison, C., & Wulff, K. (1998). Church-based emotional support, negative interaction, and psychological well-being. *Journal for the Scientific Study of Religion, 37*, 725–741.

Krause, N., Morgan, D. L., Chatters, L. M., & Meltzer, T. (2000). Negative interaction in the church: Insights from focus groups with older adults. *Review of Religious Research, 41*, 510–533.

Krause, N., & Wulff, K. M. (2005). Church-based social ties, a sense of belonging in a congregation, and physical health status. *International Journal for the Psychology of Religion, 15*(1), 73–93.

Landecker, W. S. (1951). Types of integration and their measurement. *American Journal of Sociology, 56*, 332–340.

Lincoln, K. D. (2007). Financial strain, negative interactions and mastery: Pathways to mental health among older African Americans. *Journal of Black Psychology, 33*(4), 439–462.

Lincoln, K. D., Chatters, L. M., & Taylor, R. J. (2005). Social support, traumatic events and depressive symptoms among African Americans. *Journal of Marriage and the Family 67*(3), 754–766.

Lincoln, K. D., Chatters, L. M., Taylor, R. J., & Jackson, J. S. (2007). Profiles of depressive symptoms among African Americans and Caribbean Blacks. *Social Science and Medicine, 65*(2), 200–213.

Lincoln, C. E., & Mamiya, L. H. (1990). *The Black church in the African American experience*. Durham, NC: Duke University Press.

Mavandadi, S., Rook, K. S., & Newsom, J. T. (2007). Positive and negative social exchanges and disability in later life: An investigation of trajectories of change. *Journal of Gerontology: Social Sciences, 62B*(6), S361–S370.

McCutcheon, A. L. (1987). *Latent class analysis*. Sage University Paper Series on Quantitative Applications in the Social Sciences. Beverly Hills, CA: Sage.

McLachlan, G. J., & Peel, D. (2000). *Finite mixture models*. New York: Wiley.

Meiser, T. H., & Ohrt, B. (1996). Modeling structure and chance in transitions: Mixed latent partial Markov-Chain models. *Journal of Educational and Behavioral Statistics, 21*, 91–109.

Muthén, B. O, & Muthén, L. K. (2000). Integrating person-centered and variable-centered analysis: Growth mixture modeling with latent trajectory classes. *Alcoholism: Clinical and Experimental Research, 24*, 882–891.

Newsom, J. T., Nishishiba, M., Morgan, D. L., & Rook, K. S. (2003). The relative importance of three domains of positive and negative social exchanges: A longitudinal model with comparable measures. *Psychology and Aging, 18*, 746–754.

Newsom, J. T., Rook, K. S., Nishishiba, M., Sorkin, D. H., & Mahan, T. L. (2005). Understanding the relative importance of positive and negative social exchanges: Examining specific domains and subjective appraisals. *Journal of Gerontology: Psychological Sciences, 60*, P304–P312.

Nye, F., & Rushing, W. (1969). Toward family measurement research. In J. Hadden & E. Borgatta (Eds.), *Marriage and family* (pp. 133–140). Itasca, IL: F. E. Peacock.

Pargament, K. I., Silverman, W. H., Johnson, S. M., Echemendia, R. J., & Snyder, S.

(1983). The psychosocial climate of religious congregations. *American Journal of Community Psychology, 11,* 351–381.

Rook, K. S., & Pietromonaco, P. (1987). Close relationships: Ties that heal or ties that bind? In W. H. Jones & D. Perlman (Eds.), *Advances in personal relationships* (Vol. 1, pp.1–35). Greenwich, CT: JAI Press.

Seeman, T., & Chen, X. (2002). Risk and protective factors for physical functioning in older adults with and without chronic conditions. *Journal of Gerontology: Social Sciences, 57,* S135–S144.

Sorkin, D. H., & Rook, K. S. (2006). Dealing with negative social exchanges in later life: Coping responses, goals, and effectiveness. *Psychology and Aging, 21,* 715–725.

Tanne, D., Goldbourt, U., & Medalie, J. H. (2004). Perceived family difficulties and prediction of 23-year stroke mortality among middle-aged men. *Cerebrovascular Diseases, 18,* 277–282.

Taylor, R. J., & Chatters, L. M. (1986). Church-based informal support among elderly Blacks. *The Gerontologist, 26,* 637–642.

javascript:popup('A1988R388100008')Taylor, R. J., & Chatters, L. M. (1988). Church members as a source of informal social support. *Review of Religious Research, 30,* 193–203.

Taylor, R. J., Chatters, L. M., & Jackson, J. S. (2007a). Religious and spiritual involvement among older African Americans, Caribbean Blacks, and Non-Hispanic Whites: Findings from the National Survey of American Life. *Journal of Gerontology: Social Sciences, 62B,* S238–S250.

Taylor, R. J., Chatters, L. M., & Jackson, J. S. (2007b). Religious participation among older Black Caribbeans in the United States. *Journal of Gerontology: Social Sciences, 62B,* S251–S256.

Taylor, R. J., Chatters, L. M., & Levin, J. S. (2004). *Religion in the lives of African Americans: Social, psychological, and health perspectives.* Thousand Oaks, CA: Sage.

Taylor, R. J., Jackson, J. S., & Chatters, L. M. (1997). *Family life in Black America.* Thousand Oaks, CA: Sage.

Taylor, R. J., Lincoln, K. D., & Chatters, L. M. (2005). Supportive relationships with church members among African Americans. *Family Relations, 54,* 501–511.

Wiesner, M., & Windle, M. (2004). Assessing covariates of adolescent delinquency trajectories: A latent growth mixture modeling approach. *Journal of Youth and Adolescence, 33,* 431–442.

Zlotnick, C., Kohn, R., Keitner, G., & Grotta, S. A. (2000). The relationships between quality of interpersonal relationships and major depressive disorder: Findings from the National Comorbidity Survey. *Journal of Affective Disorders, 59*(3), 205–215.

PART V / Global, Cross-National, and Cross-Ethnic Issues

Who Will Care for the Young and the Old?

Although there are disparities among countries in population aging, with some developing countries still considered young and some developed countries deemed to be old, these differences will not last long, as the speed of demographic change is increasing. The demographic transition, as well as globalization of the econonomy and transnational migration, has implications for who will care for the young and the old in an aging society.

Marshall addresses the issue of global aging as a serious policy concern but disagrees that cutbacks in state resources and an increasingly thin family culture (due to decreased fertility and geographic dispersion) will rise to the level of crisis for older adults and the societies they inhabit. Dannefer and Siders discuss the impact of globalization for transnational families, noting the constrained choices faced by dispersed family members who are compelled to rely on each other (mostly economically) as a form of "induced solidarity." Marcum and Treas examine attitudes toward public spending on youth and elders in 27 countries. The authors find that all nations support public spending on both the young and the old, affirming the intergenerational contract; however, in contrast to the age neutrality of other nations, liberal-market nations, including the United States, tend more to support spending on the elderly only, suggesting strains in solidarity across age groups. Finally, Markides, Angel, and Peek seek to understand the differences in health outcomes and caregiving arrangements for elderly Hispanics (many of whom have migrated from Mexico to the United States) compared to the elderly of other ethnic groups in America. They find that despite being of lower socioeconomic standing, the Hispanic elderly fair far better than their socioeconomic counterparts in other ethnic groups, due largely to the high levels of intergenerational solidarity (both structural and associational) they experience at the family and community level. As a whole, these chapters show that the intergenerational solidarity paradigm is relevant at macro as well as micro levels of analysis.

CHAPTER TWELVE

Global Aging and Families

Some Policy Concerns about the Global Aging Perspective

Victor W. Marshall

The concept of global aging has recently become widely used in social gerontology. This chapter reviews the concept of globalization, critically addresses the political undertones of the general policy discourse about globalization and aging, suggests some major consequences of global aging for families, and calls for an expansion of current thinking about families and aging to accommodate not only globalization but also the politics underlying globalization and aging discourse.

If you live long enough and labor in the vineyards of gerontology, you see new ideas and concerns, seemingly emanating from nowhere, rise to capture the gerontological imagination. Many current scholars in gerontology were active or had retired from service before the terms "eldercare" or "caregiver burden" were invented and before "elder abuse" became an important practice, policy, and research concern. We attended gerontology conferences where perhaps a third of the papers dealt with the debate between activity theory and disengagement theory, and we witnessed the loss of interest in that debate. We saw the rise, and then the fall, of political, then media, and then research interest in criminal victimization of the elderly (Cook, 1981; Cook & Skogan, 1984). We lived through a time before health and health care came to dominate the research (and research funding), the publication, and the conference agendas of gerontology and where social and economic issues—poverty, income security, and retirement, for example—had a larger role to play. When a new topic, or a new buzzword, arises in the field, we ought to pay attention.

I am intrigued by the recent appearance, and growth in popularity, of the term "global aging." The term seems to come from nowhere but to be everywhere. In the academic writings of social gerontology, this includes chapter or volume mention in the second (but not the first) edition of *The Encyclopedia of Aging* (Phillipson & Vincent, 2007), *The Cambridge Handbook of Age and Ageing* (Kalache, Barreto, & Keller, 2005), a text by Estes, Biggs, and Phillipson (2003), and an edited collection by Baars, Dannefer, Phillipson, and Walker (2006) as well as significant analytical treatment in journal articles by such luminaries as Dale Dannefer (2003), Peter Townsend (2006), and Alan Walker (2005; Walker & Deacon, 2003). Outside the strictly academic realm, global aging and the globalization of aging enter prominently into policy discourse, a topic I will address in a later section of this chapter. Finally, global aging receives attention in the recent writing of Vern Bengtson, whom we are honoring through this book.

Bengtson's book, edited with Ariela Lowenstein under the title *Global Aging and Challenges to Families* (2003), addresses globalization in the context of the family—which is of course an obvious context for Vern Bengtson. The scope of global aging is very narrowly interpreted in this volume. For the most part, it appears simply to refer to comparative international aging. In their introductory chapter, Bengtson, Lowenstein, Putney, and Gans (2003, p. 17) list five research issues for a future agenda, only one of which touches on globalization, and it is "How shall we address diversity in family structures and social norms in view of global social changes." This is surely a big enough research question to drive a large future research program. However, the possibilities for research are much greater if a broader approach to globalization is taken. In this paper I first introduce a broader conceptualization of globalization and then focus on selected aspects of the global politics of aging. I then return to the question of the family in the context of global aging.

What Is Global Aging?

In the past decade, we have seen a dramatic increase in attention to something called "global aging." This is not just a concern with aging around the globe or an interest in comparative aging, although looking at aging in other countries is certainly related to the concept as it is used today. Global aging is related to globalization more generally, so let us first consider that concept. Phillipson and Vincent's chapter on "Globalization and Aging," in the 2007 edition of *The Encyclopedia of Gerontology*, provides a simple definition of globalization as referring "to those mechanisms, actors, and institutions that link together individuals and groups across different nation-states" (Phillipson & Vincent, 2007, p. 630). That can serve as a starting point, and importantly, what it describes goes well beyond a comparative international sociology of aging to consider linkages across nation-states to be a defining characteristic of globalization.

I turn to the International Monetary Fund for a more detailed definition of this concept. The IMF website (IMF, 2002) offers a helpful staff paper, *Globalization: Threat or Opportunity*, in which it observes that globalization is viewed with strong emotions, both positive and negative. Economic globalization, this paper says, "refers to the increasing integration of economies around the world, particularly through trade and financial flows. The term sometimes also refers to the movement of people (labor) and knowledge (technology) across international borders. There are also broader cultural, political and environmental dimensions of globalization that are not covered here" (in the paper) (IMF, 2002).

From the IMF point of view, globalization "has come into common usage since the 1980s, reflecting technological advances that have made it easier and quicker to complete international transactions—both trade and financial flows. It refers to an extension beyond national borders of the same market forces that have operated for centuries at all levels of human economic activity" (IMF, 2002).[1]

The global aspects have to do with the increasing recognition that "the economy" can no longer be bounded within a nation state. The state of one nation's economy is related to that of other nations, because we live in an economic system that is increasingly characterized by multinational corporations, global production, and global distribution systems. Because population aging does not occur uniformly in all the nations of the world, it is possible that differential aging, in global terms, will affect market economies. The organization of global market economies has implications for nation-states in a world system, and hence it becomes a question of political economy.

The term "global aging" also looks at different parts of the world as a holistic system, but it focuses on international demographic changes and their impact on a number of phenomena, such as health and family supports for the growing number and proportion of older people in most societies of the world, and the global implications of the patterns of these changes. However, the term's focus is mostly in the economic realm and is mostly concerned with asking (and trying to answer) two basic questions: (1) What is the impact of global aging on the economies of different countries at various levels of economic development? and (2) Can the nations of the world afford to support the needs of a growing population of old citizens? Within that political economy we can speak of a global politics of aging, and within that context it is also possible to address implications for the family.

The Global Politics of Aging

How did global aging get onto the policy agenda? What are the interests, or perhaps the motives, of those who push the idea of global aging? Why, in the past decade, have we seen more and more newspaper and magazine articles about a "crisis" of global aging? Why is an agency such as the United States Central Intelligence Agency (CIA) interested in global aging? I don't have all the answers to these questions, but in this paper I want to explore these questions and share with you the concerns I have about this increasingly popular concept. At the outset, it is quite clear that global aging did not get on the policy agenda because of aging and family issues. More direct economic concerns raised the profile of global aging. Concerns about global aging take on a most dramatic tone when it is recognized that economic conditions affect international stability. This concern is evident in two significant initiatives that I will now briefly describe.

The CIA and the Geopolitics of Aging

The first is the release of a policy paper by the United States Central Intelligence Agency under the title *Long-Term Global Demographic Trends: Reshaping the Geopolitical Landscape* (CIA, 2001).[2] Prepared by the Rand Corporation and based on a strategic planning conference with "experts from academia, the business world, and the Intelligence Community," the report asserts that "global demographic trends will have far-reaching consequences for the key elements of national power: economic, military, and political within the larger global community. Allies and rivals will cope differently—some better than others" (CIA, 2001, p. 3).

This American report begins with a powerful summary of global demographic changes, which it sees as potentially threatening to American security and power. By 2020, the world population will have grown to 7.8 billion, of whom only 4% will be Americans and just 13% from the Western Hemisphere. Of the world's population, 5% will be from Western Europe, 7% from Eastern Europe and the former Soviet Union, 3% from the Middle East, 16% from Africa, and fully 56% from Asia. These regions will vary greatly in the extent to which their populations are "old" or "young," and this has great potential for global differentiation of economies. The report also notes that by 2020, "the world will be older and far less Caucasian, and it will be far more concentrated in urban areas" (CIA, 2001, p. 5); that by 2015, for the first time, more than half the world's population will live in cities; and that by 2050, the size of the population aged 65 and over will have tripled to about 1.5 billion people, or 16% of the total. Nevertheless, many countries will see significant "youth bulges," and the countries projected to have the largest proportion of youth will be Pakistan, Afghanistan, Saudi Arabia, Yemen, and Iraq.

While countries such as these face great economic challenges creating productive work for large youth and young adult populations, the countries that are currently the economic engines of the world face a far different problem, this CIA report alleges, because of the impact of the aging of their populations on the economy. Whereas the "young" countries may see great unrest due to continuing poverty and the challenge of meeting the needs of rapid population growth, the "old" countries, struggling economically because of their aging population, will be less able to deal with geopolitical flashpoints in the younger countries. The strategic issues, again from the very American position of the CIA, are starkly given in a "key findings" table that appears in the report, with the three bullets reading "Our allies in the industrialized world will face an unprecedented crisis of aging"; "The aging challenge could reduce Japan's economic power"; and "An older Europe will be less willing to face up to global hot spots."

This report does not mince words. It says, "the industrialized world will record an unprecedented crisis of aging beginning early next decade and reaching critical mass in the mid-2020s" (CIA, 2001, p. 7). In crisis mode, the CIA report cites OECD predictions that population aging will lead to decreases in GDP growth rates in the developed world. For example, "all things equal, the impact of aging on GDP growth rates will be a decrease in Europe to 0.5 percent, in Japan to 0.6 percent, and in the United States to 1.5% in the years 2025–50" (CIA, 2001, p. 7). Additionally, "the average bill for public pensions and health care in Japan and Europe will grow by 9 to 16 percent of GDP over the next three decades" (CIA, 2001, p. 7).

The Global Aging Initiative of the Center for Strategic and International Studies

The second significant initiative concerning global aging is in fact called the "Global Aging Initiative Program" and was begun in 1999 by the Center for Strategic and International Studies (CSIS), in Washington, DC.[3] An overview of the program found on the CSIS web page in 2001 gives its rationale:

> Over the next three decades, Japan, Western Europe, and the United States will each undergo unprecedented demographic transitions characterized by a dangerous combination of rising elderly populations and flat or, in many cases, negative labor force growth. As a result, all face the danger of large structural deficits, declining savings, and slower economic growth. That this transformation initially will be limited to the world's leading economies suggests an important strategic dimension. These nations account for two-thirds of world GDP and play a dominant role in global security and economic stabilization arrangements. How the advanced nations adapt to the new realities of aging has far-reaching consequences not only for the aging nations themselves, but also for global economic growth, international financial markets, and the larger global community" (CSIS, 2001).[4]

As with the CIA report, the CSIS Global Aging Initiative is concerned not only with economic issues but also with global security issues. Given the preponderance of major, international corporate executives in the composition of the Commission on Global Aging, established to run this program, we might conclude that security in this case means security of global capitalism. The commission was initially led by three honorary cochairs, including a former president of Deutsche Bundesbank (which functions as a major global investment bank), a former prime minister of Japan, and Walter Mondale, former vice president of the United States. Mondale later resigned from the commission. The 82 additional commission members, who were "senior government officials and business leaders, with the support of subject experts" (CSIS, 2001), include politicians; investment bankers, insurers, and pension fund executives; major drug company executives; and representatives of the IMF, the OECD, the World Bank, and the International Chamber of Commerce and of think tanks such as the American Enterprise Institute. The subject experts (other than politicians and business leaders) included a few academics and a representative from the AARP.

In a number of conferences held around the world, and through working papers and other publications, the Global Aging Program has communicated a message very similar to that of the CIA report. Some of the reports (England, 2001a,b; Schieber, Hewitt, Tuljapurkar, Li, & Anderson, 2000) are based on the program's own commissioned demographic forecasts because, as the Global Aging Initiative's director of research puts it, "Official forecasts, at best, mildly underestimate longevity gains and mildly overestimate improvements in fertility. At worst, they are rosy scenarios that significantly understate the long-range fiscal challenge" (England, 2001a, p. 2).

As a sociologist, I am familiar with the use of corporate interlocks as a means for capital to steer policy and practice. The Commission on Global Aging looks a lot like such a board, and it has the capacity to promote its version of voodoo, or apocalyptic, demography (Gee, 2000; Robertson, 1997) before the public. For example, a "special report on global aging" from *The Guardian* (a UK newspaper), based on the report of a CSIS conference held in Tokyo, is headlined, "Ageing populace is killing economy, says study" (Watts, 2001). This story begins, "The rapid ageing of the developed world is pushing the global economy towards the edge of a demographic abyss, an international panel warned yesterday." Its report from Tokyo, the story said, concluded "that urgent action was needed by world leaders to prevent protracted 'aging recessions' and financial turmoil" and that "The major social crises of the twenty-first century will be the byproduct of labour shortages" (Watts, 2001). These in turn are caused by population aging accompanied by a larger older, non-working population and fewer people in the workforce. The conference organizer is reported as Paul Hewitt.

The next example, one of many I could give, is a policy paper issued by Goldman Sachs and authored by Maureen Culhane of the Strategic Relationship Management Group. Called "Global Aging: Capital Market Implications," it may or may not be related to the fact that Robert D. Hormats, vice chairman of Goldman Sachs International, is on the CSIS Commission on Global Aging. At any rate, it gives more or less the same picture but focuses on world capital markets as influenced by global aging. It sees aging as having a positive effect on capital markets for the next decade but paints a crisis scenario over a longer time frame of fifty years. Demographics is seen as "the problem," and "the culprits are low fertility rates and increased life expectancies" (Culhane, 2001, p. 2). The report suggests that "GDP growth could slow dramatically for countries with shrinking working age populations" (Culhane, 2001, p. 2), and it suggests that no single solution will solve these problems but that a menu of solutions is required. This includes "changing the promise" and reducing retirement benefits, moving to more privatized pension schemes while abandoning or reducing PAYGO systems, and keeping people in the labor force longer.

To take a final example, the day after my return from the Valencia Forum on Aging in 2002, a conference at which a number of plenary speakers and conference attendees were at pains to argue against this alarmist scenario, my local newspaper in North Carolina carried an AP wire service report under the heading, "Senior-youth ratio could bring crisis" (Sokolovsky, 2002). This was not a report based on the Valencia Forum, which had just ended, nor was it a report based on the World Assembly on Aging, which was just about to begin in Madrid. But it was datelined Madrid. Clearly, it emanated from a press release, and it quoted "Paul Hewitt of the Center for Strategic and International Studies in Washington" as follows: "By the mid-2020s, virtually the entire developed world will be one big Argentina unless some serious reforms are made." Hewitt is the member of the Commission on Global Aging who organized the Tokyo conference.

There are, then, powerful voices arguing that there is a crisis of global aging, implicating in part the aging of the labor force and making a number of suggestions to keep older workers in the labor force longer to ameliorate the problem.

A less strident tone, suggesting that we face challenges rather than a crisis, is set by a report of the AARP. This report, *Global Aging: Achieving Its Potential* (2001), does paint a rosier picture than the two I have just noted, but it is one that I find more credible.

Global Aging: The AARP Stance Concerning the Alleged Crisis

Let me now focus on one aspect of the crisis theme, concern about the economic burden of increasingly large proportions of the population who are nonproductive because they are not in the workforce, coupled with fewer people in the productive years of the life course (for other concerns, see Marshall, 2002). The AARP report, *Global Aging: Achieving Its Potential*, is one of a number of sources documenting an alternative scenario: that there are certainly challenges to be faced, but not a crisis, due to global population aging. Interestingly, former vice president Mondale, who resigned from cochairmanship of the Global Aging initiative of CSIS, wrote the foreword to the AARP report. He notes that "too often, aging issues are used as an excuse to promote a particular agenda, such as the privatization of important social protection programs.

As shown in this report, however, valuable programs like Social Security and Medicare are sustainable in the long term, provided that we understand the challenges and take reasonable measures to address them" (AARP, 2001, p. v).

The AARP report points out that population aging does not in itself create a larger number of old dependents; rather, it does so in conjunction with statutory or normative retirement, creating a growing pool of people who are not working for pay (AARP, 2001). Many analysts seem to assume that people are not productive unless they are working for pay. This is a concern for industrialized countries with growing proportions of old people, but it is also a concern for the countries that will be experiencing larger youth populations because they will also see increases in the proportion of the population who are in the retirement years. Moreover, postponement of entry to paid employment has also been a feature of modernizing societies, and this too reduces the proportion of the total population that is in paid employment (AARP, 2001).

Population aging is not the only reason why people are not productive (in terms of being in the paid labor force). There is great cross-societal variability in labor force participation at any age, depending on such things as the duration of education that precedes entry to paid labor (or the extent of withdrawals from work into education that might be staged across the life course); patterns of female labor force participation at various ages; and, not least, unemployment rates. Public policy can focus on increasing labor force participation of older people or, for example, on making it easier for women with family care responsibilities to work, or on reducing unemployment rates, or on increasing the normative hours of work per week, or on decreasing the number and length of paid holidays and statutory vacation entitlements. All these things can increase the hours of productive work. As the AARP report notes (2001, p. 8), increased female labor force participation will offset the effects of population aging on the economy in countries like Ireland and Italy. European countries, with persistently high unemployment rates, have more room to move through reducing unemployment than, for example, the United States, which has much lower unemployment rates.

Is There Really a Crisis Caused by Global Population Aging?

My direct answer to this question is that there is not a crisis caused by global population aging. There is, however, serious cause for concern and strategic planning. The CIA report and the activities and reports of the CSIS Global Aging Initiative have raised the profile of population aging issues, just as the Americans for Generational Equity (AGE) organization raised the profile of global aging issues in the mid-1980s (Bengtson & Achenbaum, 1993; Marshall, Cook, & Marshall, 1993).[5] We have to accept the challenges without panicking, and I would argue, we have to be wary of the uses to which apocalyptic demography can be put in attacking the welfare state and fostering support for individualistic solutions when collective solutions are likely to work better.

We need a much stronger, but also a much broader, research data base that considers the issues through lenses in addition to those of economics, demography, and strategic security. There are major differences of opinion and interpretation on a number of issues, including the basic demographic projections. Various working or position papers from CSIS and its Global Aging Initiative show clearly that different assumptions lead to different demographic scenarios. The scenarios they use are less optimistic than those commonly used by governments or other agencies such as OECD (England, 2001a,b). Similarly, various papers disagree in predicting the impact of population aging on economic indicators. For example, a report by the AARP (2001, p. 7) suggests that U.S. Bureau of Labor Statistics projections of older persons' labor force participation use overly pessimistic assumptions, and AARP substitutes its own simulations based on its own assumptions.

There is also great disagreement about what variables should be included in economic models and about economic projections. England (2001b, p. 4) recognizes these differences and goes further to note that:

> When one looks at the issues of aging and the economy, the uncertainties are compounded. One has to consider how people will behave in situations that have no historical precedent. How long will people live in 2050? At what age will they become disabled on average? Will people retire later than they do now—or retire earlier? One has to consider the likely behavior of elected officials in the future—a highly speculative exercise. For example, how will governments in any given country respond to the increasing costs of benefits for the elderly? Will they raise taxes, borrow more or cut benefits?

These are important questions, and I would add that the answers lie less in the realm of economics than in sociology, political science, medicine, and public health—yet it is primarily economists and business people who are ringing the alarm bells about the aging crisis.

Academic gerontologists need to be aware that a great deal of aging policy discussion is not going on within the house of gerontology but in a broader world in which the strongest voices are more concerned with the preservation of international economic markets than with the well-being of older people (or people of any age). Svihula and Estes (2007) have sought to interpret American social security policy and politics in light of sets of values and ideological positions manifested through and advocated by not only political actors but also experts from academia, the financial and consulting sectors, and policy think tanks positioned across the ideological spectrum. Equal consideration should be given to ideological factors operating at a global level. An understanding of global aging is a central task of what Alan Walker (2005) calls the "international political economy of aging." Such a specialty field would examine global inequalities in aging and the effects of economic development on older people in different economic contexts; the role that international government organizations (IGOs) such as the World Bank, as well as transnational corporations, have on the global political economy as it affects different age groups; the continuing role of the nation state but also the emerging role of supranational regional structures (such as NAFTA, ASEAN, and APEC); and the role of the United Nations itself and international nongovernmental organizations in advocating for policy change. Understanding the politics of global aging should therefore be a large part of the research agenda in social gerontology.

Globalization and the Family

And where is the family in all this? Phillipson & Vincent (2007, p. 631) assert that "the focus on globalization confirms the importance of locating individuals within the orbit of social and economic structures, with these increasingly subject to forces acting beyond the boundaries of the nation-state." The family is, of course, the structure, both social and economic, that most immediately touches on the lives of people, including as they age into the later years. The demographic transition, which creates differential demographic pressures in societies, is very much a family affair. Economic changes influence fertility behavior, which spins out as different rates of population aging that in turn have implications for economic growth or decline. Global economic relationships are also associated with international migration and with urbanization in underdeveloped countries, a major factor in the decline of three-generational family residency patterns (Haber, 2006; Kalache, Barreto, & Keller, 2005).

Phillipson and Vincent, drawing on notions of the risk society, observe that "at one level, the risks associated with aging—the threat of poverty, the need for long-term care, the likelihood of serious illness—are relatively unchanged. What has changed is that the duty and the necessity to cope with these risks are being transferred to individual families (women carers in particular) and individual older people (notably with respect to financing for old age)" (Phillipson & Vincent, 2007. p. 631). Of course, financing old age is very much a family affair as well. As Lowenstein (2005, p. 408) has observed, "ageing policies of most countries . . . regard families and service systems as alternatives that tend to counteract (substitute), not complement."

The globalization of work has numerous effects on financial well-being and sometimes on family structure. Most obvious, and noted by these authors, is global migration, both permanent and of the migrant workforce, which often separates the generations yet can allow migrant workers to send home financial resources to help both elder parents and children. For example, a recent study conducted for the Inter-American Development Bank estimated that about 12.6 million Latin America-born immigrants (of which most would have emigrated from Mexico to the United States) generated about $460 billion in income in 2005, of which 90% was left in the United States but about $45 billion, or 10%, flowed home to their native countries (Barrett & Bachelet, 2006). So we have a dilemma with globalization in terms of the family. Using Bengtson's framework, as a "structural arrangement," geographical proximity is reduced by these global working arrangements, leading to a decrease in associational solidarity and in many types of functional exchanges (such as direct care) but making possible the provision of financial assistance to the older generation by the younger, migrant generation. There are a host of issues in this area that could fruitfully be engaged with the "Bengtson typology" of family solidarity (Bengtson & Mabry, 2006; Bengtson & Schrader, 1982). To make matters more complicated, for nonmigrants in the receiving country, this pattern can have adverse effects. The presence of migrant workers, whether legal or illegal, depresses wages (especially the working poor), with the potential to force families into poverty (see Marshall, 2006, for a discussion in relation to North America).[6]

Drawing on Hochschild (2000), Mittelman and Tambe (2000), and others, Estes, Biggs, and Phillipson (2003) describe the emergence of "global families" resulting from international migration, with generations separated and people moving back and forth between origin and receiving destinations as they age, economic marginalization of women, and the emergence of international caregiving networks. Global migration can have some benefits. For example, cultural diversity can enrich the quality of life, and, as noted above, overseas earnings remitted to origin countries play a huge role in enhancing living standards. But the many negative effects on family life, including the increased burden on women to provide family care (to kin of all ages) are worthy of note.

Returning to the explicit globalization, family, and aging work of Vern Bengtson, in the conclusion to their edited book, Lowenstein and Bengtson address the challenges posed by global aging to families in the twenty-first century. As they point out:

> despite this situation of flux in modern societies [characterized by globalization], the couple and family orientation of social life and the value attached to sociability make the family a main reference point in the aging process, and the needs of the elderly are best understood within the context of the family. Solidarity between generations has long been at the forefront as an enduring characteristic of families. . . . Intergenerational bonds among adult family members may be even more important today than in earlier decades because individuals live longer and thus can share more years and experiences with other generations" (Lowenstein & Bengtson, 2003, p. 372).

Yet, as we have seen, family life can be threatened by the economic forces and social consequences of globalization. The work reported in Bengtson and Lowenstein's book is to a great extent premised on two theoretical perspectives, which also underlay the OASIS[7] project on which most of the book rests. As they note, "the research presented here is based primarily on the theoretical perspectives of the life course and modernization. Thus, the focus of the volume is on the outcomes of . . . changes . . . in demography and in family forms, households, and behaviors—and their impact on the personal and familial life course of elders and their families and the quality of life of all concerned" (Lowenstein & Bengtson, 2003, p. 373). Had Bengtson, Lowenstein, and their colleagues adopted a different theoretical perspective, such as that of political economy[8] or "the new critical theory," the OASIS project would have been very different.

I suggest that there is a great deal more to be researched and understood about globalization and aging. This is true in general and in relation to aging in a family context. The aging individual is properly placed in a family context, but there are broader contexts related to globalization that influence family life. Let me suggest three.

First, the challenges of coping with an older population lead those who take the "crisis perspective" to advocate for cutbacks in state resources that provide financial and health care security. Instead, they argue that the family should assume more of the care burden (see also Marcum and Treas, Chapter 14). At the same time, the intergenerational family is coming to be more and more like the thin, beanpole structure that Bengtson has described (Bengtson & Mabry, 2006; Bengtson, Rosenthal, & Burton, 1995). Moreover, the economic aspects of globalization include destabilization of working patterns and an increase in contingent labor force patterns. These, in turn, introduce complexity in intergenerational relations, such as greater diversity in intergenerational financial support patterns.

Second, families in virtually all countries will be affected by the need for people to work longer, due to population aging, decreased fertility, and greater geographical dispersion of families. The move to delay the timing of retirement is now almost universal (Marshall, 2006, 2009) as even nations still classified as developing face labor shortages.[9] The nature of family life in the so-called retirement years will change, with both men and women working for a few years at least beyond now-conventional retirement ages, often in flexible work arrangements.

Third, we may see increased normative pressures being deliberately developed by nation-states to increase fertility rates. As Culhane (2001) put it, for the crisis mongers, demography is the problem, with the two culprits being low fertility rates and increased life expectancy.[10] We might wish to reflect on how two factors once lauded as good, and indeed the objectives of much public policy, came to be viewed as negative. On the positive side, these pressures will in many nation-states be accompanied by social policy changes to make it easier for mothers and fathers to remain in the work force because of easier and less costly access to child care and more flexible workforce arrangements (so-called flexicurity policies)[11] that will facilitate flexible working hours, phased retirement, parental leave, and so forth.

These three factors have the potential to strongly affect family life, albeit in ways that are not entirely clear. There is thus a continuing research agenda in the area of global aging and the family. It should be clear that the Bengtson legacy has provided an enduring set of analytical categories to understand changes in family life in relation to aging and intergenerational relationships. His foray, in recent years, into global aging is to be welcomed, but to continue this work will require extending the concepts to accommodate the greater dispersion of members of intergenerational families, changes in the operationalization of family solidarity in a global context, and changing pressures on families to assume more of the risk in a "risk society." We need a clearer understanding of the economic and political interests and ideologies that are at play whenever any individual or other social actor invokes the concept of global aging.[12] This understanding will be required if we are to avoid forming public policy (as it affects aging families) based on an unrealistic invocation of crisis.

ACKNOWLEDGMENTS

This chapter, based on a paper presented at a Festchrift for Vern L. Bengtson on September 28–29, 2007, at the University of Southern California, Los Angeles, expands on a paper presented at the meeting of the Southern Gerontological Society in Orlando, Florida, in 2002 and an address to the Valencia Forum on Aging in 2002. See also Kelly and Marshall (2007) for a brief discussion of some of these issues.

NOTES

1. The lag time between general introduction of the term and its appearance in the discourse of social gerontology is a sad commentary on our field.

2. See also John Vincent's description of this report (2006, esp. pp. 263–264).

3. For a related treatment of these two issues, see Kelly & Marshall (2007).

4. This page could not be retrieved in April 2008. However, current information about the CSIS Global Aging Initiative, its rationale, and the program's current members, activities, and publications can be found at www.csis.org/gai. CSIS is very transparent, and its website provides access to its numerous reports, conference notices, press releases, etc.

5. Paul Hewitt, who had been a management intern for AGE founder Senator Durenberger, became the AGE president and executive director. Hewitt is the same person who later became director of the CSIS Global Aging program. He spent a period as deputy commissioner for policy in the Social Security Administration during the George W. Bush regime and remains a member of the CSIS Commission on Global Aging.

6. In her finely textured account of older African Americans and Latino migrants in New York, Katherine Newman (2003) also notes that later waves of Hispanic migrants came to New York in different, and more difficult, economic times. The decline of manufacturing thus affected their economic lives and consequently their family lives over time.

7. Lowenstein led the OASIS project Old Age and Autonomy: The Role of Service Systems and Inter-Generational Family Solidarity. This comparative study was conducted in Israel, Germany, Spain, the UK, and Norway.

8. One chapter in the Bengtson and Lowenstein volume addresses issues in the political economy of aging. Aboderin (2003) critiques modernization theory for its

failure to address material constraints on family support provision as well as its failure to investigate mechanisms. Her work can be interpreted as drawing on the political economy perspective (as noted explicitly in Aboderin, 2006; see also Marshall & Clarke, 2007).

9. *The Economist* magazine for July 28, 2007 (p. 11) notes that "Worries about a population explosion have been replaced by fears of decline," noting predictions that the global population will peak at around 10 billion (currently 6.5 billion), and it argues that states should implement a number of strategies. "The best way to ease the transition towards a smaller population would be to encourage people to work for longer, and remove the barriers that prevent them from doing so."

10. The CIA report discussed above is blunt and clear about the economic and military concerns for "the U.S. and its allies" of differential fertility rates among the developed and relatively underdeveloped societies.

11. "Flexicurity" refers to deliberate policy attempts to enhance labor market flexibility while at the same time providing security. The approach is being taken in several policy circles in Europe and through the Policy Research Initiative (PRI) of the Canadian government. See, for example, Côté (2005), Hunsley (2006), and various papers at the project website: http://policyresearch.gc.ca/page.asp?pagenm=pri_index.

12. This is the same kind of exercise that Bengtson encouraged when president of the Gerontological Society of America and in a conference dedicated to examining the then-current concept of "generational equity" (Bengtson & Achenbaum, 1993). Indeed, some of the players who advocated the generational equity perspective have been involved in the politics of global aging as well, including corporate backers of AGE and the CSIS Global Aging Initiative and Paul S. Hewitt, a key player in both AGE and that initiative.

REFERENCES

AARP. (2001). *Global aging: Achieving its potential.* Washington, DC: AARP.
Aboderin, I. (2003). "Modernization" and economic strain: The impact of social change on material family support for older people in Ghana. In V. L. Bengtson & A. Lowenstein (Eds.), *Global aging and challenges to families* (pp. 284–302). New York: Aldine de Gruyter.
Aboderin, I. (2006). *Intergenerational support and old age in Africa.* Piscataway, NJ: Transaction Publishers.
Baars, J., Dannefer, D., Phillipson, C., & Walker, A. (Eds.). (2006). *Aging, globalization, and inequality: The new critical gerontology.* Amityville, NY: Baywood Publishing.
Barrett, B., & Bachelet, P. (2006, October 21). Migrants export billions home. *The News and Observer,* Raleigh, NC, p. 1.
Bengtson, V. L., & Achenbaum, W. A. (Eds.). (1993). *The changing contract across generations.* New York: Aldine de Gruyter.

Bengtson, V. L., & Lowenstein, A. (Eds.) (2003). *Global aging and challenges to families.* New York: Aldine de Gruyter.

Bengtson, V. L., Lowenstein, A., Putney, N. M., & Gans, D. (2003). Global aging and the challenge to families. In V. L. Bengtson & A. Lowenstein (Eds.), *Global aging and challenges to families* (pp. 1–24). New York: Aldine de Gruyter.

Bengtson, V. L., & Mabry, J. B. (2006). Intergenerational relationships. In R. Schulz, with L. S. Noelker, K. Rockwood, & R. L. Sprott (Eds.), *The encyclopedia of aging: A comprehensive resource in gerontology and geriatrics* (4th ed., p. 609–615). New York: Springer.

Bengtson, V. L., Rosenthal, C. J., & Burton, L. M. (1995). Paradoxes of families and aging. In R. H. Binstock & L. K. George (Eds.), *Handbook of aging and the social sciences* (4th ed., pp. 253–282). San Diego, CA: Academic Press.

Bengtson, V. L., & Schrader, S. S. (1982). Parent-child relations. In D. Mangen & W. Peterson (Eds.), *Handbook of research instruments in social gerontology* (Vol. 2, pp. 115–185). Minneapolis, MN: University of Minnesota Press.

Center for Strategic and International Studies (CSIS). (2001). Program overview, Global Aging Program. Retrieved April 6, 2008 (http:/www.csis.org/gai).

Central Intelligence Agency (CIA). (2001). *Long-term global demographic trends: Reshaping the geopolitical landscape.* United States: Central Intelligence Agency. Retrieved April 7, 2008 (https://www.cia.gov/library/reports/general-reports-1/Demo_Trends_For_Web.pdf).

Cook, F. L. (1981). Crime and the elderly: The emergence of a policy issue. In D. A. Lewis (Ed.), *Reactions to crime.* Beverly Hills, CA: Sage.

Cook, F. L., & Skogan, W.G. (1984). Evaluating the changing definition of a policy issue in Congress: Crime against the elderly. In H. Rogers (Ed.), *Public policy and social institutions.* Greenwich, CT: JAI Press.

Côté, S. (2005). *Population aging and labour market reforms in OECD countries.* Working Paper Series 003, Population Aging and Life-Course Flexibility Project. Ottawa: Policy Research Initiative.

Culhane, M. M. (2001, February 8). *Global aging: Capital market implications.* Chicago, IL: Goldman Sachs Strategic Relationship Management Group.

Dannefer, D. (2003). Toward a global geography of the life course. In J. Mortimer & M. Shanahan (Eds.), *Handbook of the life course* (pp. 647–659). New York: Kluwer Academic/Plenum Publishers.

England, R. S. (2001a). *The fiscal challenge of an aging industrial world. A white paper on demographics and medical technology.* Washington, DC: Center for Strategic and International Studies.

England, R.S. (2001b). *A new era of economic frailty? A white paper on the macroeconomic impact of population aging.* Washington, DC: Center for Strategic and International Studies.

Estes, C. L., Biggs, S., & Phillipson, C. (2003). *Social theory, social policy and ageing: A critical introduction.* Maidenhead, England: Open University Press.

Gee, E. M. (2000). Population and politics: Voodoo demography, population aging, and Canadian social policy. In E. M. Gee & G. Gutman (Eds.), *The overselling of population aging. Apocalyptic demography, intergenerational challenges, and social policy* (pp. 5–25). Don Mills, Ontario: Oxford University Press.

Haber, C. (2006). Old age through the lens of family history. In R. H. Binstock & L. K. George (Eds.), *Handbook of aging and the social sciences* (6th ed., pp. 59–75). Amsterdam: Elsevier.

Hochschild, A. (2000). Global care chains and emotional surplus value. In W. Hutton & A. Giddens (Eds.), *On the edge: Living with global capitalism*. London: Cape.

Hunsley, T. (2006). *Encouraging choice in work and retirement*. Project Report. PRI Project, Population Aging and Life Course Flexibility. Ottawa: Policy Research Initiative.

International Monetary Fund (IMF). (2002). Globalization: Threat or opportunity? Issue Brief, April 12, 2000, corrected 2002. Retrieved April 6, 2008 (http://www.imf.org/external/np/exr/ib/2000/041200to.htm).

Kalache, A., Barreto, S. M., & Keller, I. (2005). Global ageing: The demographic revolution in all cultures and societies. In M. L. Johnson, V. L. Bengtson, P. G. Coleman, & T. B. L. Kirkwood (Eds.), *The Cambridge handbook of age and ageing* (pp. 30–46). Cambridge, UK: Cambridge University Press.

Kelly, C., & Marshall, V. W. (2007). Politics of aging. In James E. Birren (Ed.), *Encyclopedia of gerontology* (2nd ed., Vol. 2, pp. 370–378). Amsterdam: Elsevier.

Lowenstein, A. L. (2005). Global ageing and challenges to families. In M. L. Johnson, V. L. Bengtson, P. G. Coleman, & T. B. L. Kirkwood (Eds.), *The Cambridge handbook of age and ageing* (pp. 403–412). Cambridge, UK: Cambridge University Press.

Lowenstein, A. L., & Bengtson, V. L. (2003). *Global aging and challenges to families*. New York: Aldine de Gruyter.

Marshall, V. W. (2002). New perspectives worldwide on ageing, work and retirement. *Keynote address, Valencia Forum on Aging*, April 2002.

Marshall, V. W. (2006). Investing in human capital for North America: Adaptation opportunities and barriers. *Paper presented at "Labor Markets in North America: Challenges and Opportunities of an Aging Population," Commission for Labor Cooperation*, Mexico City, November 13, 2006.

Marshall, V. W. (2009). Theory informing public policy: The life course perspective as a policy tool. In V. L. Bengtson, M. Silverstein, N. Putney, & D. Gans (Eds.), *Handbook of Theories of Aging* (2nd ed., pp. 573–593). New York: Springer.

Marshall, V. W., & Clarke, P. (2007). Theories of aging: Social. In James W. Birren (Ed.), *Encyclopedia of gerontology* (2nd ed., Vol. 2, pp. 621–630). Amsterdam: Elsevier.

Marshall, V. W., Cook, F. L., & Marshall, J. G. (1993). Conflict over intergenerational equity: Rhetoric and reality in a comparative context. In V. L. Bengtson & W. A. Achenbaum (Eds.), *The changing contract across generations* (pp. 119–140). New York: Aldine de Gruyter.

Mittelman, J. H., & Tambe, A. (2000). Global poverty and gender. In J. H. Mittelman (Ed.), *The globalization syndrome: Transformation and resistance*. Princeton, NJ: Princeton University Press.

Newman, K. S. (2003). *A different shade of gray: Midlife and beyond in the inner city.* New York: The New Press.

Phillipson, C., & Vincent, J. (2007). Globalization and aging. In J. E. Birren (Ed.), *Encyclopedia of gerontology* (2nd ed., pp. 630–635). Amsterdam: Elsevier.

Robertson, A. (1997). Beyond apocalyptic demography: Towards a moral economy of interdependence. *Ageing and Society, 17,* 425–446.

Schieber, S. J., Hewitt, P. S., Tuljapurkar, S., Li, N., & Anderson, M. (2000). Demographic risk in industrial societies. Independent population forecasts for the G-7 countries. An analysis for the Commission on Global Aging. *World Economics, 1*(4), 1–46.

Sokolovsky, J. (2002, April 7). Senior-youth ratio could bring crisis. *The News & Observer,* Raleigh, NC, p. 13A.

Svihula, J., & Estes, C. L. (2007). Social security politics: Ideology and reform. *Journal of Gerontology: Social Sciences, 62B*(2), S79–S89.

Townsend, P. (2006). Policies for the aged in the 21st century: More "structured dependency" or the realization of human rights? *Ageing & Society, 26*(2), 161–179.

Vincent, J. A. (2006). Globalization and critical theory: Political economy of world population issues. In J. Baars, D. Dannefer, C. Phillipson, & A. Walker (Eds.), *Aging, globalization, and inequality: The new critical gerontology* (pp. 245–276). Amityville, NY: Baywood.

Walker, A. (2005). Towards an international political economy of ageing. *Ageing & Society, 25*(6), 815–839.

Walker, A., & Deacon, B. (2003). Economic globalisation and policies on ageing. *Journal of Societal and Public Policy, 2*(2), 1–18.

Watts, J. (2001, August 30). Ageing populace is killing economy, says study. *Guardian Unlimited.* Retrieved April 6, 2008 (http://www.guardian.co.uk/Archive/Article/0,4273,4247445,00.html).

CHAPTER THIRTEEN

Social Change, Social Structure, and the Cycle of Induced Solidarity

Dale Dannefer and Rebecca A. Siders

R ecently, the cover of the *New York Times* Sunday magazine featured a Filipino woman with the caption, "200 million migrants worldwide sent home $300 billion last year." The article, entitled "A Good Provider Is One Who Leaves," describes how families are simultaneously sustained economically and strained socially and emotionally by the absence of a parent who is participating in the rapidly growing arrangement of transnational labor migration. The article is timely. Presently, approximately 10% of Filipino citizens— 89 million people—live and work abroad on a permanent basis, with only very few occasionally returning home to see their spouses and children. Nevertheless, these migrant workers are called modern-day heroes since they send home approximately $15 billion each year, which equates to a seventh of the country's gross domestic product (Choy, 2003; DeParle, 2007).

The Philippines, of course, is only one country where extended periods of parent absenteeism linked to economic opportunities have become institutionalized. It has become an increasingly common style of family life in other regions of the world including Asia, West Africa, Eastern Europe, Latin America, and parts of the Middle East (Burawoy & Blum, 2000). Transnational migration is becoming an increasingly frequent topic of social research. One example of research on this phenomenon is the work of Phillipson, Ahmed, and Latimer (2003), which focused on Bangladeshi women living in London and explored the changes in the family and community life introduced by transnational migration.

Closer to home, consider Robert Courtney Smith's ethnography *Mexican New York* (2006). Smith has referred to this project as "life-course ethnography," since it has lasted for almost two decades and is still ongoing. In it, Smith documents bidirectional migration between New York City and rural Mexico as a permanently institutionalized, intergenerational practice in which families operate with different dynamics, role expectations, and kinds of solidarity when they are in New York City than when they are in rural Mexico.

Although transnational labor migration is not a new phenomenon, its rapid and sustained growth has established it as a concomitant of globalization (for globalization, see Marshall, Chapter 12). Yet, transnational labor migration is only one manifestation of the social forces that are restructuring the family as an institution.

The Second Demographic Transition and the Transformation of Families in Late Modernity

While globalization is clearly having profound and worldwide effects on families, in the developed world, perhaps equally profound changes are captured by the term "second demographic transition" (SDT). The SDT entails a reversal of the twentieth-century trend in Europe and North America toward greater homogeneity and in some respects normativity and stability in numerous dimensions of family life as well as the life course (e.g., Dannefer & Patterson, 2007; Hogan, 1981; Uhlenberg, 1974). Compared to earlier cohorts, baby boomers married late, delayed childbearing, and divorced more often (Lesthaeghe & Neidert, 2006; Van de Kaa, 2002). They also adopted alternative family forms: "The single life," single parenthood, and same-sex relationships as the basis of families have all become more prevalent and accepted lifestyles. Multigenerational households have been produced by the return of "boomerang children," by circumstances compelling grandparents or others to function as surrogate parents, and by elder care needs.

With cohorts whose members' lives entail such diverse family transitions at such variable ages, the likely result will be an increasingly kaleidoscopic picture of family structures, histories, and relationships. Just as is the case with transnational families, this picture strains the boundaries and premises of established understandings of the family.

What is driving the deinstitutionalization of the family? One of the forces behind these trends in the family is a change in cultural values that gives individuals a new level of freedom of choice; another force is the changing opportunity structure derived from shifts in the labor market and the economy (Hughes and Waite, 2007). The latter force is likely to affect families with resources differently than those without resources.

What are the consequences of deinstitutionalization for the everyday experience of family life and the lives of individuals? We suggest that this freedom of choice poses a challenge for individuals due to the unavailability of cultural rulebooks for new and complex kin relationships; new family forms lead to perplexing expectations that entail experiences of chaos, powerlessness, and stressful role ambiguities. Forces that push the boundaries of families also raise questions about the boundaries of the very definition of the term "family." And, given the extensive range of forces and increasing diversification of family forms and experiences involved, is it possible to develop anything like a coherent explanatory model for family change? These are the questions that this chapter seeks to address.

Family Transformation and Social Processes

The broad social forces creating both new opportunities and new challenges are being experienced in powerful yet distinctly different ways by families living under different economic and cultural regimes. Is it possible to conceptualize social processes in ways that cut across this social and cultural diversity? Our answer to this question is in the affirmative. However, it is an answer that requires some reconsideration of dominant assumptions in the research on the family. In this chapter, we focus on three issues that cut across cultural and economic contexts. These are (1) the nature of choice and agency underlying these transformations of family life; (2) the important role of economic factors (including social class) in shaping family outcomes; and (3) the need to examine more closely the actual mechanisms through which observed family patterns and outcomes are produced in the first place—that is, in the microinteraction of everyday life.

Forces Accounting for Transformations of Family Life

As we mentioned above, one of the forces behind the shifting character of the family is often assumed to be the "choices" people make. After all, family affiliation is, ideally, a matter of personal discretion and choice, and it is recognized—implicitly if not explicitly—in the research literature—that family formation and endurance have an element of volition. Thus, choice and agency are often emphasized in life-course analysis and in family and life-course research.

Some individuals undeniably have more options than others. Even if that is true, people are "making choices" all the time, even when options are few and less than ideal. The Filipino mothers and fathers engaged in transnational migration—the good providers who leave—have obviously made choices, even if hard ones. More than likely, they would have made a different choice if their circumstances were different. Researchers studying labor migration have been among those who have encouraged examining the effect of structural factors on these choices. Studies of migrant nurses, for example, commonly refer to push and pull factors to describe structural conditions that drive transnational migration. Pull factors include things like high remuneration, job satisfaction, safe work environment, or professional development opportunities, whereas push factors include poor quality of life, high crime, political repression, lack of education, and insufficient employment opportunities in the country of origin (Kingma, 2007; Ong & Azores, 1994).

As Marx said, "men [people] make history, but not under conditions of their own choosing" (1972 [1852]). Choices are typically constrained, and they cannot be understood outside the context of constraints (Dannefer, 1999). Therefore, choice alone really does not explain very much. Constraints typically involve differentials in power and resources, especially economic resources. This is, of course, manifestly true in the case of the good providers who leave.

But beyond the level of conscious decision making, economic circumstances have deeper effects on individuals and families. It is clear from numerous lines of research that economic strain and adversity contribute to stress and dissatisfaction in family life (Conger & Elder, 1994; Conger et al., 1990; Mills, Grasmick, Morgan, & Wenk, 1992; Dannefer & Patterson, 2007; Voydanoff & Majka, 1988). These stressors are often enduring and can be transmitted and reproduced intergenerationally, thus providing continuity in patterns either of stability or of disruption.

More generally, the importance of family and community is emphasized in many of the ethnographic and qualitative studies on Filipino nurse migrants. The social cost of separation from the family is paramount, especially for those leaving children behind (see Parrenas, 2005, and Pyle, 2006). Departing nurses count on mothers, husbands, or other family members to take care of their children. Even if surrogate parents function well, asking women to place the economic survival of their family ahead of their bond with their children is an inherently contradictory personal and social demand. Such demands have major implications not only for the provider who leaves but also for the children and families left behind (Parrenas, 2005; Zimmerman, Litt, & Bose, 2006).

Numerous commentators have observed that the SDT also may simultaneously reflect both diversity and choice, on one hand, and uncertainty and vulnerability on the other. The SDT will likely increase stresses on families as risks accumulate, especially if the secular trend toward increasing inequality continues (Dannefer & Patterson, 2007; Greenspan, 2007; Hughes & Waite, 2007). We propose that the increase in both the diversity of family structures and the precariousness of family relationships will require researchers to pay increasing attention to economic resources as well as other constraining factors. In mainstream American families no less than in minority or transnational families, economic resources play a significant role in the shaping of family patterns, strengths, and tensions. Of course, that is why social class is such a powerful predictor of family stability, values, and lifestyle.

The Interaction of Resources with Family Processes

In the simpler mid-twentieth-century days, prior to the clear emergence of the forces described by the SDT and the expansion of global migration, the effects of social class differentials were recognized, robust, and powerful.

The effects of social class are mediated through family in complex ways. This means, of course, that one cannot understand the effects of either family or social class without looking at both of them together. Although we have some sense of this for ethnic and religious variation and life history (e.g., Elder & Liker, 1982), it is also true for other factors, such as how marriage and family intersect with where one is in the life course. For example, an analysis of the effects of education on depression using National Longitudinal Survey data reveals a clear divergence based on education, a clear pattern of cumulative advantage and disadvantage. Yet multivariate analyses of these same data showed that much of the education effect is mediated through the experience of marriage and families (Patterson, Falletta, Burant, & Dannefer, 2007). For example, the effect becomes even more pronounced for those who were alone, whereas it diminishes sharply for those who married during the 10-year period of data collection. If such diversity and complexity can be accepted as characterizing family life, where does the cumulative advantage and disadvantage come from? What is actually going on in the lives of families?

The Constitution of Family Structure in Everyday Social Interaction: The Cycle of Induced Solidarity

Although we are continuing to learn about the degree to which family patterns are organized by broader forces, families are private entities, and we have little detailed information on the actual dynamics that occur in everyday family life. Yet almost all of the accumulated data on families, from whatever source, is ultimately the product of relentless, everyday social interaction—which is also the primary meeting ground of agency and structure.

We propose that the Cycle of Induced Incompetence, first introduced in Bengtson's early work (1973), provides a valuable heuristic framework for analyzing such dynamics, because it maps the fundamental interactional processes through which self and personhood are constructed in social relations. Applying the principles of labeling theory, Bengtson created a diagram to demonstrate the cycle through which the sociogenesis of individual age-related incompetence is produced. Beginning with a social definition of vulnerability, the diagram shows how that definition can become a self-fulfilling prophecy that is reified by others and then internalized by the actor.

But this schematic is actually a more general model of human and social processes than is implied by the focus on the production of incompetence. It is important to remember that the processes of labeling, reality construction, and internalization that underlie the model operate just as much in the reproduction of affirmation and success as they do in the production of deviance and decline. More often than anything else, they likely operate in the production of normality and solidarity.

At least as prevalent in social reality, then, is what may be called the Cycle of Induced Solidarity (figure 13.1). Such sentiments do not just spring from nowhere. Like induced incompetence, they are generated in the ongoing dynamics of social interaction—just as feelings of exclusion and rejection are generated when something triggers the start of a cycle of incompetence. Figure 13.1 shows that the same dynamic that generates feelings of incompetence also generates solidarity and affirmation. The cycle begins with increased vulner-

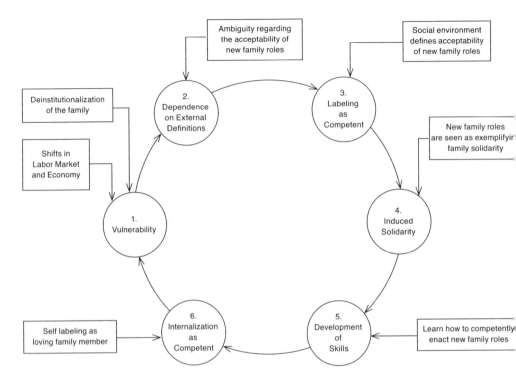

Figure 13.1. The cycle of induced solidarity. Adapted from Bengtson's "Cycle of Induced Dependence" (1973).

ability due to the creation of new family roles that lack cultural guidelines. It proceeds with a dependence on external definitions because of ambiguous norms regarding the acceptability of unconventional family forms. Next, the social environment imbues these new family forms and roles with acceptability, leading to induced solidarity and ultimately the internalization of feelings of competence among family actors.

We suggest that in order to understand how the outcomes measured in survey, interview, and epidemiological data collection are produced, it is necessary to examine everyday interaction in family contexts. Doing so can help provide new insights concerning forces that constitute both solidarity and conflict within families.

ACKNOWLEDGMENTS

The authors wish to thank Sandra Barnes, Gary Deimling, and David Warner for comments on an earlier draft of this paper.

REFERENCES

Bengtson, V. L. (1973). *The social psychology of aging.* Indianapolis, IN: Bobbs-Merrill.

Burawoy, M., & Blum, J. A. (2000). *Global ethnography: Forces, connections, and imaginations in a postmodern world.* Berkeley, CA: University of California Press.

Choy, C. C. (2003). *Empire of care: Nursing and migration in Filipino American history.* Durham, NC: Duke University Press.

Conger, R., & Elder, G. H. (1994). *Families in troubled times: Adapting to change in rural America.* New York: Aldine de Gruyter.

Conger, R., Elder, G. H., Lorenz, F. O., Conger, K. J., Simons, R. L., Whitbeck, L. B., Huck, S., & Melby, J. N. (1990). Linking economic hardship to marital quality and instability. *Journal of Marriage and the Family, 52,* 643–656.

Dannefer, D. (1999). Freedom isn't free: Power, alienation and the consequences of action. In J. Brandstadter & R. M. Lerner (Eds.), *Action and self development* (pp. 105–131). Thousand Oaks, CA: Sage.

Dannefer, D., & Patterson, R. S. (2007). The Second Demographic Transition, aging families, and the aging of the institutionalized life course (commentary). In K. W. Schaie & P. Uhlenberg (Eds.), *Social structures: Demographic changes and the well-being of older persons* (pp. 212–229). New York: Springer.

DeParle, J. (2007). A good provider is one who leaves. *New York Times Magazine,* April 22, p. 50.

Elder, G. H., & Liker, J. K. (1982). Hard times in women's lives: Historical influences across forty years. *The American Journal of Sociology, 88,* 241–269.

Greenspan, A. (2007). *The age of turbulence: Adventures in a new world.* New York: Penguin Group.

Hogan, D. P. (1981). *Transitions and social change: The early lives of American men.* New York: Academic Press.

Hughes, M. E., & Waite, L. J. (2007). The aging of the Second Demographic Transition. In K. W. Schaie & P. Uhlenberg (Eds.), *Social structures: Demographic changes and the well-being of older persons* (pp. 179–211). New York: Springer.

Kingma, M. (2007). Nurses on the move: A global overview. *Health Services Research, Part II, 42*(3), 1281–1298.

Lesthaeghe, R. J., & Neidert, L. (2006). The "Second Demographic Transition" in the U.S.: Exception or textbook example? *Population and Development Review, 32*(4), 669–698.

Marx, K. (1972 [1852]). The eighteenth brumaire of Louis Bonaparte. In R. C. Tucker (Ed.), *The Marx-Engels reader* (pp. 436–525). New York: W. W. Norton.

Mills, R. J., Grasmick, H. G., Morgan, C. S., & Wenk, D. (1992). Effects of gender, family satisfaction, and economic strain on psychological well-being. *Family Relations,* *41*(4), 440–445.

Ong, P., & Azores, T. (1994). The migration and incorporation of Filipino nurses. In P. Ong, E. Bonacich, & L. Cheng (Eds.), *The Asian immigration in Los Angeles and global restructuring* (pp. 164–196). Philadelphia, PA: Temple University Press.

Parrenas, R. S. (2005). *Children of global migration: Transnational families and gendered woes.* Stanford, CA: Stanford University Press.

Patterson, R. S., Falletta, L., Burant, C., and Dannefer, D. (2007). Education, marriage and health: The dynamics of cumulative advantage/disadvantage in young adulthood. *Paper presented at the annual meeting of the Gerontological Society of America.* San Francisco, CA.

Phillipson, C., Ahmed, N., & Latimer, J. (2003). *Women in transition: A study of the experiences of Bangladeshi women living in Tower Hamlets.* Bristol, UK: The Policy Press.

Pyle, J. L. (2006). Globalization, transnational migration, and gendered care work: Introduction. *Globalization, 3*(3), 283–295.

Smith, R. C. (2006). *Mexican New York: Transnational lives of new immigrants.* Berkeley, CA: University of California Press.

Uhlenberg, P. (1974). Cohort variations in family life cycle experiences of U.S. females. *Journal of Marriage and the Family, 36,* 284–292.

Van de Kaa., D. J. (2002). The idea of a Second Demographic Transition in industrialized countries. *Paper presented at the 6th welfare policy seminar of the National Institute of Population and Social Security.* Tokyo, Japan.

Voydanoff, P., & Majka, L. C. (1988). *Families and economic distress: Coping strategies and social policy.* Thousand Oaks, CA: Sage.

Zimmerman, M. K., Litt, J. S., & Bose, C. E. (2006). *Global dimensions of gender and carework.* Stanford, CA: Stanford Social Sciences.

CHAPTER FOURTEEN

The Intergenerational Social Contract Revisited

Cross-National Perspectives

Christopher Steven Marcum and Judith Treas

> I dare say that if we passed through life backwards, adults would insist on conditions in childhood be made far more appealing.
> SAMUEL PRESTON (1984, P. 466)

Population aging is a global phenomenon. In what Bengtson and colleagues (2003) call a "population explosion" and what Myers (2007) calls a "third demographic transition," older people the world over are growing more numerous and living longer. With strong expectations of early retirement in developed nations (Kääriäinen & Lehtonen, 2006; Doling & Horsewood, 2003; Pienta & Hayward, 2002), the ratio of older adults to working-aged people constitutes a deficit of providers. The eventual workforce exodus from mass retirement may reverse intergenerational wealth transfers, which have traditionally flowed from older to younger people (Delong, 2002; Lee, 1994). Population aging has posed a particular challenge to the welfare state as expenditures are allocated across generations on an increasingly smaller tax base. The changing tax base is likely to be a major issue facing families and states alike into the twenty-first century (Lowenstein & Bengtson, 2003).

The state of intergenerational relations in various countries is a backdrop for the challenges ahead. In this paper, we take stock of attitudes toward state support for children and older people. We address the question of state support orientations across different welfare regimes, that is, across nation states characterized by different approaches to the provision of social welfare. Concerns are often voiced that population aging will either demand a draconian scaling back of government commitments to old age support or prompt a political mobilization of older adults that preserves their retirement prerogatives at the expense of public support for children. In light of these issues, we are particularly interested in the level of public endorsement for the long-standing intergenerational contract of state support for both young and old. Similarly, we examine the extent of approval for government support of older adults without provisions for children. Lastly, because a neoliberal ideology of market fundamentalism has been broadly promulgated in recent decades, we are keen to determine how many individuals have embraced a position that disapproves of government spending on young and old alike.

The Challenge to Individuals and the State

Society's dependents are increasingly concentrated in older age groups. Early retirement trends during the 1990s (Gruber and Wise, 1997), coupled with low fertility, threaten to raise the overall support ratio in virtually every developed nation (Fougère & Mérette, 1999). State policies have encouraged working-aged people to have more children, albeit with little effect. This demographic situation places greater demand on working-aged adults to support both themselves and preceding and succeeding generations. If the demands on the working-aged, the so-called "sandwich generation" (Miller, 1981), exceed their capacity to support society's dependents, states will confront painful and challenging conflicts over the allocation of public resources. States are faced with a particularly delicate situation in regard to generational spending.

Elders and children compete for limited resources from states. Older adults have been reasonably effective in mobilizing to protect their interests (Binstock, 2000; Preston, 1984). Children, however, cannot compete for themselves and are represented largely by parents. This places middle-aged adults in a fiscal and political squeeze, making it unclear where their own self-interest lies. They are burdened with maintaining the interests of their young children, looking out for their own future well-being into old age, and addressing the needs of their parents. Furthermore, middle-aged adults end up with the biggest stake in generational spending because they foot the bill. Demographer Dowell Myers (2004, 2007), however, makes a case for investments in children as benefiting everyone, because the young are future taxpayers who will support the old and those who are soon to be old. How a state treats children reflects the nature and extent of the public's egalitarian values, family philosophy, and willingness to encourage women's employment outside the home.

Esping-Andersen (1999), the Danish sociologist, has explained that the government needs to ensure social protection for both the young and the old through the welfare state because traditional systems of economic support for these groups are in decline. Institutional support and self-support are gradually replacing support provided by the family in general and by women in particular. However, policymakers in democratic states respond to voters and organized interests. This dynamic is a potential source of intergenerational conflict because individuals tend to react to their social world in ways that are most salient to themselves. Indeed, Hasenfeld and Rafferty (1989) found that people who support the welfare state tend to be those who are most disadvantaged. Their findings also suggest that age-related self-interest influences views of welfare programs. Older adults are less likely than younger people to support the welfare state in general, but are more likely to support social spending on programs that would be beneficial to their own age group, such as universal health care and old age pensions.

Despite the recent Obama youth mobilization in the United States (see Lynch, 2008, for a discussion), much research has shown that older people tend to be more politically active than their younger counterparts (Binstock, 2000; Goerres, 2007). The consequences of older people's disproportionate political influence have not gone unnoticed by researchers. Preston (1984) linked social indicators of differences between children and older people with fiscal and social policy changes from the 1960s to the mid-1980s in the United States. Nearly every well-being measure rose for the elderly but fell for children. This appeared to coincide, at least anecdotally, with cuts in children's programs and stability or improvements in programs for older adults. Like Preston, Coale (1986) pointed out that the relative increases in quality of life and political influence for older people have been matched with deprivations for children in the United States. However, in a cross-national comparison, Pampel (1994) found that European countries exhibit no such pattern. In fact, elderly poverty shows a modest positive association with child poverty across Western nations (Brady, 2004). As this suggests, in countries with developed welfare states, the well-being of older adults and children share much in common. Furthermore, by the early twenty-first century, older adults came to have a higher risk of poverty than children in some nations (Förster & d'Ercole, 2005).

Newacheck and Benjamin (2004) are concerned that social welfare spending will be driven by politics and macroeconomic trends rather than by the needs of children and the elderly. They suggest that posing the question of generational spending as a polarizing issue—that is, wedging a gap between young and old—obscures the problem of dependency. Walker (1993) raised the question of whether the issue of intergenerational equity was largely a ploy to undermine Social Security in the United States. Indeed, Parrott, Reynolds, and Bengston (1997) ask whether the gerontocratic takeover of spending programs is really a myth seeded by the media's preoccupation with a few well-known research articles that suggest the older cohorts are winning out at the expense of children. Similar concern regarding the social construction of age inequality has been raised by Binstock (1983) and Minkler (1991). Indeed, many of these questions and concerns were raised in a 1993 volume edited by Bengtson and Achenbaum, *The Changing Contract across Generations*, which concludes that the possibility of intergenerational conflict is genuine but leaves open the question of threats to the welfare state (Quadagno, Achenbaum, & Bengtson, 1993).

These arguments point to a particular feature of social life that Bengtson (1993) has famously called the intergenerational social contract. In what follows, we describe the intergenerational social contract and assess where individuals from different contexts stand on the state's role in support of young and old.

The Intergenerational Social Contract

For decades, Vern Bengtson has been at the forefront of framing the issues of generations at both the macro and micro levels. At the macro level, he has called attention to the "contract across generations and age groups" as a set of norms that guide behavior and interaction through the life course (1993, p. 4). The intergenerational social contract is an implicit agreement between society's providers and dependents. It guides and reinforces norms of entitlement and responsibility. In particular, as Bengtson emphasizes, the contract lays out the rules for the exchange of care between generations.

At the micro level, Bengtson and associates (Bengtson, Olander, & Haddad, 1976) have emphasized the concept of functional solidarity. With significant implications for the intergenerational social contract, functional solidarity is "the exchange of material and instrumental support and assistance between generations" (Mabry, Giarrusso, & Bengtson, 2004, p. 95). While functional solidarity is forwarded as a relation between individuals, the concept is also applicable to macrostructures such as support for generational equity in state spending. The concept of functional solidarity across generations is useful for understanding attitudes toward state spending because it acts as a lubricant for a potentially frictive economic relation implied by the dependency ratio.

At least since Spencer (1879), social theorists have been interested in the redistribution of resources across generations, examining one or more aspects of the intergenerational contract. The benefits and burdens prescribed by the contract have, at times, been unevenly distributed across generations (Bengtson, Marti, & Roberts, 1991). Naturally, one of the major factors shaping how the contract impacts individuals is the age structure. For most developed nations today, this means elders constitute the majority stakeholders.

In the past, the intergenerational contract held that citizens had mutual obligations to each other. These obligations were met through diverse public and private initiatives, including public education, health care for the poor and elderly, child labor laws, and social insurance against the risk of becoming impoverished through bad luck or illness (Reich, 1999).

More recently, different states have added or removed obligations and entitlements in response to changes in ideology or economic conditions. In the United States, for example, a neoliberal philosophy of market fundamentalism has been the dominant policy perspective for the past two decades (Somers & Block, 2005). Market fundamentalism is "the idea that society as a whole should be subordinated to a system of self-regulating markets" (Somers & Block, 2005, p. 261) and that individuals should be responsible for themselves and their families. This is in stark contrast to Scandinavian states where the state is charged with reducing market-based inequalities and where various government benefits, such as public child care, are considered as universal entitlements (Leira, 2002). At this point, it is worth discussing the sociopolitical context of the intergenerational social contract.

The Welfare State and the Intergenerational Social Contract

The welfare state itself can be characterized as an institutionalization of the intergenerational social contract (Esping-Andersen, 2002b; Thomson, 1989; Walker, 1993). Different welfare state regimes with their differing approaches to social welfare provisions provide a context within which individuals' attitudes and behavior toward social spending are shaped. Given the diversity in welfare state regimes (see Myles & Quadagno, 2002, for a review), it is useful to review the state types and the ways in which their approaches toward welfare provisioning might shape public opinion regarding the intergenerational social contract. Although welfare state typologies have come in for debate and criticism (Arts & Gellisen, 2002; Orloff, 1993), they constitute a valuable heuristic device for comparative theorizing. In addition to the three capitalist welfare regimes first described by Esping-Andersen (1990)—liberal, conservative, and social democratic—we also consider postsocialist states of Eastern Europe and Southern European welfare regimes.

Liberal States

Countries generally recognized as belonging to this group include Australia, Canada, the United States, the United Kingdom, and New Zealand (Esping-Andersen, 1990). In general, these welfare states are characterized by comparatively low state spending; limited, means-tested welfare programs; and policies designed not to interfere with the free market. As the United States shows, social security old age benefits, for example, may only be mildly progressive and redistributive. The dominant laissez-faire ethos leaves the family largely responsible for providing care to the young and old alike. Since they do not take a stand for or against women's labor force participation, the liberal states provide little in the way of public child care (Gornick, Meyers, & Ross, 1998). The question of generational equity and the intergenerational social contract is particularly contentious in liberal countries, possibly because of the low provision of universalistic benefits and the higher degrees of individualism in their cultures (Walker, 1993). The principles of market fundamentalism have also resonated in these states, as evidenced by the restrictive U.S. welfare reforms of 1996. Thus, compared to other welfare regimes, we would expect public opinion in the liberal states to be less likely to adhere to the intergenerational contract of state support for young and old. We would expect these populations to be comparatively likely to reject state support altogether or to limit it to the politically mobilized population of older adults.

Conservative States

Western European countries like Germany, Austria, and the Netherlands (Esping-Andersen, 1990) have devoted substantial shares of GDP to social spending, but benefits, being based on occupation and status, tend to preserve market inequalities. Because the taxation, employment, and welfare policies of conservative states have favored "traditional" families with a male breadwinner and female homemaker (Forssén & Hakorvirta, 2002; Gustafsson, 1994), there is limited government support for child care, and children in female-headed families are at a disadvantage. Given their long-standing old age support programs and their conventional attitudes about maternal responsibility for children (Treas and Widmer, 2000), we might expect these countries to be more inclined than others to favor government support for older adults but not for children.

Nordic Social Democratic States

The generous welfare schemes of Nordic social democratic states emphasize universal entitlements to a host of public programs. In addition to well-developed old age provisions, children benefit from child allowances and from public child care to encourage their mothers to work for pay (Leira, 2002). To use the term of Esping-Andersen (1999), the social democratic states of Scandinavia are the most advanced in terms of defamilialization, whereby the state assumes caregiving and support responsibilities that would otherwise fall to the family. Given their strong egalitarian ideology and their history of support for young and old, we would not expect the social democratic states to favor one age group over the other, much less retreat from state provisions for dependents. In sum, we would expect strong support for the intergenerational social contract in social democratic countries.

Post-Socialist States

Eastern European states with a legacy of communism under the former USSR may also exhibit strong support for equitable social spending on the young and the old. Under socialism, citizens could count on state support from cradle to grave, including public child care, guaranteed employment, universal health care, and old age pensions. An egalitarian gender ideology promoting maternal employment translated to notably high levels of public child care. As these transition economies have struggled, however, they have often had to cut public spending by rewriting the social contract (e.g., reducing benefits and tying them more closely to earnings). Lipsmeyer (2003) warns that postsocialist countries are not homogeneous in terms of public attitudes toward state spending. As these countries transition toward capitalism, people are exposed to more individualistic values, including the ideology of market fundamentalism, which may reduce the effect of their socialist legacy. Therefore, we cautiously anticipate support for the intergenerational social contract in such states.

Southern European States

Identified as a distinctive welfare regime type (Caspers & Mitchell, 1993; Ferrera, 1996), Mediterranean countries such as Spain and Italy have familistic cultures and were slow to develop either a welfare state or a formal service sector. Their welfare systems are characterized by dualistic schemes (differing provisions for regular-sector and irregular-sector workers), institutional fragmentation (separate plans for various occupational groups), and clientelism (welfare serving political purposes). Given their traditional culture of generational interdependence and the absence of individualistic, market fundamentalist objections to state welfare provisions found in the United States, we might expect Southern European states, in particular, to embrace the social contract doctrine of state support for young and old.

For various reasons, we hypothesize that the citizens of social democratic, postsocialist, and Southern European countries will be most likely to embrace the intergenerational social contract exemplified in approval of state support for both children and older adults. We hypothesize that those in liberal welfare states will be less likely to embrace the social contract and more likely to favor either no state support for either age group or support limited to older adults. As for those in conservative states, we anticipate that they will be more likely to agree with state support for older adults than for children.

Individual Factors and the Intergenerational Social Contract

Besides the likely influence of context, we also anticipate that views of state support for young and old will be shaped by the characteristics of individuals. Absent overriding norms of intergenerational solidarity, principles of self-interest suggest that people are more oriented toward their own immediate needs than to those of others. That is, younger people might want to secure services for child care while older people might want to ensure that they are provided a decent living standard. However, given the context of increasing demand on working-aged groups to provide for both children and the aged, it might be more reasonable to expect that more young and middle-aged people would seek state support for both classes of dependents to alleviate that pressure.

These self-interest arguments extend to the effects of gender on support for the welfare state, in general, and state spending orientation, in particular. Past research has shown that women demonstrate more support for the welfare state than men. Some researchers suggest that the reason for the gender gap is that women are more likely to be recipients of benefits (i.e., as homemakers, single mothers, or widows) (Hernes, 1984; Sainsbury, 1996). Blekesaune and Quadagno (2003) argue that women have more self-interest in the welfare state because of their greater risk of being caregivers throughout the life course; women often transition into the paid workforce when the state provides for caregiving services. Following these arguments, we would expect that women would have a greater propensity to support spending at both ends of the life course, thus embracing an intergenerational orientation. Additionally, Charles and Cech (2010) found that welfare regime context matters in shaping women's caregiving ideals. In particular, postsocialist states, which traditionally provided universal child care, tend to display greater support for maternal employment. Of course, individuals with more limited economic resources, whether measured by education or social class, are known to be more supportive of social welfare (Hasenfeld & Rafferty, 1989).

Finally, it follows that attitudes toward spending on the young and the old may be shaped by household and family composition. The great diversity in household and family structure—ranging from single-generation households to extended multigenerational "beanpole" families (Bengtson, Rosenthal, & Burton, 1990)—implies multiplex expectations about how social contract orientations might be related to various family attributes. For example, having a living parent may compel one to support state spending on older people (and perhaps on children as well to relieve some of the pressure from being in the sandwich generation). Alternatively, having a living parent may be a valued resource to parents, shifting orientations away from spending altogether to leave more earned income to be spent as the family sees fit. Likewise, having young children may entrench parents into an orientation that supports spending on child care only, or it may shift parents to support intergenerational spending. We therefore consider each scenario as a competing hypothesis of how family and household composition affect social contract orientation.

If self-interest dominates, we would expect older adults and those with surviving mothers to be more likely to favor support of older adults only over an intergenerational orientation. Similarly, younger adults with children present in the household are hypothesized to be less likely to favor alternatives to an intergenerational orientation toward government spending. Following prior research, we would also expect those with more limited socioeconomic resources (less educated, lower social class) or greater need (larger household size) to be less likely to endorse the alternatives to the more inclusive intergenerational contract orientation. Similarly, women, and perhaps those who are not currently married, are expected to be less disposed to options that do not offer support of young and old alike.

Data and Methods

Our data were drawn from the International Social Survey Programme's (ISSP) 2001 Social Network II module. This dataset consists of responses from individuals in a variety of social contexts, including 30 samples from the population of 27 countries (Klein & Harkness, 2001).2 The ISSP has an approximately representative national sample design and is widely used in social science and policy research. A common survey instrument is fielded by independent survey organizations in participating countries, often as part of other ongoing surveys.

Variables

Our dependent variable measures social contract orientation. This is a latent construct inferred by combining two items from the ISSP that measure attitudes toward social support for older people and children, respectively. Respondents were asked to indicate whether they think that the government definitely should support, probably should support, probably should not support, or definitely should not support spending programs that would (1) provide child care for everyone who wants it or (2) provide a decent standard of living for the old.

These items were used to construct four binary response variables that indicate whether the respondent was more *family/market oriented* (did not support either), *intergenerationally oriented* (supported both), *older adult only oriented* (supported the old but not the young), or *child only oriented* (supported the young but not the old). Collectively, these binary variables constitute a measure of social contract orientation.

Our primary interest here is to evaluate the relationship between social contract orientation and social context. The analysis incorporates individual and household-independent variables with indicators of the state regime type. Individual and household factors consist of age, sex, marital status, level of education, self-identified social class, household size, whether the respondent has a surviving parent, and whether the respondent has a child under 18 years of age. The state factors are measured at the country level and include dummies for welfare regime types.

Roughly 35% of the cases were missing on at least one variable, representing less than 4% of the data. Most missing data appeared to be non-systematic and fell close to a random baseline. Missing data were imputed using multiple imputation methods, including the MICE package for R as well as Bayesian inference. We omitted cases where respondents were missing on four or more out of eight independent variables. Responses missing on the dependent variables were not imputed to avoid bias and were omitted. The ISSP did not collect information about household size in Brazil or South Africa. Additionally, data were not sufficient for Northern Ireland. We therefore omit responses from these three countries in the multivariate analysis. Our final sample size is $n = 21,168$.

Analysis

First we examine the marginal distributions for the social contract orientations within countries. This provides us with a general summary of the cross-national patterns and differences in contract orientation. Second, to understand what factors help shape an individual's orientation, we conduct a weighted multinomial logistic regression of the probability of contract orientation on individual, household, and state-context factors.

Results

First we turn to the distribution of the four spending orientations by welfare regime type as shown in figure 14.1. The figure clearly shows the exceptionalism of liberal welfare states, which have the lowest proportion of their populations that are intergenerationally oriented and the highest proportion that are older adult only oriented and family/market oriented.

Consistent with expectations, support for the intergenerational social contract is most tenuous in liberal regimes, where only 55% favor government provisions for both the young and old compared to more than three-quarters in other regimes. As hypothesized, the family/market orientation also gains the most traction in liberal countries (this is especially true in the United States); however, it is still a minority position, embraced by less than 7% of liberal countries. Support for older adults only is relatively high in liberal countries (38%). The welfare state appears well entrenched in these liberal regimes insofar as it reflects the popularity of old age support programs. As hypothesized, postsocialist and Southern European states, like social democratic ones, demonstrate very high levels of support for the intergenerational orientation. Surprisingly, conservative regimes seem to be about as strongly supportive of the intergenerational social contract as are social democratic regimes.

The country-specific proportions of support for different social contract orientations are shown in the appendix (table 14A.1). In most countries, the largest

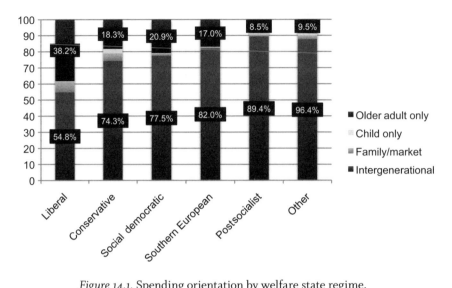

Figure 14.1. Spending orientation by welfare state regime.

share of people report being intergenerationally oriented, or supportive of spending on young and old alike. This is a nearly universal orientation among a few populations, such as Russians (96%), Spaniards (96%), and Israeli Arabs (97%), but the intergenerational orientation is not embraced by majorities in the United States, Australia, New Zealand, or Switzerland.

The older adult only orientation is the next most popular, garnering the most support in the United States, Australia, New Zealand, and Switzerland. Despite the dissemination of the ideology of market fundamentalism, the family/market orientation, which disapproves of spending on young and old, is a minority position in all countries. Although the family/market orientation attracts 16% of Americans, 10% of the Japanese, and 9% of the Swiss, support tends to be considerably lower in other countries (e.g., 2% in Denmark). Least popular in all but a handful of countries is the position of spending on children to the neglect of the old. Although 7% of the Japanese and 5% of West Germans favor the child only orientation, it finds even less favor elsewhere.

Conservative states are the most heterogeneous, and postsocialist, social democratic, Southern European, and other states are relatively uniform in their distributions, reflecting their strong support of government spending on both children and older adults.

Overall, we find strong endorsement for intergenerational benefits across societies. In these aging populations, there is no evidence of any substantial constituency willing to abandon support for older adults in order to favor children in the distribution of state resources. Nor is there support for a neoliberal market fundamentalism that would have the state withdraw from social welfare responsibilities. On the other hand, in some places, especially liberal regimes like the United States, enthusiasm for state support of only older adults points out that government responsibility for the living standards of older people has been thoroughly institutionalized. Despite widespread support for the intergenerational contract, older adults appear to be better positioned in a resource competition than do children. It is the liberal states that appear most vulnerable to intergenerational conflict, because a high acceptance of public pensions is coupled with an undercurrent of skepticism that the state has a rightful role in social welfare provisions to children.

We now turn to our multivariate analysis to examine how individual-level characteristics and welfare state regime together predict the probability of social contract orientation. The multinomial regression simultaneously estimates the log-odds of having a child only orientation, an older adult only orientation, and a family/market orientation, each versus an intergenerational orientation—controlling for individual. Table 14A.2 reports the coefficients of the multinomial logistic regression of government spending orientation on individual/ household factors and state regime membership.

Advancing age increases the odds of having older adult only and family/ market orientations compared to an intergenerational orientation. In real terms, an average 65-year-old is 38% more likely than an average 25-year-old to have an older adult only orientation versus an intergenerational orientation. (Additional analyses, not shown, ruled out the possibility of an inverse U-shaped relationship between age and having an intergenerational orientation).

All of the contrasts demonstrate a significant gender effect. Net of other factors, women are more likely than men to have an intergenerational orientation. Marital status has little effect on the orientation. Never-married people are an exception, however, and are less likely than married people to have an older adult only orientation (versus an intergenerational orientation). A test for the interaction between the presence of young children and marital status revealed no statistically significant effect net of other factors.

As anticipated, compared with college completion, less education is associated with a greater likelihood of having an intergenerational orientation. The less educated are also likely to be poorer, which may increase their needs and support for state sponsored care at all life stages. The effects of relative social class, in general, substantiate the idea that the poorest people have greater needs and demonstrate greater support for state-sponsored care across the life course. Compared to people from middle-class backgrounds, people from a lower-class background are 27% less likely to have a child only orientation, 40% less likely to have a family/market orientation, and 13% less likely to have an older adult only orientation (versus having an intergenerational orientation). The middle-class groups are a bit more variable than expected, with both the lower middle class and the upper middle class being more likely than the middle-class group to have an orientation that is not intergenerational.

Contrary to expectations, there are few significant effects of household composition on spending preferences. Neither household size nor having a surviving parent significantly predicts a particular welfare state orientation. Those with young children in the home are less likely than people without young children to have a family/market orientation and an adult only orientation, this last effect representing a 31% decrease in likelihood compared to an intergenerational orientation.

Controlling for the microlevel factors, the effects of the welfare state regime contrasts are consistent with our descriptive findings. Those living in liberal welfare state regimes are less likely to have an intergenerational orientation and more likely to have family/market and older adult only orientations compared to those in each of the other welfare regimes. This is consistent with the notion that liberal welfare states are at once more free-market oriented and also wedded to old age entitlement. People living in Nordic social democratic states are most strongly intergenerational in their spending orientations. Surprisingly, people in conservative states are more likely than people in liberal states to support spending solely on children; previous studies have shown that most people under both regimes do not support state-sponsored child care (Gustafsson, 1994).

The overall conclusion is that liberal states are exceptional, being more likely than virtually any other regime type to embrace alternatives to the intergenerational social contract. These results may reflect the neoliberal market fundamentalism ethos of liberal states. They also support the theory that the intergenerational social contract would be more embedded in societies with (1) a history of social support across the life course, (2) a culture of intimate intergenerational family relations, or (3) a legacy of socialism. These results suggest that the intergenerational social contract is more tenuous in liberal states than under other welfare regimes.

Discussion

Our findings suggest a public more committed to an intergenerational social contract than to orientations that favor only one age group or private solutions to dependent support (see also Marshall, Chapter 12). Despite the political groundswell for market solutions in recent decades, there is no evidence of much support for a retreat from the welfare state. The greatest prevalence of the family/market orientation is found in the United States, where individualism has always been a strong cultural influence and where market fundamentalism has co-opted social welfare (Gilbert, 2002; Somers & Block, 2005). In embracing the family/market orientation, the U.S. minority is followed by Japan, where economic growth has been prioritized over the development of the welfare state.

Esping-Andersen (2002a), Daniel and Ivatts (1998), and Leira (2002), among others, have suggested that the social contract should be reworked to incorporate more spending on children. Our results suggest that there may be a greater receptivity to a focus on functional solidarity that emphasizes needs and obligations throughout the life course, rather than singling out any particular age group. Thus, the intergenerational social contract that has demonstrated such usefulness as a theoretical concept also shows great promise for framing public policy discussion.

Policy recommendations aimed at improving intergenerational solidarity are on the right track. The overwhelming prevalence of the intergenerational social contract orientation within and between nations and the relative sparsity of support for alternative orientations is good news for intergenerational solidarity. With a few exceptions, predominantly in liberal welfare states, overwhelming majorities in each country examined here support government responsibility for both young and old. This is consistent with the intergenerational social contract. However, if push comes to shove in allocating scarce resources in an increasingly difficult demographic context—that is, the lifeboat situation—children may be at greater risk than older adults. Those who only approve of government support for one population typically choose older adults over children.

Despite a large body of literature that emphasizes significant attitudinal differences for individuals in different welfare state regimes (Esping-Andersen, 1990; Edlund, 1999; Svallfors, 1996), we find that welfare state regime is not a strong predictor of social contract orientation, except for liberal states. The findings for the liberal states do raise warnings about their willingness to address the resource pressures on aging populations in ways that avoid intergenerational conflict and ensure the well-being of the next generation.

Table 14A.1. Marginal distribution of social contract orientation by country

	Inter-generational	Family/ market	Child only	Older adult only	n
Liberal States					
Australia	0.429	0.070	0.006	0.495	1,352
Canada	0.569	0.038	0.006	0.387	1,115
Great Britain	0.682	0.024	0.005	0.289	912
New Zealand	0.442	0.073	0.007	0.478	1,146
Northern Ireland	0.779	0.014	0.002	0.204	1,407
United States	0.388	0.160	0.012	0.440	1,149
Grand means	0.548	0.063	0.006	0.382	
Conservative states					
Austria	0.710	0.022	0.013	0.255	1,011
France	0.824	0.030	0.016	0.129	1,398
Germany, West	0.837	0.024	0.046	0.092	936
Israel Arabs	0.966	0.020	0.000	0.014	154
Israel Jews	0.787	0.033	0.016	0.164	1,053
Japan	0.685	0.104	0.074	0.137	1,321
Switzerland	0.391	0.093	0.028	0.488	1,001
Grand means	0.743	0.047	0.028	0.183	
Social democratic states					
Denmark	0.808	0.018	0.003	0.171	1,293
Finland	0.837	0.014	0.002	0.147	1,439
Norway	0.681	0.007	0.004	0.308	1,560
Grand means	0.775	0.013	0.003	0.209	
Southern European States					
Cyprus	0.587	0.004	0.000	0.409	1,006
Italy	0.915	0.009	0.002	0.074	999
Spain	0.957	0.011	0.004	0.028	1,214
Grand means	0.820	0.008	0.002	0.170	
Postsocialist states					
Czech Republic	0.712	0.029	0.014	0.245	1,200
Germany, East	0.945	0.009	0.028	0.017	433
Hungary	0.919	0.009	0.004	0.068	1,524
Latvia	0.874	0.017	0.003	0.106	1,000
Poland	0.899	0.007	0.005	0.089	1,221
Russia	0.962	0.003	0.005	0.031	2,000
Slovenia	0.946	0.006	0.011	0.038	1,077
Grand means	0.894	0.011	0.010	0.085	
Other states					
Brazil	0.933	0.007	0.002	0.057	2,000
Chile	0.943	0.008	0.003	0.047	1,504
Philippines	0.752	0.063	0.040	0.145	1,200
South Africa	0.827	0.026	0.016	0.131	2,563
Grand Means	0.864	0.026	0.015	0.095	

Table 14A.2. Log-odds from the multinomial regression of contract orientation on individual, household, and state factors

Variable	Child only			Family/market			Older adult only		
	Log-odds	SE	Pr(> |t|)	Log-odds	SE	Pr(> |t|)	Log-odds	SE	Pr(> |t|)
Intercept	-3.609	0.430	0.000	-1.202	0.250	0.000	-0.145	0.130	0.263
Individual and Household Factors									
Age	0.007	0.010	0.197	0.008	0.000	0.018	0.008	0.000	0.000
Female	-0.276	0.120	0.025	-0.179	0.080	0.029	-0.095	0.040	0.018
Married (ref)									
Widowed	-0.286	0.280	0.312	-0.206	0.180	0.258	-0.116	0.090	0.174
Divorced/separated	-0.269	0.240	0.271	-0.206	0.150	0.177	0.090	0.070	0.190
Never married	-0.043	0.190	0.826	-0.226	0.130	0.084	-0.135	0.060	0.033
Completed college/university (ref)									
Incomplete primary education	-1.400	0.320	0.000	-1.398	0.240	0.000	-0.519	0.100	0.000
Complete primary education	-0.394	0.220	0.078	-0.611	0.170	0.000	-0.560	0.090	0.000
Incomplete secondary education	-0.786	0.220	0.000	-0.689	0.130	0.000	-0.052	0.070	0.430
Complete secondary education	-0.179	0.180	0.312	-0.221	0.120	0.057	0.047	0.060	0.453
Incomplete college education	-0.405	0.200	0.047	-0.398	0.120	0.001	-0.237	0.070	0.000
Middle class (ref)									
Lower class	-0.313	0.190	0.095	-0.497	0.120	0.000	-0.130	0.050	0.011
Low er middle class	0.495	0.170	0.003	0.366	0.130	0.004	0.225	0.060	0.000
Upper middle class	0.255	0.200	0.204	0.294	0.130	0.026	0.259	0.070	0.000
Upper class	0.189	0.320	0.549	0.605	0.190	0.002	-0.026	0.130	0.841
Household population	-0.008	0.040	0.849	0.013	0.030	0.674	-0.005	0.020	0.741
Children <18	-0.022	0.160	0.889	-0.373	0.110	0.000	-0.128	0.050	0.012
Surviving parent	-0.160	0.130	0.211	-0.103	0.090	0.226	-0.011	0.040	0.795
State factors									
Liberal states (ref)									
Social democratic states	-2.307	0.620	0.000	-2.367	0.200	0.000	-1.582	0.080	0.000
Conservative states	0.845	0.240	0.000	-1.308	0.110	0.000	-1.579	0.060	0.000
Southern European states	-1.973	0.440	0.000	-3.122	0.220	0.000	-1.586	0.070	0.000
Postsocialist states	-0.858	0.260	0.001	-2.829	0.140	0.000	-2.318	0.060	0.000
Other states	0.193	0.280	0.490	-1.598	0.160	0.000	-2.094	0.090	0.000

Note: Standard errors are robust against the clustering effect of grouped data (respondents who are not independent because they are sampled within countries).

REFERENCES

Arts, W. A., & Gellisen, J. (2002). Three worlds of welfare capitalism or more? A state-of-the-art report. *Journal of European Social Policy, 12*, 137–158.

Bengtson, V. L. (1993). Is the "contract across generations" changing? Effects of population aging on obligations and expectations across age groups. In V. L. Bengtson & W. A. Achenbaum (Eds.), *The changing contract across generations* (pp. 3–24). New York: Aldine de Gruyter.

Bengtson, V. L., Lowenstein, A., Putney, N. M., & Gans, D. (2003). Global aging and the challenge to families. In V. L. Bengtson & A. Lowenstein (Eds.), *Global aging and the challenges to families* (pp. 1–24). Hawthorne, NY: Aldine de Gruyter.

Bengtson, V. L., Marti, G., & Roberts, R. E. L. (1991). Age group relations: Generational equity and inequity. In K. Pillemer & K. McCartney (Eds.), *Parent-child relations across the lifespan* (pp. 253–278). Hillsdale, NJ: Lawrence Erlbaum Associates.

Bengtson, V. L., Olander, E. B., & Haddad, A. A. (1976). The generation gap and aging family members: Toward a conceptual model. In J. F. Gubrium (Ed.), *Time, roles, and self in old age* (pp. 237–263). New York: Human Sciences Press.

Bengtson, V. L., Rosenthal, C., & Burton, L. (1990). Paradoxes of families and aging. In R. Binstock & L. George (Eds.), *Handbook of aging and the social sciences* (pp. 234–259). New York: Academic Press.

Binstock, R. H. (1983). The aged as scapegoat. *The Gerontologist, 23*, 136–143.

Binstock, R. H. (2000). Older people and voting participation: Past and future. *The Gerontologist, 40*(1), 18–31.

Blekesaune, M., & Quadagno, J. (2003). Public attitudes toward welfare state policies: A comparative analysis of 24 nations. *European Sociological Review, 19*(4), 415–427.

Brady, D. (2004). Reconsidering the divergence between elderly, child, and overall poverty. *Research on Aging, 26*(5), 487–510.

Caspers, F. G., & Mitchell, D. (1993). Worlds of welfare and families of nations. In F. G. Castles (Ed.), *Families of nations: Patterns of public policy in western democracies* (pp. 23–45). Sudbury, MA: Dartmouth Publishing Company.

Charles, M., & Cech, E. (2010). Beliefs about maternal employment. In J. Treas & S. Drobnic (Eds.), *Dividing the domestic: Men, women, and household work in cross-national perspective* (pp. 147–163). Stanford, CA: Stanford University Press.

Coale, A. J. (1986). Demographic effects of below-replacement fertility and their social implications. *Population and Development Review, 12* (Supplement: Below-replacement fertility in industrial societies: Causes, consequences, policies), 203–216.

Daniel, P., & Ivatts, J. (1998). *Children and social policy.* New York: Palgrave.

Delong, J. B. (2002). A history of bequests in the United States. In A. H. Munnell & A. E. Sunden (Eds.), *Death and dollars: The role of gifts and bequests in America* (pp. 64–90). Washington, DC: Brookings Institution Press.

Doling, J., & Horsewood, N. (2003). Home ownership and early retirement: European experience in the 1990s. *Journal of Housing and the Built Environment, 18*(4), 289–308.

Edlund, J. (1999). Trust in government and welfare regimes: Attitudes to redistribution and financial cheating in the USA and Norway. *European Journal of Political Research, 35*, 341–370.

Esping-Andersen, G. (1990). *The three worlds of welfare capitalism*. Cambridge, UK: Cambridge: Polity Press.

Esping-Andersen, G. (1999). *Social foundations of postindustrial economies*. Oxford, UK: Oxford University Press.

Esping-Andersen, G. (2002a). A child-centred social investment strategy. In G. Esping-Andersen (Ed.), *Why we need a new welfare state* (pp. 26–67). New York: Oxford University Press.

Esping-Andersen, G. (2002b). *Why we need a new welfare state*. New York: Oxford University Press.

Ferrera, M. (1996). The Southern model of welfare in social Europe. *Journal of European Social Policy, 6*(17), 12–37.

Forssén, K., & Hakorvirta, M. (2002). Family policy, work incentives, and the employment of mothers. In R. Sigg & C. Behrendt (Eds.), *Social security in the global village* (pp. 297–309). New Brunswick, NJ: Transaction Publishers.

Förster, M., & d'Ercole, M. M. (2005). *Income distribution and poverty in OECD countries in the second half of the 1990s*. OECD Social, Employment, and Migration Working Papers 22. Paris: OECD.

Fougère, M., & Mérette, M. (1999). Population ageing and economic growth in seven OECD countries. *Economic Modelling, 3*(3), 411–427.

Gilbert, N. (2002). *Transformation of the welfare state*. New York: Oxford University Press.

Goerres, A. (2007). Why are older people more likely to vote? The impact of ageing on electoral turnout in Europe. *The British Journal of Politics and International Relations, 9*(1), 90–121.

Gornick, J. C., Meyers, M. K., & Ross, K. E. (1998). Public policies and the employment of mothers: A cross national study. *Social Science Quarterly, 79*, 35–54.

Gruber, J., & Wise, D. (1997, August). *Social security programs and retirement around the world*. Working Paper 6134. Cambridge, MA: National Bureau of Economic Research.

Gustafsson, S. (1994). Childcare and types of welfare states. In D. Sainsbury (Ed.), *Gendering welfare states* (pp. 45–61). London: Sage.

Hasenfeld, Y., & Rafferty, J. A. (1989). The determinants of public attitudes toward the welfare state. *Social Forces, 67*(4), 1027–1048.

Hernes, H. (1984). Women and the welfare state: The transition from private to public dependence. In H. Holter (Ed.), *Patriarchy in a welfare state*. Oslo, Norway: Universitetsforlaget.

Kääriäinen, J., & Lehtonen, H. (2006). The variety of social capital in welfare state regimes: A comparative study of 21 countries. *European Societies, 8*(1), 27–57.

Klein, S., & Harkness, J. (2001). *ISSP study monitoring 2001*. Report to the ISSP General Assembly on monitoring work undertaken for the ISSP by Zuma, Germany. Retrieved September 28, 2012 (http://www.gesis.org/issp/overview/reports).

Lee, R. (1994). Population age structure, intergenerational transfer, and wealth: A new approach, with applications to the United States. *The Journal of Human Resources, 29*(4), 1027–1063.

Leira, A. (2002). Childcare as a social right: Family change and policy reform. In *Working parents and the welfare state: Family change and policy reform in Scandinavia* (pp. 132–149). New York: Cambridge University Press.

Lipsmeyer, C. S. (2003). Welfare and the discriminating public: Evaluating entitlement attitudes in post-Communist Europe. *The Policy Studies Journal, 31*(4), 545–564.

Lowenstein, A., & Bengtson, V. (2003). Challenges of global aging to families in the twenty-first century. In V. L. Bengtson & A. Lowenstein (Eds.), *Global aging and the challenges to families* (pp. 371–377). Hawthorne, NY: Walter de Gruyter.

Lynch, F. R. (2008). Immigrants and the politics of aging boomers: Renewed reciprocity or "Blade Runner" society? In J. Treas & F. Torres-Gil (Eds.), *Generations, 32*(4), 64–72.

Mabry, J. B., Giarrusso, R., & Bengtson, V. L. (2004). Generations, the life course, and family change. In J. Scott, J. Treas, & M. Richards (Eds.), *The Blackwell companion to the sociology of families* (pp. 87–105). Boston, MA: Blackwell.

Miller, D. A. (1981, September). The "sandwich" generation: Adult children of the aging. *Social Work, 13*, 419–423.

Minkler, M. (1991). Generational equity and the new victim blaming. In M. Minkler & C. Estes (Eds.), *Critical perspectives on aging* pp. 67–79. Amityville, NY: Baywood.

Myers, D. (2004). Cohorts and socioeconomic progress. In R. Farley & J. Haaga (Eds.), *The American people: Census 2000* (pp. 139–166). New York: Russell Sage.

Myers, D. (2007). *Immigrants and boomers: Forging a new social contract for the future of America.* New York: Russell Sage Foundation.

Myles, J., & Quadagno, J. (2002, March). Political theories of the welfare state. *Social Science Review,* 34–37.

Newacheck, P. W., & Benjamin, A. E. (2004). Intergenerational equity and public spending. *Health Affairs, 23*(5), 142–146.

Orloff, A. S. (1993). Gender and the social rights of citizenship. *American Sociological Review, 58*, 303–328.

Pampel, F. C. (1994). Population aging, class context, and age inequality in public spending. *The American Journal of Sociology, 100*(1), 153–195.

Parrott, T. M., Reynolds, S. L., & Bengtson, V. L. (1997). Aging and social welfare in transition: The case of the United States. *Scandinavian Journal of Social Welfare, 6*, 168–179.

Pienta, A. M., & Hayward, M. D. (2002). Who expects to continue working after age 62? The retirement plans of couples. *The Journals of Gerontology Series B: Psychological and Social Sciences, 57*, 199–208.

Preston, S. H. (1984). Children and the elderly: Divergent paths for America's dependents. *Demography, 21*(4), 435–457.

Quadagno, J., Achenbaum, W. A., & Bengtson, V. L. (1993). Setting the agenda for research on cohorts and generations: Theoretical, political, and policy implications. In V. L. Bengtson & W. A. Achenbaum (Eds.), *The changing contract across generations* (pp. 259–272). Hawthorne, NY: Aldine de Gruyter.

Reich, R. B. (1999). Broken faith: Why we need to renew the social compact. *Generations, 22*(4), 19–24.

Sainsbury, D. (1996). *Gender, equality and welfare states.* Cambridge: Cambridge University Press.

Somers, M. R., & Block, F. (2005). From poverty to perversity: Ideas, markets, and institutions over 200 years of welfare debate. *American Sociological Review, 70,* 260–287.

Spencer, H. (1879). The rights of children and the true principles of family government. In B. Meyer (Ed.), *Aids to family government: Or, from the cradle to the school according to Froebel* (pp. 169–182). New York: M. L. Holbrook.

Svallfors, S. (1996). Worlds of welfare and attitudes to redistribution: A comparison of eight Western nations. *European Sociological Review, 13*(3), 283–304.

Thomson, D. W. (1989). The welfare state and generation conflict: Winners and losers. In P. Johnson, C. Conrad, and D. W. Thomson (Eds.), *Workers versus pensioners: Intergenerational justice in an ageing world* (pp. 33–56). Manchester, UK: Manchester University Press.

Treas, J., & Widmer, E. (2000). Married women's employment over the life course: Attitudes in cross-national perspective. *Social Forces, 78*(4), 1409–1436.

Walker, A. (1993). Intergenerational relations and welfare restructuring: The social construction of an intergenerational problem. In V. L. Bengtson & W. A. Achenbaum (Eds.), *The changing contract across generations* (pp. 141–165). Hawthorne, NY: Aldine de Gruyter.

CHAPTER FIFTEEN

Aging, Health, and Families in the Hispanic Population

Evolution of a Paradigm

Kyriakos S. Markides, Ronald J. Angel, and M. Kristen Peek

The "multiple hierarchy stratification" perspective emerged as a distinct paradigm in the 1970s that viewed ethnic minority status as a source of inequality on par with other sources of inequality based on social class, gender, and age (Bengtson, 1979). Specifically, ethnic minority status was thought to converge with low social class, female gender, and old age to produce a confluence of inequality at the lower end of the stratification continuum. A cluster of poor older women from minority populations occupied the bottom of the status hierarchy. A cluster of upper-class or middle-class White men who were middle-aged or younger occupied the top of the status hierarchy, and other combinations fell somewhere in the middle. Evidence in support of such a perspective was easily obtained using such traditional indicators of social stratification as income, political power, and prestige. However, examination of how the four structural factors operated simultaneously was limited by the absence of sufficiently large and ethnically heterogeneous samples.

The simpler "double jeopardy" hypothesis highlighted the double disadvantage of being old and a minority group member in terms of social policy initiatives targeting underserved populations. Dowd and Bengtson (1978), who were among the first to test the viability of this hypothesis, suggested that the double jeopardy hypothesis would be supported if the disadvantages of minorities (relative to members of the majority) observed in middle age became greater in old age. Although the authors acknowledged that ideally longitudinal data would have to be employed, such longitudinal data were not available at that time, making it necessary to base generalizations on cross-sectional data. Dowd and Bengtson's (1978) cross-sectional data from Los Angeles on middle-aged and older Blacks, Mexican Americans, and Anglos yielded partial support for the hypothesis, showing that the income and health disadvantage of Blacks and Mexican Americans increased from middle age to old age. No such patterns were observed with respect to social interaction with family and friends or life satisfaction. Others examining cross-sectional data (Ferraro, 1987; Markides, 1983; Ward, 1983) did not find support for widening differences between Blacks and Non-Hispanic Whites in income and health. While the double jeopardy hypothesis was perhaps sound conceptually, it had met with mixed support in the empirical world. Some of the evidence indeed supported the "age as leveler" hypothesis that differences between groups diminish in old age.

As stated earlier, one problem in testing for the presence of double jeopardy was reliance on cross-sectional data. Since Blacks (and perhaps other minorities at that time) experienced higher early mortality than Whites, the few Blacks who survived to advanced old age were hardy and in relatively good health. The Black/White mortality crossover that illustrated this phenomenon was generally accepted in the literature as genuine (Kitagawa & Hauser, 1973; Manton, 1980; Manton, 1982). All this led to a focus on "selective survival" as the process by which health and income inequalities—but also inequalities in other outcomes, such as psychological well-being, suicide, and institutionalization rates—were manifest between ethnic groups in old age (Markides & Machalek, 1984).

Social Determinants of Health and Well-Being in the Older Hispanic Population

Research on the Hispanic/Latino population of the United States has received increased attention in large part because Hispanics constitute the largest ethnic-minority population and are expected to reach over 100 million by the middle of the twenty-first century, representing approximately 25% of the total population. Recognizing the growing number of elderly Hispanics—a rapidly rising component of the older population—the Hispanic Established

Population for the Epidemiological Study of the Elderly (Hispanic EPESE) was begun in 1992. Hispanic EPESE is an ongoing longitudinal study of the health of older Mexican Americans from the southwestern United States. It was originally funded by the National Institute on Aging (NIA) in 1992 and modeled after the previous EPESE studies conducted in East Boston, New Haven, Connecticut, rural Iowa, and North Carolina, but that did not include a significant number of older Hispanics.

Baseline interviews were conducted with 3,050 Mexican Americans aged 65 and over during 1993–1994. The subjects were selected using area probability sampling procedures and were representative of approximately 500,000 people living in Texas, New Mexico, Colorado, Arizona, and California. These subjects were followed up with in 1995–1996 (n = 2,438), 1998–1999 (n = 1,980), 2000–2001 (n = 1,683), and 2004–2005 (n = 1,167), when they were aged 75 and older. An additional representative sample of 902 Mexican Americans also aged 75 and older from the same region was added in 2004–2005. This combined sample of 2,069 Mexican Americans aged 75 and over was followed up with approximately two and a half to three years later during 2007. A total of 1,541 subjects, now aged approximately 78 and over, were reinterviewed in person or by proxy. During 2010–2011, 1,078 subjects now aged 80 and over were followed up with and interviewed.

To date the study has generated over 250 publications and has provided important information on medical conditions, disability, mortality, emotional and cognitive function, formal and informal health care utilization, and related issues. A central goal of the Hispanic EPESE in conjunction with related projects was to document and explain differentials in health between Hispanics and those of other ethnicities. Although Hispanics as a group are generally disadvantaged socioeconomically, they appear to have a relatively favorable health profile, which is often referred to in the literature as the "Hispanic Paradox" (Crimmins, 2007; Riall et al., 2007; Franzini, Ribble, & Keddie, 2001; Hummer et al., 2007; Markides & Eschbach, 2005; Markides & Coreil, 1986; Palloni & Morenoff, 2001). Realization of this phenomenon has brought with it a reevaluation, though not necessarily a refutation, of the multiple jeopardy hypothesis with regard to aging and health.

The existence of an epidemiologic paradox with respect to the overall health status of the United States Hispanic population was first identified over two decades ago by Markides and Coreil (1986), who focused on evidence with respect to southwestern Hispanics who were mostly of Mexican origin. As originally conceived, the health status of southwestern Hispanics was thought to be more comparable to the health status of Non-Hispanic Whites than to that of African Americans, with whom the Hispanics were similar socioeconomically (see also Hayes-Bautista, 1992; Vega & Amaro, 1994).

Among the hypothesized reasons for this epidemiologic paradox were certain cultural practices, strong family supports, and selective migration. Beginning in the 1990s, evidence was found suggesting the existence of a mortality advantage among Mexican Americans as well as among other Hispanic populations. This mortality advantage was present among both men and women and was greatest at old age. Although there was some evidence that selective migration back to Mexico may bias mortality rates downwards among older Mexican Americans (Abraido-Lanza, Dohrenwend, Ng-Mak, & Turner, 1999; Palloni & Arias, 2004), such a "salmon bias" cannot explain the overall mortality advantage (Hummer et al., 2007; Markides & Eschbach, 2005) because very few older people of Mexican origin appear to go back to Mexico in their older years. (See also Markides, Salinas, & Wong, 2010.) Perhaps the most definitive test of the salmon bias was recently performed by Turra & Elo (2008) using Social Security data on Medicare beneficiaries. The existence of a salmon bias was confirmed, but it was too small to explain the mortality advantage of Hispanics.

The Hispanic EPESE has investigated a variety of social determinants of well-being in the older Mexican-American population, including neighborhoods, marriage, living arrangements, and religion. These are discussed below.

Neighborhood Context and Health

Neighborhood socioeconomic environments are thought to influence health by influencing the socioeconomic position and life chances of individuals and families (Robert, 1999). In addition, disadvantaged neighborhoods are more likely to have poor housing quality (Troutt, 1993), fewer recreational facilities (Macintyre, Maciver, & Sooman, 1993), and poor air and water quality (Bullard, 1990). Poor neighborhoods have poor public services (Robert & House, 2000), poor access to quality health care (Smedley, Stith, & Nelson, 2002), and high rates of crime and violence (Sampson, Raudenbush, & Earls, 1997).

A question we set out to investigate was the extent to which neighborhoods where older Mexicans live can help explain their relatively good health outcomes, at least with respect to mortality. Is there an advantage to living in a heavily Mexican American neighborhood despite high rates of poverty? To investigate this hypothesis we linked Hispanic EPESE subjects to census tract information using 1990 United States census data. We were interested in finding out whether the percentage of Mexican Americans in a neighborhood according to the census might be associated with mortality over a seven-year period from baseline through 2000–2001 (Eschbach et al., 2004).

Logistic regression models adjusted for age and gender revealed that higher percentages of Mexican Americans in the census tract were associated with lower prevalence of stroke, cancer, and hip fracture. There was also a linear trend of decreasing mortality rate by increasing percentage of Mexican Americans. The relationship persisted in hazard model analysis that adjusted for individual demographic and socioeconomic characteristics, baseline medical conditions and disability, and neighborhood percentage living in poverty. Thus, despite high rates of neighborhood socioeconomic disadvantage, heavily Mexican American neighborhoods appear to have a protective effect on the health of Mexican Americans, adding support for a cultural effect on mortality in this population. These communities may have social support systems that offset the negative effects of socioeconomic disadvantage (Eschbach et al., 2004).

Other analyses using baseline data generally support the above findings and conclusions. Older Mexican Americans living in heavily Mexican American neighborhoods reported better self-rated health (Patel et al., 2003) and lower rates of depressive symptomatology (Ostir, Eschbach, Markides, & Goodwin, 2003). These findings suggest that the community context, over and above individual characteristics, might help explain the apparent health advantages of Mexican Americans (Markides & Eschbach, 2005).

Marriage and Health

Previous research has indicated a strong connection between being married and positive health outcomes (e.g., Ross, Mirowsky, & Goldsteen, 1990). There is also evidence that spouses' health statuses are similar or "concordant" (Tower & Kasl, 1996a,b; Townsend, Miller, & Guo, 2001; Umberson, 1987). This notion of concordance has important public health implications for long-term formal and informal care if, in fact, spouses experience health declines together. If there is evidence for concordance in health declines, then interventions can be more effectively targeted toward the affected spouses (e.g. by providing support groups or connecting spouses to formal services). However, concordance is not well understood, especially among older couples (Tower & Kasl, 1996a). Individuals who are married show some concordance over time in health behaviors and health outcomes (Umberson, 1987), but this research is limited and has been based primarily on Non-Hispanic White adults (Townsend, Miller, & Guo, 2001).

One way to address concordance is to examine the association between the presence of health events and general health in one spouse and the other spouse's health status. For instance, one type of evidence for concordance in health between spouses would be apparent if a decline in the health of the incident spouse were associated with a decline in the health of the affected spouse. To address the connection between spouses' health more extensively in older ethnic couples, we examined the relationship between health events and physical functioning in one spouse and the health of the other spouse over a two-year to five-year period in older Mexican Americans. These analyses resulted in eight publications with outcomes ranging from well-being to prevalence or incidence of disease to mortality. Select findings are summarized below.

One article examined two issues with respect to well-being. We hypothesized that Mexican American husbands' and wives' emotional well-being would be strongly associated. We found evidence that husbands' depressive symptoms, life satisfaction, and self-rated health are predictive of the same in their wives. However, we did not find the reverse to be true. We originally expected that part of the gender difference might be due to immigrant status, since previous research has indicated that immigrant Mexican American women have higher rates of depressive symptoms and that they may experience greater social isolation, which could lead to a greater dependence on husbands. However, in these analyses, nativity status did not have a significant effect. One possibility is that nativity has less of an effect on the well-being of older Mexican American women. In the Hispanic EPESE sample, those women who were not born in the United States have been in the United States for an average of 40 years. This long time period may serve to "wash out" some of the effects of nativity (Stimpson, Peek, & Markides, 2006).

Another study focused on concordance of blood pressure and incidence of several health conditions predicted by the same health condition of the spouse. We found similarities in blood pressure when examining both systolic and diastolic hypertension as well as hypertension defined as currently taking blood pressure medications (Peek & Markides, 2003). We hypothesized that couples may have high concordance in blood pressure because of similar health behaviors, especially if they have been married for a long time. Consistent with this notion, we found evidence of strong concordance in blood pressure in older married couples, 90% of whom had been married for more than 30 years.

We also investigated the hypothesis that chronic conditions of one spouse presented a risk factor for the same condition in the other spouse. Little research had been conducted on the concordance of health among spouses, and the research that does exist has largely focused on depression or depressive symptoms. Findings from this study provided evidence that some chronic conditions are concordant among older Mexican American spouses even after adjusting for age, education, U.S. nativity, blood pressure, BMI, smoking, and alcohol consumption. Of the six conditions tested, only stroke was not a statistically significant risk factor for both husbands and wives. The husband's risks for being diagnosed with hypertension, diabetes, arthritis, and cancer were significantly increased when the wife was diagnosed with the corresponding condition (Stimpson & Peek, 2005). The wife's risks for being diagnosed with hypertension, arthritis, and cancer were significantly increased when the husband was diagnosed with the corresponding condition. This pattern suggests that marital partners are an important influence on health, especially among older couples.

Finally, we assessed the association between widowhood and mortality among older Mexican Americans (Stimpson et al., 2007). The results suggest that widowhood puts men at higher risk for mortality, but it does not seem to have the same risk for women. Overall, our findings are consistent with other studies by finding increased risk of death for husbands. The primary difference with our finding is that the length of time that husbands are at risk of death is extended. Most studies find the risk of death after widowhood levels out within 24 months, but our study of Mexican Americans revealed that the risk of death after losing a spouse levels out by 33 months, which may suggest that Mexican American men have a longer trajectory of risk of death related to widowhood than Non-Hispanic Whites and that Mexican American men may take longer to adjust to the loss of a spouse.

Living Arrangements and Health

The Hispanic EPESE clearly showed that the economic situation of older Mexican Americans is closely associated with family living arrangements, a fact which may influence their morbidity and mortality risks. Several manuscripts using Hispanic EPESE data show that older Mexican Americans are more likely than other groups to live with children, a fact that reflects both cultural preferences and economic necessity (Angel, Angel, & Markides, 2000; Lee & Angel, 2002).

Living with children also appears to be part of a community orientation.

Older Mexican Americans appear to benefit from participating in the community and its social life; as such, engagement is clearly important to the maintenance of good health among older Mexican Americans. In general, the Hispanic EPESE data reveal the complex and nuanced association among culture, social structure, health care use, and health outcomes (Angel & Angel, 1997; Angel, Angel, & Hill, 2008).

The Hispanic EPESE provides an opportunity to examine changes in living arrangements as a function of declining health as well as to examine differences based on age at migration (Angel, Angel, Lee, & Markides, 1999). The data show that older foreign-born Mexican-origin individuals are more likely to live with family than the native-born for economic and health reasons (Angel, Angel, McClellan, & Markides, 1996) and that individuals who immigrated late in life are more likely than the native born or those who came to the United States as children or young adults to live with children, especially in the case of declining health (Angel, Angel, & Markides, 2000).

Despite suffering from higher rates of functional dependency than other ethnic groups, older Mexican Americans are much less likely than other groups to use assisted-living facilities or nursing homes. Frail and disabled elderly Mexican Americans resist the use of formal long-term care services not only because families desire to keep loved ones at home but also because they are unable to afford nursing home care (Angel & Angel, 1997; Angel, Angel, McClellan, & Markides, 1996). The high value placed on family in Mexican culture contributes to an increased probability of home-based care.

Subjects in the Hispanic EPESE express a strong desire to live within an extended-family household in the event of diminished capacity (Angel, Angel, McClellan, & Markides, 1996). This is especially true for late-life migrants (Angel, Angel, & Markides, 2000). Even among unmarried older adults, who often lack social support, a decline in functional capacity rarely results in institutionalization (Angel, Angel, Aranda, & Miles, 2004; Angel, Angel, & Markides, 2000). However, the data also show that marital status is still an important predictor of long-term care utilization. Among those whose health declined, widows were more likely than widowers to use community-based long-term care services (Angel, Douglas, & Angel, 2003). The data also reveal that cognitive and functional decline were strong predictors of institutionalization, despite overall low levels of use (Angel, Douglas, & Angel, 2003; Angel, Angel, Aranda, & Miles, 2004). Although many older individuals qualified for Medicaid nursing home benefits, they were more likely to be cared for in the community than in a nursing home. Those who died in a nursing home were those without any family or social support. For this latter group, institutionalization occurred despite their desire to remain in the home.

These and other findings from the Hispanic EPESE data present a complex picture in which aspects of social structure, particularly economic constraints, interact with cultural factors to influence social support, physical and mental health, and functional capacity (Hill, Angel, Ellison, & Angel, 2005; Hill, Burdette, Angel, & Angel, 2006). Despite a favorable mortality experience, older Mexican Americans suffer from significant rates of disability, for which they do not necessarily receive adequate care (Angel & Angel, 1997). Future analyses of the Hispanic EPESE promise to help illuminate the complex association among health insurance coverage, social engagement, and living arrangements in the determination of health levels among older Mexican Americans.

Religion and Health

Religious involvement appears to have beneficial effects on the health of older Mexican Americans. Analysis of eight years of longitudinal data revealed that those individuals who attended church regularly had a far lower mortality risk than those who never attended religious services, even after controlling for physical health risk factors including self-rated health, depressive symptoms, cognitive functioning, cardiovascular health, activities of daily living, health behaviors, and social support (Hill, Angel, Ellison, & Angel, 2005). Frequent church attendance also lowered fear of falling over time. (Reyes-Ortiz et al., 2006).

Another analysis using four waves of data found that church attendance was associated with slower decline in cognitive function (Hill, Burdette, Angel, & Angel, 2006). Among subjects with clinically significant depressive symptomatology, infrequent church attendance was associated with greater decline in cognitive function scores compared with frequent attendance (Reyes-Ortiz et al., 2008).

Finally we examined the importance of church attendance before strokes in older Mexican Americans who reported having had a stroke and experiencing residual physical limitations due to stroke. We found that frequent church attendees reported lower declines in disability over time after a stroke than did less frequent attendees. The same was true with respect to a performance measure of lower body function (Berges, Kuo, Markides, & Ottenbacher, 2007).

The above findings with respect to the positive influence of church attendance are not unique to older Mexican Americans. Moreover, we do not mean to imply that church attendance captures the importance of religious feelings (although this cannot be precluded). More likely, church attendance is a major measure of social engagement and community participation for older Mexican Americans. These findings are consistent with the neighborhood findings summarized earlier, which suggest that high Hispanic concentration in the neighborhood has positive associations with good health and mental health. Presumably one way in which Hispanic concentration operates is by providing more opportunities for older Mexican Americans to be socially engaged.

Multigenerational Mexican American Families

One of the first studies to provide a detailed examination of intergenerational relationships in Mexican American families is the Three-Generations Study of Mexican Americans. This study, funded in 1980 by the National Institute on Aging, was a natural outgrowth of our work on older Mexican Americans in San Antonio in the late 1970s and was modeled to a large extent after Bengtson's Study of Three Generations in Southern California (Markides & Martin, 1983). The sample consisted of 375 three-generation lineages, amounting to 1,125 subjects. Each lineage consisted of an older person (aged 65–80 years), a middle-aged child, and an adult (aged 18 years and over) married or previously married grandchild, all living within 50 miles of San Antonio. In 1992–1993, the investigators reinterviewed 624 of the original subjects, or 56% of the original sample.

The survey sought to describe the extended family of older Mexican Americans by obtaining information on relations between generations based on frequency of contact, amount of intergenerational social support, and strength of affectual ties. The intention was to go beyond examining reports from older people to also examine reports of their children and grandchildren. The design of the Southern California three-generation study provided a convenient model. The study also used some measures of intergenerational solidarity similar to those developed in the Southern California study (Bengtson & Schrader, 1982), although the San Antonio study was conceptualized primarily as a study of intergenerational relationships and to a lesser extent as a study of generational differences or gaps.

When this study was conducted, the literature emphasized the warmth and supportive qualities of the Mexican American family, particularly toward older family members. Our research was the first to provide evidence challenging such conceptions. For example, we found that older Mexican Ameri-

324   *Global, Cross-National, and Cross-Ethnic Issues*

cans were considerably more likely than older Anglos to report unfulfilled expectations of filial responsibility: Mexican Americans perceived a gap between expectations and reality that was not reported by Anglos in the Southern California study, who seemed more satisfied with their relationships with their children. We hypothesized that the discrepancy between expectations and reality was based on the fact that older Mexican Americans grew up in an agrarian culture whereas their children had grown up in a complex urban society. Perhaps "acculturation" of the younger generation was influencing relationships between the generations, something that was replicated in other immigrant groups such as the Vietnamese.

In another analysis we investigated levels of different forms of intergenerational solidarity across different generation pairs. Overall, "associational solidarity" was highest between the middle and younger generations, slightly lower between the middle and older generations, and considerably lower between the older and younger generations. Feelings of affection were similarly strong between adjacent generations and lower between nonadjacent generations (Markides & Krause, 1985). As predicted in this familistic culture, we showed the almost exclusive reliance by elders on family members for help and a high degree of reciprocity between the oldest generation and their middle-aged children (Markides, Boldt, & Ray, 1986).

However, there was little evidence of positive associations between measures of intergenerational solidarity and psychological well-being after other important measures were controlled. In fact, high levels of association with children were significantly related to higher levels of depressive symptoms in older family members. We speculated that this finding may result from the older family members' dependency on their children (see also Mutran & Reitzes, 1984). We subsequently found that a high level of reliance on children for help was associated with lower well-being in the older generation. We also found that middle-aged persons, especially women, who were heavily relied on by their parents or their children tended to report lower psychological well-being, something also reported in other familistic cultures such as Italian Americans (Cohler, 1983).

Several analyses examined the influence of family relationships and health. We examined the association between marriage and health (Farrell & Markides, 1985). In one study, no relationship was found between widowhood and physical health in the oldest generation, but both widowhood and divorce seemed to have negative consequences in the younger two generations, supporting the notion that there are differences in "on-time" and "off-time" transitions. Another analysis focusing on gender differences in illness and health behavior revealed that while employment had greater additive effects than nurturant roles, the combination of the two proved more significant among women (Krause & Markides, 1987). The effects of multiple roles were especially pronounced among divorced and separated women, for whom employment was associated with less illness. However, the positive effects of employment disappeared in nonmarried women with preschool children at home.

Conclusion

In this chapter we reviewed selected research findings related to ethnicity, aging, and health that are rooted in two broad traditions: multiple stratification hierarchies and multigenerational families. Specifically, the contributions of two research programs on Mexican Americans were used to highlight the evolution of the field of ethnicity within the study of aging (see also Burton, Welsh, & Destro, Chapter 4). The ongoing Hispanic EPESE study in particular may bear little resemblance to Bengtson's main contributions to social gerontology, yet his early conceptual work on the role of age in multiple jeopardy had a profound influence on its development. And one could not dispute his essential contribution to Mexican American family studies by providing a design blueprint and measurement protocols for assessing intergenerational relationships. The notion that ethnicity is a multidimensional force still resonates in more contemporary research on aging. Minority ethnic background is variably a risk factor for negative outcomes (poverty, low use of formal service, family strain) and a resource for improved quality of life (heightened family support and social/church engagement) in old age.

As a multipurpose study, the Hispanic EPESE has made contributions to a variety of important areas related to the well-being of older Hispanics. We began by identifying a paradox in the health of Mexican Americans (and to some extent other Hispanic populations): Despite generally lower living standards, Mexican Americans appear to enjoy relatively good health and are thought to live longer than the general population. Our findings with respect to mortality, depressive symptomatology, self-rated health, and disability lend some support to the hypothesis that more homogeneous Mexican American neighborhoods are sociocultural environments that may offset the negative effects of poverty and poor living conditions on the health of older Mexican Americans. The mechanisms that make these environments protective are not well understood. Clearly they relate to cultural and linguistic familiarity, family, and availability of social institutions that might promote social engagement. Our data show that the church may be such an institution. We found that frequent church attendance was consistently associated with lower mortality, slower decline in cognitive function, lower depressive symptomatology, lower fear of falling, and better recovery from the effects of a stroke. Again, we do not believe that these beneficial influences are a reflection of religious feelings. Rather, they most likely reflect the benefits of social participation and social engagement. Thus, in addition to the family, the church is a very important vehicle for social engagement and social support for older Mexican Americans.

One aspect of family support and family influence is the marital unit. Our findings on the influence of the health and well-being of one spouse on the other spouse were less consistent than findings among older Non-Hispanic Whites. Depressive symptoms, life satisfaction, and self-rated health of husbands were associated with these variables in wives, controlling for wives' characteristics. The reverse was not true. It is possible that relations with children and other members of the extended family are more important for older males in the Mexican American community and may thus buffer the negative effects of their wives' poor health and low psychological well-being on their own health and well-being.

We have also shown that because of limited financial resources older Mexican Americans are much less likely than the general population to use assisted living facilities or nursing homes. This is so despite the fact that older Mexican Americans have considerably higher rates of disability than older Non-Hispanic Whites. Lower rates of institutionalization increase the burden in the community, typically on the immediate family. The extremely limited financial resources of older Mexican Americans often make them dependent on family, especially adult children, and often result in shared living arrangements that further magnify financial dependence on the extended family.

The multigenerational study of the 1980s and 1990s similarly found great strengths in mature Mexican American families in terms of social support and coresidence of the elderly, but it also showed great vulnerabilities, including heightened obligations, unfulfilled expectations, and elevated burden of care, in part contradicting the stereotypical and overly simplistic notion that elders are without unmet needs in familistic cultures.

At our last wave of data collection in 2010–2011, we also interviewed 925 family informants, two-thirds of whom were children of our very old subjects. Informants provided information on the subjects' health, health care, family, and financial situation. The data provide an opportunity for dyadic analyses.

For instance, it will be possible to detect the burden that advanced old age and impairment puts on the physical, psychological, and financial resources of Mexican American family members. Such an addition to the sample closes the circle by bridging stratification and family domains of research in aging minority populations that have their roots in the early works of Bengtson and other pioneering social gerontologists.

Postscript by Kyriakos Markides

In approaching the development of a chapter on minority aging early in my career (Markides, 1983), I looked for a way to organize the material and a way to give a conceptual foundation to the chapter. I was lucky to rediscover three papers that helped me to do that: Dowd & Bengtson's paper "Aging in Minority Populations: An Examination of the Double Jeopardy Hypothesis" (*Journal of Gerontology*, 1978); Ward's then-unpublished paper "The Stability of Racial Differences across Age Strata" (1980, later published in 1983); and Bengtson's chapter "Ethnicity and Aging: Problems and Issues in Current Social Science Inquiry" (1979). Bengtson's writings had a direct impact on empirical and conceptual developments related to aging and ethnicity. As such, this is a personal thank-you to Vern for helping give direction to the early work of an inexperienced and generally unmentored young scholar. Vern's influence has had a lasting impact on my career and the work I have subsequently conducted on minorities and more specifically on aging in the Mexican American population.

REFERENCES

Abraido-Lanza, A. F., Dohrenwend, B. P., Ng-Mak, D. S., & Turner, J. B. (1999). The mortality paradox: A test of the "salmon bias" and healthy migrant hypotheses. *American Journal of Public Health, 89*(10), 1543–1548.

Angel, R. J., & Angel, J. L. (1997). *Who will care for us? Aging and long-term care in multicultural America.* New York: New York University Press.

Angel, J. L., Angel, R. J., Aranda, M. P., & Miles, T. P. (2004). Can the family still cope? Social support and health as determinants of nursing home use in the older Mexican-origin population. *Journal of Aging and Health, 16*, 338–354.

Angel, J. L., Angel, R. J., & Markides, K. S. (2000). Late life immigration, changes in living arrangements and headship status among older Mexican-origin individuals. *Social Science Quarterly, 81*, 389–403.

Angel, R. J., Angel, J. L., & Hill, T. D. (2008). A comparison of the health of older Hispanics in the U.S. and Mexico: Methodological challenges. *Journal of Aging and Health*, 20(1), 3–31.

Angel, R. J., Angel, J. L., Lee, G.-Y., & Markides, K. S. (1999). Age at migration and family dependency among older Mexican immigrants: Recent evidence from the Mexican American EPESE. *The Gerontologist*, *39*, 59–65.

Angel, J. L., Angel, R. J., McClellan, J. L., & Markides, K. S. (1996). Nativity, declining health, and preferences in living arrangements among elderly Mexican Americans: Implications for long term care. *The Gerontologist*, *36*, 464–473.

Angel, J. L., Douglas, N., & Angel, R. J. (2003). Gender, widowhood, and long-term care in the older Mexican American population. *Journal of Women and Aging*, *15*, 89–103. Reprinted in C. L. Jenkins (Ed.), *Widows and divorcees in later life: On their own again*. Binghamton, NY: The Haworth Press.

Bengtson, V. L. (1979) Ethnicity and aging: Problems and issues in current social science inquiry. In D. E. Gelfand & A. J. Kutzik (Eds.), *Ethnicity and Aging* (pp. 9–31). New York: Springer.

Bengtson, V. L., & Schrader, S. S. (1982). Parent child relationships. In D.J. Mangen & N. A. Peterson (Eds.), *Research instruments in social gerontology* (Vol. 2 , pp. 115–185). Minneapolis, MN: University of Minnesota Press.

Berges, I. M., Kuo, Y.-F., Markides, K. S., & Ottenbacher, K. (2007). Attendance at religious services and physical functioning after stroke among older Mexican Americans. *Experimental Aging Research*, *33*(1), 1–11.

Bullard, R.D. (1990). *Dumping in Dixie: Race, class and environmental quality*. Boulder, CO: Westview Press.

Cohler, B. (1983). Autonomy and interdependence in the family of adulthood: A psychological perspective. *The Gerontologist*, *23*, 33–39.

Crimmins, E. (2007) Compression of morbidity. In K.S. Markides (Ed.), *Encyclopedia of health and aging* (pp. 114–115). Thousand Oaks, CA: Sage.

Dowd, J. J., & Bengtson, V. L. (1978). Aging in minority populations: An examination of the double jeopardy hypothesis. *Journal of Gerontology*, *33*, 427–436.

Eschbach, K. S., Ostir, G. V., Patel, K. V., Markides, K. S., & Goodwin, J. S. (2004). Neighborhood context and mortality among older Mexican Americans: Is there a barrio advantage? *American Journal of Public Health*, *94*(10), 1807–1812.

Farrell, J., and Markides, K. S. (1985). Marriage and health: A three-generation study of Mexican Americans. *Journal of Marriage and the Family*, *47*, 1029–1036.

Ferraro, K. F. (1987) Double jeopardy to health for Black older adults. *Journal of Gerontology*, *42*, 528–533.

Franzini, L., Ribble, J. C., & Keddie, A. M. (2001). Understanding the Hispanic paradox. *Ethnicity and Disease*, *11*, 496–518.

Hayes-Bautista, D. E. (1992). Latino health indicators and the underclass model: From paradox to new policy models. In A. Furino (Ed.), *Health Policy and the Hispanic* (pp. 32–47). Boulder, CO: Westview Press.

Hill, T., Angel, J. L., Ellison, C., & Angel, R. J. (2005). Religious attendance and mortality: An eight-year follow up of older Mexican Americans. *Journal of Gerontology: Social Sciences*, *60B*, S102–S109.

Hill, T. D., Burdette, A. M., Angel, J. L., & Angel, R. J. (2006). Religious attendance and cognitive functioning among older Mexican Americans. *Journal of Gerontology: Psychological Sciences, 61,* P3–P9.

Hummer, R. A., Powers, D. A., Pullum, S. G., Grossman, G. L., & Frisbie, W. P. (2007). Paradox found again: Infant mortality among the Mexican-origin population in the United States. *Demography, 44,* 441–458.

Kitagawa, E. M., & Hauser, P. M. (1973). *Differential mortality in the United States: A study in socioeconomic epidemiology.* Cambridge, MA: Harvard University Press.

Krause, N., & Markides, K. S. (1987). Gender roles, illness, and illness behavior in Mexican American population. *Social Sciences Quarterly, 68,* 102–121.

Lee, G.-Y., & Angel, R. J. (2002). Living arrangements and supplemental security income use among elderly Asians and Hispanics in the United States: The role of nativity and citizenship. *Journal of Ethnic and Migration Studies, 28,* 553–563.

Macintyre, S., Maciver, S., & Soonan, A. (1993). Area, class, and health: Should we be focusing on places or people? *Journal of Social Policy, 33,* 213–234.

Manton, K. G. (1980). Sex and race specific mortality differentials in multiple cause of death data. *The Gerontologist, 20,* 480–493.

Manton, K. G. (1982). Differential life expectancy: Possible explanations during the later ages. In R. C. Manuel (Ed.), *Minority aging* (pp. 55–74). Westport, CT: Greenwood.

Markides, K. S. (1983). Minority aging. In M. W. Riley, B. B. Hess, & K. Bond (Eds.), *Aging and society: Selected reviews of recent research* (pp. 15–37). Hillsdale, NJ: Lawrence Erlbaum Associates.

Markides, K. S., Boldt, J. S., & Ray, L. A. (1986). Sources of helping and intergenerational solidarity: A three-generations study of Mexican Americans. *Journal of Gerontology, 41,* 506–511.

Markides, K. S., & Coreil, J. (1986). The health of southwestern Hispanics: An epidemiologic paradox. *Public Health Reports, 101,* 253–265.

Markides, K. S., & Eschbach, K. (2005). Aging, migration, and mortality: Current status of research on the Hispanic paradox. *Journal of Gerontology: Social Sciences, 60B,* 68–75.

Markides, K. S., & Krause, N. (1985). Intergenerational solidarity and psychological well-being among older Mexican Americans: A three-generations study. *Journal of Gerontology, 40,* 390–392.

Markides, K. S., and Machalek, R. (1984). Selective survival, aging and society. *Archives of Gerontology and Geriatrics, 3,* 207–222.

Markides, K. S., Martin, H. W., & Gomez, E. (1983). *Older Mexican-Americans: A study in an urban barrio.* Center for Mexican-American Studies Monograph. Austin, TX: The University of Texas Press.

Markides, K. S., Salinas, J., & Wong, R. (2010). Aging and health among Hispanics/ Latinos in the Americas. In D. Dannefer & C. Phillipson (Eds.), *Handbook of social gerontology* (pp. 150–163). Thousand Oaks, CA: Sage.

Mutran, E., & Reitzes, D. C. (1984). Intergenerational support activities and well-being among the elderly: A convergence of exchange and symbolic interaction perspectives. *American Sociological Review, 49,* 117–139.

Ostir, G. V., Eschbach, K., Markides, K. S., & Goodwin, J. S. (2004). Neighborhood composition and depressive e symptoms among older Mexican Americans. *Journal of Epidemiology and Community Health, 57,* 987–992.

Palloni, A., & Arias, E. (2004). Paradox lost: Explaining the Hispanic adult mortality advantage. *Demography, 41,* 385–415. Washington, DC: National Center for Health Statistics.

Palloni, A., & Morenoff, J. (2001). Interpreting the paradoxical in the "Hispanic Paradox." Demographic and epidemiological approaches. In M. Weinstein, A. Hermalin, & M. Soto (Eds.), *Population health and aging* (pp. 140–174). New York: New York Academy of Sciences.

Patel, K. V., Eschbach, K., Rudkin, L. L., Peek, M. K., & Markides, K. S. (2003). Neighborhood context and self-rated health in older Mexican Americans. *Annals of Epidemiology, 13,* 620–628.

Peek, M. K., & Markides, K. S. (2003). Blood pressure concordance among older Mexican American married couples. *Journal of the American Geriatrics Society, 93,* 433–435.

Reyes-Ortiz, C. A., Ayele, H., Mulligan, T., Espino, D. V., Berges, I., & Markides, K. S. (2006). Higher church attendance predicts lower fear of falling in older Mexican Americans. *Aging and Mental Health, 10*(1), 13–18.

Reyes-Ortiz, C. A., Berges, I. M., Raji, M. A., Koenig, H. G., Kuo, Y.-F., & Markides, K. S. (2008). Church attendance mediates the association between depressive symptoms and cognitive functioning among older Mexican Americans. *Journal of Gerontology: Medical Sciences, 63A*(5), 480–486.

Riall, T. S., Eschbach, K. A., Townsend, C. M. Jr., Nealon, W. H., Freeman, J. L., & Goodwin, J. S. (2007). Trends and disparities in regionalization of pancreatic resection. *Journal of Gastrointestinal Surgery, 11*(10), 1242–1251.

Robert, S. A. (1999). Socioeconomic position and health: The independent contribution of community socioeconomic context. *Annual Review of Sociology, 25,* 489–516.

Robert, S. A., & House, J. S. (2000). Socioeconomic inequalities in health: Integrating individual-, community-, and societal-level theory and research. In G. Albrecht, S. Scrimshaw, & R. Fitzpatrick (Eds.), *Handbook of social studies in health and medicine.* Thousand Oaks, CA: Sage.

Ross, C. E., Mirowsky, J., & Goldsteen, K. (1990). The impact of the family on health: The decade in review. *Journal of Marriage and the Family, 52,* 1059–1078.

Sampson, R. J., Raudenbush, S. W., Earls, F. (1997). Neighborhoods and violent crime: A multilevel study of collective efficacy. *Science, 277,* 918–924.

Smedley, B. D., Stith, A. Y., & Nelson, A. R. (Eds.). (2002). *Unequal treatment: Confronting racial and ethnic disparities in health care.* Washington, DC: National Academy Press.

Stimpson, J. P., Kuo, Y. F., Ray, R., Raji, M. A., & Peek, M. K. (2007). Risk of mortality related to widowhood in older Mexican Americans. *Annals of Epidemiology, 17*(4), 313–319.

Stimpson, J. P., & Peek, M. K. (2005). Concordance of chronic conditions in older Mexican-American couples. *Preventing Chronic Disease, 2,* serial online.

Stimpson, J. P., Peek, M. K., & Markides, K.S. (2006). Depression and mental health among older Mexican American spouses. Aging & Mental Health, 10(4), 386–392.

Tower, R. B., & Kasl, S. V. (1996a). Depressive symptoms across older spouses: Longitudinal influences. *Psychology and Aging, 11,* 683–697.

Tower, R. B., & Kasl, S. V. (1996b). Gender, marital closeness, and depressive symptoms in elderly couples. *Journals of Gerontology, Series B: Psychological Sciences and Social Sciences, 51,* 115–129.

Townsend, A. L., Miller, B., & Guo, S. (2001). Depressive symptomatology in middle-aged and older married couples: A dyadic analysis. *Journals of Gerontology, Series B: Psychological Sciences and Social Sciences, 56,* S352–S364.

Troutt, D. D. (1993). *The thin red line: How the poor still pay more.* San Francisco, CA: Consumers Union of the United States.

Turra, C. M., & Elo, I. T. (2008). The impact of salmon bias on the Hispanic mortality advantage: New evidence from social security data. *Population Research and Policy Review, 27,* 515–530.

Umberson, D. (1987). Family status and health behaviors: Social control as a dimension of social integration. *Journal of Health and Social Behavior, 28,* 306–319.

Vega, W. A., & Amaro, H. (1994). Latino outlook: Good health, uncertain prognosis. *Annual Review of Public Health, 15,* 39–67.

Ward, R. A. (1983). The stability of racial differences across age strata. *Social Science Research, 67,* 312–323.

Short Biography of Vern L. Bengtson

Vern L. Bengtson earned his Ph.D. at the University of Chicago under the guidance of Bernice Neugarten and Robert Havighurst in the Committee for Human Development. Bengtson's first and only academic post was at the University of Southern California in the Davis School of Gerontology and the Department of Sociology. While at USC, Bengtson established one of the most long-term research and training programs in social gerontology. His scholarly interest in the "generation gap" spawned one of the most enduring studies in the social sciences: the Longitudinal Study of Generations, a study of families that spans four generations, collecting data beginning in 1971 and continuing for four decades. At the study's conceptual core were intergenerational solidarity, a construct that describes the emotional, normative, structural, and behavioral factors that bind the generations, and life course dynamics, which locate families at the intersection of personal biography and historical time. In retirement, Bengtson continues his research into the intergenerational transmission of religiosity across generations.

Contributors

W. Andrew Achenbaum
University of Houston
Houston, Texas

Duane F. Alwin
The Pennsylvania State University
University Park, Pennsylvania

Ronald J. Angel
University of Texas
Austin, Texas

Simon Biggs
The University of Melbourne
Melbourne, Australia

Linda M. Burton
Duke University
Durham, North Carolina

Linda M. Chatters
University of Michigan
Ann Arbor, Michigan

Dale Dannefer
Case Western Reserve University
Cleveland, Ohio

Lane M. Destro
Roanoke College
Salem, Virginia

Glen H. Elder, Jr.
University of North Carolina
Chapel Hill, North Carolina

Roseann Giarrusso
California State University, Los Angeles
Los Angeles, California

Susan C. Harris
University of Southern California
Los Angeles, California

Malcolm Johnson
University of Bristol
Bristol, United Kingdom

Kees Knipscheer
VU University Amsterdam
Amsterdam, The Netherlands

Joy Y. Lam
University of Southern California
Los Angeles, California

Karen D. Lincoln
University of Southern California
Los Angeles, California

Ariela Lowenstein
Haifa University
Haifa, Israel

Christopher Steven Marcum
National Human Genome Research
    Institute
Bethesda, Maryland

Kyriakos S. Markides
University of Texas Medical Branch
Galveston, Texas

Victor W. Marshall
University of North Carolina
Chapel Hill, North Carolina

Steve McDonald
North Carolina State University
Raleigh, North Carolina

Frances Nedjat-Haiem
University of Southern California
Los Angeles, California

Thien-Huong Ninh
University of Southern California
Los Angeles, California

Angela M. O'Rand
Duke University
Durham, North Carolina

Petrice S. Oyama
University of Southern California
Los Angeles, California

M. Kristen Peek
University of Texas Medical Branch
Galveston, Texas

Karl Pillemer
Cornell University
Ithaca, New York

Norella M. Putney
University of Southern California
Los Angeles, California

R. Corey Remle
Francis Marion University
Florence, South Carolina

Rebecca A. Siders
Case Western Reserve University
Cleveland, Ohio

Merril Silverstein
Syracuse University
Syracuse, New York

J. Jill Suitor
Purdue University
West Lafayette, Indiana

Miles G. Taylor
Florida State University
Tallahasee, Florida

Robert Joseph Taylor
University of Michigan
Ann Arbor, Michigan

Judith Treas
University of California, Irvine
Irvine, California

Peter Uhlenberg
University of North Carolina
Chapel Hill, North Carolina

Theo van Tilburg
VU University Amsterdam
Amsterdam, The Netherlands

Whitney Welsh
Duke University
Durham, North Carolina

Index

AARP, 270, 272–74
Aboderin, I., 159, 279, 280
Abraido-Lanza, A. F., 317
Achenbaum, A., 179
Achenbaum, W. A., 194, 195, 197, 199, 206, 274, 280, 296
activities of daily living (ADL), 322
Adam, B., 205
ADD Health (The National Longitudinal Study of Adolescent Health), 81 105, 122
adoption, 31–32
adulthood, 104, 109–14, 121
adversity. *See* transitions to adulthood
African American studies, Pan-African identity, 200–202
age as leveler hypothesis, 315
age structure, transformation of, 159. *See also* population aging
aging, 176, 197, 198
Ahmed, N., 285
Ahrons, C. A., 31, 44
Akiyama, H., 60, 61, 159
Aldous, J., 12, 13, 14
Ali, A., 15
Alison, P., 20
Altergott, J., 31
Alwin, D. F., 20, 134, 136, 137, 138, 140, 141, 142, 144, 145, 146, 147, 148, 149, 150, 151, 152, 154
Amaro, H., 317
Amato, P., 31, 33, 35, 138
Amato, P. R., 111, 112
ambivalence, 2, 3, 35, 62, 164, 170, 243–44
American Association of Public Opinion Research (AAPOR), 245
American dream, mythology of, 179
Americans for Generational Equity (AGE) organization, the, 274

American Sociological Association, 193
Analysis of Variance (ANOVA), 248
Anderson, M., 271
Angel, J. L., 320, 321, 322
Angel, R. J., 214, 320, 321, 322
Angelou, M., 182
Antonucci, T. C., 60, 61, 159, 160, 242
Aquilino, W. S., 33, 36, 38, 50
Aranda, M. P., 321
Arber, S., 169
Ardelt, M., 140
Arias, E., 317
Armstrong, E. M., 105, 114, 117
Arthur, C., 202
Arts, W. A., 298
Atienza, A., 241
Atlas.ti (qualitative data analysis software), 216
attachment theory, 62
Attias-Donfut, C., 163, 164, 169
Avioli, P. S., 60, 61
Azores, T., 287

Baars, J., 266
baby boom (boomers), 71, 180; and empowerment of minorities, 202; and inclusivity, 201; and religious faith, 203
Bachelet, P., 276
Baker, L. A., 12
Bank, B. J., 15
Bank, S., 62
Barreto, S. M., 266, 275
Barrett, B., 276
Bates, B., 12
Bayesian Information Criterion (BIC) values, the, 250
beanpole: families, 301; structure, 278
Becher, T., 196

Beck, A. N., 81
Bedford, V. H., 12, 60, 61
Belansky, E. S., 15
Bengtson, V. L., 2, 3, 4, 7, 14, 26, 32, 33, 35, 37,
    38, 51, 100, 106, 107, 108, 110, 133, 134, 135,
    137, 146, 154, 159, 160, 162, 163, 165, 168,
    177, 180, 181, 194, 195, 196, 197, 198, 199,
    200, 211, 212, 215, 242, 266, 274, 276, 277,
    278, 280, 289, 290, 293, 296, 297, 301, 314,
    315, 323, 327
Benjamin, A. E., 295
Bennington College, 144, 145, 154
Bennington effect, 146–48, 154
Bennington Longitudinal Study, 131, 134,
    144–54
Bennington women, 144, 145, 146, 154
Berger, S. H., 107
Berges, I. M., 322
Berry, B. M., 37, 38, 39, 40, 48, 50, 51
Bertera, E. M., 239
Biblarz, T. J., 32, 37, 51, 180, 181, 197, 212
Biggs, S., 160, 161, 164, 165, 169, 186, 266, 276
Billingsley, A., 237
Binstock, R. H., 295, 296
biographical pain at the end of life, 4, 132,
    176–77, 178, 181, 182, 183, 184, 185
birth order, 91, 99
birth rate, national, 71, 74
Black, K. D., 26
Blair-Loy, M., 212
Blekesaune, M., 300
blended families, 31–52. See also stepfamilies
Block, F., 297, 307
Blum, J. A., 284
Boggiano, A. K., 15
Boldt, J. S., 324
Boon, S. D., 107
Booth, A., 31, 33, 35, 138
Bose, C. E., 288
Bourdieu, P., 166, 168
Brackbill, Y., 12, 13
Brady, D., 295
Brand, E., 107
Bray, J. H., 107
Brody, G. H., 12
Brokaw, T., 153
Bronte-Tinkew, J., 80
Brooks-Gunn, J., 110

Brose van Groenou, M. I., 68, 73
Brown, E. J., 107
Brown, S. L., 83
Brussoni, M. J., 107
Buchbinder, E., 110
Bullard, R. D., 317
Bumpass, L. L., 32, 33, 44
Burant, C., 288
Burawoy, M., 284
Burdette, A., 322
Burton, L., 301
Burton, L. M., 81, 86, 99, 100, 106, 107, 110,
    278

Cadge, W., 209, 213, 214
Caldwell, J., 107, 112
Cambridge Handbook of Age and Ageing (2005),
    266
Cancian, M., 80, 81, 83
capital and habitus, 168
Capoferro, C., 37
caregiving, 16, 24, 62, 93, 96, 107–8, 264
Carette, J., 188
Carlson, M. J., 79, 80, 90
Carstensen, L. L., 25
Cascio, T., 202
Casper, F. G., 299
Castro, C., 241
Castro-Martin, T., 32, 44
Caulfield, R., 107
Cavalli, A., 167
Cech, E., 301
Center for Strategic and International Studies
    (CSIS), 270
Center for Survey Research, 16
Central Intelligence Agency (CIA), 268–69
Ceria, C., 107
Chan, C., 107
Chang, Y., 107
Charles, M., 301
Charmaz, K., 88
Chase-Lansdale, P. L., 110
Chatters, L. M., 237, 238, 239, 240, 241, 242,
    243, 254, 255
Chen, X., 115, 241
Cherlin, A., 83
Cherlin, A. J., 35, 46, 49, 52, 81, 106, 107, 109,
    110

Child-rearing, parental approach, 136, 137, 220

Chodorow, N. J., 15

Choy, C. C., 284

Christian and Jewish faith-based communities, 201, 203

church-based: classes or subpopulations, 246, 255–56; interactions, 237, 239, 240–41, 246, 254; networks, 237–59. *See also* interpersonal conflict

Cicirelli Adult Attachment Scale, 19

Cicirelli, V., 109

Cicirelli, V. G., 19, 60, 62

Clark, S., 35, 52

Clarke, E. J., 4

Clarke, P., 280

Cleese, A. F., 12

Clingempeel, W., 107

Clogg, C. C., 51

closeness, emotional: grandparent-grandchild relations, 105, 107, 111, 113; grandparent-parent relations, 107; and happiness, 6; young children and adolescents, 12, 13, 21, 24

Coale, A. J., 295

Coates, D. L., 15

Cogswell, C., 83

Cohen, E., 12

Cohen, R. L., 134, 137, 140, 144, 145, 146, 147, 148, 149, 150, 151, 152, 154

Cohen, S., 12, 241

Cohler, B., 324

Cohler, B. J., 31

cohort, 68–73, 81, 131, 134–35, 137–43, 148–52, 154–55, 165–69, 171, 285

Coleman, M., 36, 39, 49

Coleman, P. G., 183

Collard, D., 168

Collins, R., 241

Colyar, J., 107

Commission on Global Aging, the, 270, 272

Committee on Human Development, University of Chicago, 195

community-dwelling mothers, 16

Conger, R., 287

Conger, R. D., 108

Connidis, I. A., 32, 33, 62, 104, 243

contact, frequency of, 59–61, 63–67, 69–74, 82, 104, 107, 111, 323

Cook, F. L., 265, 274

Cook, S. T., 80, 81

Cooley, M., 110

Cooney, T. M., 33, 38, 49, 51

Corbin, J., 88

Coreil, J., 316

coresidence, 50, 107, 326

Corsten, M., 167

Costa, P. T., Jr., 140

Côté, S., 280

Cowdry, E. V., 195

Cox, D., 38

Cramer, M. L., 202

Creasey, G. L., 106

Crimmins, E., 316

Crosnoe, R., 133, 135, 153

Crouter, A. C., 12, 13

Culhan, M. M., 271, 278

cultural gerontology, 166

custody, 33–35. *See also* grandparents, role of

Daatland, S. O., 164

Daniel, P., 307

Daniels, D., 12

Dannefer, D., 180, 266, 280, 285, 287, 288

Darkes, J., 251

Dashefsky, A., 212

Datan, N., 106

data rich and theory poor, 177

Davey, A., 13, 34

Davidman, L., 214

Davidson, G. O., 84

Davies, L., 111

Deacon, B., 266

Deater-Deckard, K., 111

death, 177, 178, 180, 184, 188

Death of a Salesman (1949), 179

deinstitutionalization, 286. *See also* second demographic transition (SDT)

de Jong Gierveld, J., 63

Del Boca, F. K., 251

Deleire, T., 105

Delong, J. B., 293

democratization, 177

DeParle, J., 284

depression, 78, 111, 112, 118, 136, 179, 184

D'Ercole, M. M., 295

Destro, L. M., 81

de Vries, C., 107

Diaz, P., 161
Dickerson, B. J., 110
Dill, B. T., 84
Dillon, M., 211, 220
Divorce, 32–33, 35, 38, 109, 110, 111, 114, 159, 225, 234
Dohrenwend, B. P., 317
Doling, J., 293
Donati, P., 161
Dornbusch, S. M., 111
double jeopardy hypothesis, 314, 315
Douglas, N., 321
Dowd, J., 212
Dows, J. J., 314, 315, 327
Doyle, W. J., 241
Driver, D., 107
du Boulay, S., 184
Duncan, G. J., 46
Dunham, C., 211
Dunhan, C. C., 168
Dunn, J., 13, 83, 102, 111
Dykstra, P. A., 63
Dyson, O., 81

Earls, F., 317
Ebaugh, H. R., 209, 213
Ecklund, E. H., 209, 212, 213
Edgell, P., 211
Edlund, J., 307
Edmunds, J., 165, 168, 169
Eggebeen, D. J., 38, 39, 40, 48, 50, 51
Ehrenberg, M. F., 83
Elder, G. H., 108
Elder, G. H., Jr., 83, 106, 107
Elins, J. L., 12, 13
Elliot, K., 60
Ellison, C., 241, 243, 322
Ellison, C. G., 214, 239, 255
Elo, I. T., 317
Encyclopedia of Aging (2007), 266
England, P., 80
England, R. S., 271, 274
Eschbach, K. S., 316, 317, 318
Esping-Andersen, G., 295, 297, 298, 299, 307
Estes, C. L., 266, 275, 276
ethnic identity, family, 213
ethnographic analysis, 88, 89, 285

ethnography, qualitative study, 79, 81, 84–89, 99, 288
extended family, 37, 59, 79, 111, 114, 159, 211, 301, 323
Eyerman, R., 168

Faber, A., 12
Facteau, L., 110
Faimberg, H., 170
Fairgrove, R., 202
Falletta, L., 288
family: arrangements, diversity of, 31; connections, 9–10; formation, 77, 287; lineage, 134–37, 146, 154, 161–65, 167–69; support, latent and manifest patterns and systems, 32; structure, 59, 61, 107, 113, 289
Family Life Project (FLP), 79. *See also* ethnography
Farrell, J., 324
fatherhood, meaning in later life, 25
Ferraro, K. F., 315
Ferrell, J., 35, 36, 39
Ferrera, M., 299
fertility: behavior, 275; patterns, 77, 79, 89, 211, 263, 271; rates, 271, 278. *See also* multiple partner fertility (MPF)
filial responsibility, 324
financial: assistance, 34–35, 37–41, 276; favoritism, 25; need, 50; obligations, 35–36; resources, 111; status, 40; transfers, 10, 31–32, 36–40, 49–51. *See also* intergenerational transfers
Finch, J., 164
Fingerman, K. L., 13, 82
Firebaugh, G., 138, 140
Fischer, C. S., 220
Flacks, R., 147
Flaherty, M. J., 110
Foner, A., 163, 205
forces accounting for transformation of family life, 286–88
Forssén, K., 298
Förster, M., 295
Fougère, M., 294
Fragile Family and Child Well-Being Study, 80, 90
Frank, L., 195
Franzini, L., 316

Fuller-Thompson, E., 105, 107
Furstenberg, F., 83
Furstenberg, F. F., 104, 105, 106, 107, 109, 110
Furstenberg, F. F., Jr., 35, 38, 41, 49, 50, 79, 80, 83, 90

Ganong, L. H., 36, 39, 49
Gans, D., 159, 266
Garces-Foley, K., 215
Garver, P., 110
gay/lesbian/bisexual/transgender studies, 200, 201
Gee, E. M., 271
Gellisen, J., 298
gender differences, 106, 120
generation: concept of, 131, 133–34, 137, 146, 154–55, 160, 165, 168; G, 134, 141; global, 165, 169; M, 165; sandwich, 294, 301; X, 180
generational: connections in religion, spirituality, and aging, 2, 193, 199, 198, 200, 204, 206; consciousness, 166–71; differences, 196, 198; habitus, 167; identity, 155, 167–68, 170; interdependence, 135, 162–63; logics, social, 134–35, 154; negotiation, 168; succession, 131, 137, 155
Generational Intelligence (GI), 131, 159, 170–71
generations: as historical location, 137–40, 141, 142, 152, 153; as historical participation, 10, 140–44, 154, 155; as kinship positions, 135–37, 152
geopolitics of aging. *See* global politics of aging
George, L. K., 62, 241
Gerena, M., 212
Gerontological Society of America, the, 193
gerotranscendence, theory of, 187–88
Gerstel, N., 212
Giarrusso, R., 26, 108, 242, 296
Gilbert, N., 307
Gilleard, C., 167
Gilligan, C., 15
Gladstone, J. W., 109, 110
Glass, J., 211
Glenn, N. D., 140
global aging, 159, 165, 265–67, 270, 272, 275, 279, 293
Global Aging: Achieving Its Potential, 272
"Global Aging: Capital Market Implications," 271

Global Aging and Challenges to Families (2003), 266
global aging crisis, 274
Global Aging Initiatives of the CSIS (Center for Strategic and International Studies), 270–71
global politics of aging, 265, 269, 274
globalization, 204, 263–67, 284, 285, 288; and economy, 267, 268; and family aging and intergenerational relationships, 275–78, 295, 325
Globalization: Threat or Opportunity, 267
Goerres, A., 295
Goldbourt, U., 241
Goldman, M. S., 251
Goldman Sachs policy report, 271
Goldsteen, K., 318
Gonzales, A. M., 212
Goodman, C. C., 110
Goodwin, J. S., 318
Gordon, R. A., 110
Gornick, J. C., 298
Graefe, D. R., 83
grandmothers, 3, 79, 89, 92, 198; and adversity, 110; as caregivers to grandchildren, 92, 96; and development of children, 104; and intergenerational family health, 92–99; and social support, 4, 104
grandparents, role of: and at-risk adolescents, 105; and custodial grandparenting, 105, 110; and diversity, 106, 119; and religious transmission of new roles, 198; and socioeconomic status, 107, 113; as surrogate parent, 3, 109, 114, 116, 120, 285, 288; symbolism of, 106, 119. *See also* mentoring roles of grandparents
grandparent-grandchild relations, 82–83, 104–7, 111–13; and age, 106; and emotional relationships, 82, 90, 105, 107, 111, 113; and quality of relationship, 104–5, 107, 111; and support, 82, 111; and well-being of children, 105, 118, 120
grandparent-parent relations, 107
Grasmick, H. G., 287
Gravenish, B. A., 107
Great Depression, 145, 162, 179
Greatest Generation, The, 153
Greenbaum, P. E., 251

Greenspan, A., 288
Grotta, S. A., 239
Gruber, J., 294
Guardian, the, (UK newspaper), and aging, 271
Guba, E., 88
Guo, S., 318, 319
Gur-Yaish, N., 164
Gustafsson, S., 298, 306
Guzman, L., 108, 110
Guzzo, K. B., 79
Gwaltney, J. M., 241

Ha, J., 62
Haber, C., 275
Haddad, A. A., 296
Haddad, Y. Y., 203
Hagan, J., 143
Hagestad, G., 164
Hagestad, G. O., 34, 37, 106, 108, 162, 163
Hakorvirta, M., 298
Hammer, L. B., 62
Hammill, J. G., 107
Hansford, S., 15
Hardaway, C. R., 81
Hareven, T. K., 163
Harkness, J., 302
Harknett, K., 82
Harootyan, R. A., 32, 37, 38, 199
Hasenfeld, Y., 295, 301
Haurin, R. J., 107
Hauser, P., 315
Hayes-Bautista, D. E., 317
Hayward, M. D., 293
Health and Retirement Study (HRS), 32, 41
Heatherton, T. F., 140
Heerina, S. G., 245
Heider, F., 2
Hendricks, J., 194
Henly, R. J., 105
Henry, C. S., 83
Herberg, W., 209, 213
Hernes, H., 300
Hetherington, M., 107
Hewitt, P. S., 271
Higgs, P., 167
Hill, M. S., 37
Hill, R. B., 237
Hill, T., 322

Hill, T. D., 214, 321, 322
Hispanic Established Population for the Epide-miological Study of the Elderly (Hispanic EPESE), the, 316, 320–21, 325
Hispanics/Latino population, older: and cul-ture, 321, 324; dependency, functional, 321, 323, 324; family relationships and health, 324–26; and finances, 326; foreign-born vs. native-born, 321; and "Hispanic Paradox," 315–25; neighborhood context and health, 317–18; multigenerational families, 323, 326; religion and health, 322–23
historical cohort. *See* cohort
Hochschild, A., 276
Hoffman, S. D., 38, 46, 50
Hogan, D. P., 40, 48, 50, 51, 285
Holcombe, E., 79
Homans, G. C., 2
Horowitz, A., 80
Horsewood, N., 293
House, J., 317
Hout, M., 220
Howell, D., 40
Hughes, H., 212, 213
Hughes, M. E., 105, 286, 288
Huisman, M., 63
Hummer, R., 316, 317
Hunsley, T., 280

Idler, E. L., 241
Ikramullah, E., 79
immigrants/immigration. *See* race and ethnicity
Immigration and Naturalization Act of 1965, 213
individual factors, 300, 301. *See also* Inter-generational social contract
induced solidarity, cycle of, 289, 290
Ingersoll-Dayton, B., 62
Inkeles, A., 136
interaction of resources with family processes, 288, 289
intergenerational: equity, 296; interaction, 163–64, 192, 237–59, 289; linkages, 31; stake, 109, 121. *See also* intergenerational relations; intergenerational social contract; intergenerational solidarity
Intergenerational Linkages Survey, 38

intergenerational relations, 1, 11, 14, 106, 109, 135, 147, 159–60, 170–71, 177, 178, 193, 323; and conflict, 164, 170, 295–96; and family, 98, 171; Hispanics *or* Mexican-American, 323; and social contract, 293; and ties, 4, 11; and transmission, 135, 168, 180; and relationships, 197, 212, 225; and family and cultural continuity, 212, 213; and parent-child relations, 217; and rivalry, 168

intergenerational social contract: assistance, between generations, 296; challenges to individuals and state, 294–96; instrumental support, 296; redistribution of resources across generations, 297; state or government support, 293–94; state spending, attitudes toward, 297; and social welfare, 293, 295, 296, 301; and socio-political environment, 4

intergenerational solidarity, 1–6, 26, 31–52, 168, 191, 197–98, 264, 278, 289, 323–24; affectual solidarity (emotional closeness), 9, 33–34, 50, 197, 242; associational solidarity (frequency of contact), 9, 50, 197, 242, 276, 324; Bengtson typology, 276; Bengtson's model of, 26; consensual solidarity (attitude similarity), 9, 50, 197, 242; definition of, 33; and Durkheim's concept of social solidarity, 1–2; functional solidarity (the exchange of instrumental and emotional help and support), 4, 9, 34, 36–37, 49, 197, 242, 296; and Hispanics, 323; induced solidarity, 289–90; and conflict paradigm, 1–6, 9–10, 162, 191–92; and interpersonal relations, 2; normative solidarity (feelings of family obligation), 9, 35, 51, 197, 242; structural solidarity (geographic proximity, gender, and health), 9, 50, 197, 242

intergenerational transfers: definition of, 37; of money, 37, 38, 293; of space, 37–38; of time, 37–38

International Monetary Fund (IMF), 267. *See also* globalization and economy

interpersonal conflict, 192, 239, 240, 295. *See also* church-based interactions

involvement, differential, 79–100

Ivatts, J., 307

Jackson, J., 160
Jackson, J. S., 237, 238, 241, 245, 254

Jackson-Newson, J. 13
Janke, M., 13, 34
Jendrek, M. P., 105
Jenkins, J. M., 13, 83
Johnson, C. L., 107, 108, 109
Johnson, M., 163
Johnson, M. K., 133, 135, 153
Johnson, M. L., 194, 195, 200

Kääriäinen, J., 293
Kahn, M. D., 62
Kahn, R. L., 205, 242
Kahn, S., 108
Kalache, A., 266, 275
Kaliher, G., 106
Kalil, A., 105
Kasl, S. V., 318
Kass, R. E., 250
Kataoka-Yahiro, M., 107
Katz, R., 164, 173
Kaufman, G., 14
Keddie, A. M., 316
Keitner, G., 239
Keller, I., 266, 275
Kelly, C., 279
Kennedy, C. E., 111
Kennedy, G. E., 107, 111
Kenney, C., 35, 52
Kertzer, D. I., 133, 141, 155
Keysar, A., 201
Kids Information Data System (KIDS), 90
Killian, T. S., 35, 36, 37, 38, 39, 48, 50, 51
Kim, D. Y., 209, 213
King, A. C., 241
King, R., 188
King, V., 83, 104, 107, 108
Kingma, M., 287
kinship/kin: network, 31; structure of families, 38, 146; and latent matrix, 31–32, 34, 49; and relations, 32, 34; and statuses, 31, 49; and structure, 40–41
Kirby, J. B., 110
Kitagawa, E. M., 315
Kitch, D., 13
Kivett, V., 107
Kivett, V. R., 106
Klaus, E., 13
Klein, D. M., 13

Klein, S., 302
Klerman, L., 81
Knabb, J., 82
Knipscheer, C. P. M., 63
Koenig, K. E., 147
Koh, A., 165
Kohli, M., 37
Kohn, R., 239
Kosmin, B. A., 201
Kowal, A., 12, 13
Kramer, L., 12, 13
Krause, N., 237, 239, 241, 243, 253, 254, 324, 325
Kronebusch, K., 37, 38, 50
Kuhn, T., 194
Kunemund, H., 37
Kuo, Y. F., 322
Kuypers, J. A., 26, 108

Lambert, J. D., 33, 50
Landale, N. S., 212
Landecker, W. S., 242
Landreneau, T., 15
LaRossa, R., 88
latent class analysis (LCA), 247, 250, 253
Latimer, J., 285
Lawton, L., 32, 33, 37, 38
Lazerwitz, B., 212
Leach, R., 165
Lee, G. Y., 320, 321
Lee, R., 293
Leege, D. C., 201
Lehtonen, H., 293
Leira, A., 297, 299, 307
Lesthaeghe, R. J., 285
Levin, J. S., 237, 239, 240, 254, 255
LGBT studies, 200, 201
Li, N., 271
Liberation Theology, 203
Lichter, D. T., 83
life-course theory: age-differentiated sequences, 162; aging and the life course, 131; concepts of, 181; ethnography, 285; and individual trajectories, 137; and intergenerational social contract, 296; and labeling theory, 289; and second demographic transition (SDT), 285; perspective, 52, 61–62, 72, 162, 171, 181, 188; social phenomenon, 162

life cycle, 146
life-span theory, 147, 176–77, 180, 188; and human development, 180; and intergenerational transmission, 180, 229; and longitudinal studies, 177; and nested context, 180; and processes of aging, 176
Liker, J. K., 288
Lincoln, C. E., 241
Lincoln, C. R., 214
Lincoln, K. D., 237, 239, 241, 242, 243
Lincoln, Y., 88
Lipsmeyer, C., 299
Litt, J. S., 288
Living Arrangements and Social Networks of Older Adults research program, 63
living/caregiving arrangement and health, 320–21
Livni, T., 110
Logan, C., 79
Logan, J. R., 37
longevity, 77, 271
Longitudinal Aging Study Amsterdam (LASA), 63
longitudinal data, 40
Longitudinal Study of Generations (LSOG), 3, 180, 191, 196, 215
Long-Term Global Demographic Trends: Reshaping the Geopolitical Landscape (CIA, 2001), 268
Lorenz-Meyer, D., 164
Loury, L., 111
Lowenstein, A., 110, 159, 160, 162, 164, 266, 276, 277, 293
Luescher, K., 164
Lugaila, T. A., 107
Lukose, R., 165
Lussier, L., 111
Lye, D. N., 13
Lynch, F. R., 295

Mabry, J. B., 26, 242, 276, 278, 296
Macfarlane, J., 179
Machalek, R., 315
Macintrye, S., 317
Maciver, S., 317
Maggard, S. W., 83
Mahan, T. L., 238
Majka, L. C., 287

Mamiya, L., 214
Mamiya, L. H., 241
Manlove, J., 79
Mannheim, K., 138, 139, 140, 141, 142, 143, 151,
    154, 155, 161, 165, 166
Manning, W. D., 83
Manton, K. G., 315
Marenco, A., 104
Markides, K. S., 315, 316, 317, 318, 319, 320,
    321, 322, 323, 324, 325, 327
Marks, N., 31, 33, 49
marriage, 31–32, 83, 211; cross-family analysis,
    223–25
Marshall, J. G., 274, 278
Marshall, V. W., 164, 272, 274, 276, 279, 280
Marti, G., 215, 297
Martin, H. W., 323
Martinez, E. A., 212, 213
Marty, M., 204
Marx, J., 111, 112
Marx, K., 287
Maslach, C., 15
Mavandadi, S., 237
Mayer, E., 201
Mazlish, E., 12
McAdam, D., 142
McAdoo, H. P., 212, 213
McCammon, R., 134, 140, 141, 142, 144, 154
McCammon, R. J., 138
McCluskey, K., 104
McCluskey, K. A., 138
McCluskey, A., 104
McCoy, J. K., 12
McCrae, R. R., 140
McCutcheon, A. L., 247
McDaniel, S., 160, 161
McDonald, K. B., 105, 114, 117
McGarry, K., 37, 48
McGuire, S. A., 12
McHale, S. M., 12, 13
McKeirnan, F., 183
McLachlan, G. J., 250
McLanahan, S., 80, 81, 107
McLanahan, S. S., 107
McLaughlin, D. K., 84
McMullin, J. A., 243
Medalie, J. H., 241
Meiser, T. H., 247, 254

mentoring roles of grandparents, 77, 105–9,
    111, 115, 116, 118–23
Mérette, M., 294
Merline, A., 159
Mexican American. *See* Hispanics/Latino
    population, older
Meyer, D. R., 80, 81, 83
Meyer, J. W., 162
Meyers, M. K., 298
migration, 107, 120, 275–76, 284–85, 288
Miles, T. P., 321
Miller, A., 179
Miller, B., 318, 319
Miller, D. A., 294
Mills, C. W., 99
Mills, M., 183
Mills, R. J., 287
Mills, T. L., 106
Min, P. H., 209, 213
Minkler, M., 105, 107, 296
Mirowsky, J., 318
Mistina, D., 36, 49
Mitchell, D., 299
Mittelman, J. H., 276
Modell, J., 142
modernity, late, 285
Money, A-M., 165
Morenoff, J., 316
Morgan, C. S., 287
Morgan, D. L., 237, 239, 241, 243
mortality, 3, 71, 182, 241, 318
motives, 51
Mueller, M., 104
Mueller, M. M., 106
multigenerational households, 3, 26, 35, 43,
    59, 62, 73, 107, 114, 275, 285, 301, 323, 326.
    See also mentoring role of grandparents;
    grandparenting, role of
multigenerational kinship networks, 79,
    81–82, 91, 159, 197–98
multiple hierarchy stratification, 314
multiple partner fertility (MPF), 77–79,
    80–83, 98. *See also* fertility
Murray, T. M., 162
Musick, J. S., 110
Muthén, B. O., 251
Muthén, L. K., 251
Mutran, E., 324

Mutran, E. J., 107
Myers, D., 293, 294, 298
Myers, S. M., 211, 212
Myles, J., 297

National Election Study, 134
National Institute of Mental Health, 196
National Institute on Aging (NIA), 316, 323
National Longitudinal Study of Adolescent
    Health (ADD Health), 81, 105, 122
National Longitudinal Survey data, 288
National Survey of American Life (NSAL),
    244
National Survey of Families and Households
    (NSFH), 40
National Survey of Family Growth (NSFG), 81
Neidert, L., 285
Neil, M. B., 62
Nelson, A. R., 317
Netherlands Kinship Panel Study, 60
Neugarten, B. J., 106
Neugarten, B. L., 106, 108, 109, 120
Newacheck, P. W., 295
Newcomb, T. M., 134, 137, 140, 144, 145, 146,
    147, 148, 149, 150, 151, 152
Newman K. S., 279
Newsom, J. T., 237, 238
Ng-Mak, D. S., 317
Nishishiba, M., 237, 238
Noffsinger, W. B., 13
Nordic social democratic states, 299. *See also*
    welfare state
nuclear family, 59, 62, 82
Nye, F., 242

OASIS project, 277
obligations: of family, 35–36, 38, 81, 91; of
    citizens (mutual), 297. *See also* intergenera-
    tional social contract
O'Bryant, S. L., 61
O'Connor, T. G., 13, 83
Ogburn, W. F., 205
Olander, E. B., 296
Ong, P., 287
Orht, B., 247, 254
Orloff, A. S., 298
Oropesa, R. S., 212
Ortega y Gasset, J., 142, 155

Ostir, G. V., 318
Ottenbacher, K., 322
Oyama, P. S., 165

Palloni, A., 316, 317
Pampel, F. C., 295
Pan, E., 107
parental favoritism, gender differences in: and
    birth order, 13, 21, 23; and adult children,
    12, 16, 23, 24; daughter, 15, 16, 25; and equal
    treatment, 25; and fathers, 14; financial, 25;
    and mothers, 14, 15, 25; parental, 9; pat-
    terns of, 14, 24; predictors of, 12, 13, 14–16,
    21–25; and socioemotional selectivity, 25;
    son, 15, 16, 25; and within-family differ-
    ences, 12, 13, 14, 18; and young children
    and adolescents, 12, 13, 18, 110
parent-child relationships, 11–15, 31, 34–37,
    60; in aging families, 31; closeness of, 212;
    father-child, 12, 14; in later life, 12–13, 16;
    long-term lousy, 4; mother-child, 11, 13–14,
    16; quality of, 34, 37, 217; racial/ethnic, 234;
    and religious continuity, 192; and social sup-
    port network, 10; verticalized family, 60
Pargament, K. I., 254
Park, J. Z., 212
Parke, R. D., 106, 107, 108
Parrenas, R., 288
Parrott, T. M., 296
Parsons, T., 61
Passuth, P. M., 196, 198
Patel, K. V., 318
Patterson, R. S., 287, 288, 291
Pattillo-McCoy, M., 214
Pearce, L. D., 211
Peek, M. K., 319, 320
Peel, D., 250
Pelikan, J., 205
Peterson, C. C., 104
Pew Forum on Religion and Public Life, 214
Pew Foundation, 202
Pezzin, L. E., 38, 39, 48, 50
phenomenology of generation, 169–70
Phillips, J., 164
Phillipson, C., 165, 266, 267, 275, 276, 285
Pienta, A. M., 293
Pietromonaco, P., 241
Pilcher, J., 167

Pillemer, K., 12, 13, 15, 20, 25, 164, 171
Pittman, L. D., 111, 112
polypharmacy, 179
population aging, 159, 165, 263–67, 275, 293
population explosion, 293
population growth, old and youth, 269–70
post-socialist states, 299. *See also* welfare state
Powers, R., 15, 25
Preston, M., 293, 294, 295
Price, M., 107
Problems of Ageing, The (1939), 195
Program for Research on Black Americans, 245
proximity, 61, 69, 107
Pruchno, R., 107
pull factors, 287. *See also* forces accounting for transformation of family life
push factors, 287. *See also* forces accounting for transformation of family life
Putney, N. M., 14, 159, 162, 177, 181, 266,
Pyke, K. D., 4
Pyle, J. L., 288

Quadagno, J., 296, 297, 300
qualitative data management (QDM), 88

Rabin, B. S., 241
race and ethnicity: acculturation and, 115, 209, 213, 215, 324; adaptation and, 213; assimilation and, 209, 213, 215; background in old age, 325; and differences, 109, 113–15, 120–21; and immigrants, 202, 209, 213–15, 276; and minorities, 110, 210, 232, 325; multiculturalism and, 107, 215; and multigenerational families, 3, 209, 210, 323; and religious life, 192. *See also* migration
Rafferty, J. A., 295, 301
Raftery, A. E., 250
Raines, F., 38
Raley, R. K., 32, 33
Rand Corporation, 268
Rashbash, J., 13, 83
Raudenbush, S. W., 317
Ray, L. A., 324
reciprocity, 109, 121, 164, 324
Reese, H. W., 138
Reevy, G. M., 15
regression: bivariate, 115; logistic, 318; multinomial logistic, 252

Reich, R. B., 297
Reitzes, D. C., 107, 324
religion, 4, 183–84, 191, 193, 199, 202, 209, 238, 288; Buddhism, 202; Christianity, 202; and church attendance, 214, 238, 244, 246; and demographic factors, 238, 244, 247; denomination, 238; evangelical groups, 202; faith communities, 183; and health and well-being, 198–206; Islam, 202; nondenominational churches, 202; nonorganizational religious activities, 214, 238; and racial/ethnic community, 4, 213–14, 215, 229, 234; role of, 191; and voluntary organizations, 4. *See also* death; religious transmission and ethnicity
religious: affiliation, 214; beliefs, 211; choices, individual, 211; continuity, as a predictor of the quality of intergenerational relations, 212, 217; disillusionment, 234; heritage or identity, 209, 210; identities, 214; institution and family, synergy of, 211; instruction, 4, 209–34; lags, 205; parents, 211–12; participation, 238; particularism, 215; pluralistic cohort, 191, 213; rituals, 211; switching, 233; socialization in families, 211–12; transmission across generations, 199, 201–6, 217; transmission and ethnicity, 209–34; variations, 212
remarriage, 31–33, 35, 49–52, 159
resiliency, grandparenting, 111–12, 115, 118–19, 163, 179
retirement, 265, 270, 271–72, 278, 293–94
Reyes-Ortiz, C. A., 322
Reynolds, S. L., 296
Riall, T. S., 316
Ribble, J. C., 316
Rice, C. J., 194, 195, 200
Rice, T. W., 15
Riedmann, A., 59, 60, 61
Riley, J. J., Jr., 31
Riley, M. W., 31, 61, 163, 205
Robert, S. A., 317
Roberts, R. E. L., 2, 26, 32, 37, 51, 162, 180, 181, 197, 212, 297
Robertson, A., 271
Robertson, J., 109
Roe, K. M., 107
romantic relationships, 60, 79–80, 83, 89, 91

Roof, W. C., 211
Rook, K. S., 237, 238, 241
Roos, J. P., 164, 167
Roosevelt's New Deal, 145
Roscow, I., 141
Roseberg, H., 153
Rosenmayr, L., 109
Rosenthal, C., 301
Rosenthal, C. J., 278
Ross, C. E., 318
Ross, K. E., 298
Rossi, A. S., 13, 14, 32, 33, 36, 37, 39, 48, 49, 50, 106, 162
Rossi, P. H., 13, 14, 32, 33, 36, 37, 39, 48, 49, 50, 162
Roy, K., 81
Ruiz, D. S., 105, 114
Ruiz, S., 111, 112
Rumbold, B., 186
Rushing, W., 242
Rutter, M., 179
Ryder, N. B., 138, 139, 140, 141, 144, 155, 157

Sadler, E., 186
Sainsbury, D., 300
Salinas, J., 317
salmon bias, 317
Saluter, A. F., 127
Salva, J., 13
Sampson, R., 317
Sanchez, M., 161
Sandefur, G., 107
Sarkisian, N., 212
Savla, J., 34
Schaie, K. W., 194, 197
Schieber, S. J., 271
Schlesinger, M., 37, 38, 50
Schoeni, R. F., 37, 48
Schone, B. S., 38, 39, 48, 50
Schrader, S. S., 276, 323
Schroepfer, T., 237, 239
Scott, M. E., 80
Sechrist, J., 12, 13
second demographic transition (SDT), 285, 288
Seeman, T., 241
selection effects, 123
selective survival process, 315

Selling Spirituality: The Silent Takeover of Religion (2005), 188
Settersten, R. A., Jr., 135
Sewell, W. H., Jr., 151
Shapiro, A., 33, 49, 50
Shapiro, T. M., 111
Sherkat, D. E., 211, 212
Shrestha, L., 38, 50
sibling relationships in verticalized family: age effects, 61; age peers, 60, 63, 66, 74; availability of sibling, 60, 63, 72; child relationships, 66, 71; contact, frequency of, 59–61, 63–67, 69–74; definition of, 60; education, level of, 61, 73; and horizontal family relationships, 3; inner circle, 61; outer circle, 61; proximity, 61, 69; quality of relationships, 10; racial/ethnic community, 234; roles, 61–62, 72; second tier, 61; sisters, 61; social class, 61, 73; social support network approach, 10, 64–74; structural characteristics, 59; supportive exchanges, 60–63, 65–66, 70–74
Sihula, J., 275
Silver, N. C., 107, 112
Silverman, N. L., 107, 112
Silverman, W. H., 261
Silverstein, M., 3, 14, 26, 32, 33, 37, 38, 51, 104, 110, 111, 112, 115, 242
Simmel, G., 4
Single-generation households, 301
Single-parent households, 34, 107, 109, 111
Skinner, D., 81
Skogan, W. G., 265
Skoner, D. P., 241
Smedley, B. D., 317
Smith, C., 211, 212
Smith, E. W., 110
Smith, R. C., 285
Smith, S. T., 83
Smock, P. J., 83
Snyder, A. R., 84
social capital, 105
social change, 160; generations as historical context, cemography, 137, 138; generations as historical location, culture, 140; generations as kinship position, 136; involvement, differential, 83; transformation of family life, 285–89

social generation: age differences in society, 134; concept of, 165–66; demographic transformations, 165; family, 169; generations in the family, 135; generational location, 166–67; historical generation, 166; human development and behavior, 133–34, 154; linkage, individual and society, 133–34; private sphere, 167; social location, 165–66; social structuration, 165; sociological category, 169

social gerontology, 1, 4, 176, 196, 265, 274, 277

social movements or organizations, 135, 154

Social Psychology of Aging, The, 180, 196

social structures, 168, 284

social units, 176

Sokolovsky, J., 272

Soldo, B. J., 37

Soloman, J. C., 111, 112

Somers, M. R., 297, 307

Soonan, A., 317

Sorkin, D. H., 238

Southern European states, 299, 300. *See also* welfare state

Speck, P., 183

Spencer, H., 297

spirituality: fourth age, 176, 186; definition of, 186, 204; effect of on health and well-being, 198, 206; and search for meaning approach, 186–87; and spiritual concern, 182; and spiritual transformation, 188; as spiritual, not religious, 202

Spitze, G. D., 37

spouse, horizontal family relationships, 3, 10

Stallings, M., 108

Steinhour, M., 12, 13

stepfamilies, 32, 33–34, 35, 38–43, 83, 121. *See also* blended families

Stern, G., 202

Stierman, K. L., 108

Stimpson, J. P., 319, 320

Stith, A. Y., 317

Stolba, A., 111, 112

Stolzenberg, R., 212

Stoneman, Z., 12

Strauss, A., 88, 89

stress, 25

Structure of Scientific Revolutions, The (1962), 194

successful aging, 187, 188

Suitor, J. J., 12, 13, 15, 20, 25

Svallfors, S., 307

Sweet, J., 32, 44

Sweet, J. A., 32, 33, 44

Symer, M. A., 108

Tabory, E., 212

Tambe, A., 276

Tanne, D., 241

Taylor, R. J., 237, 238, 239, 240, 241, 242, 243, 254, 255

teen childbearing, 109–11, 114

Temporary Assistance for Needy Families (TANF), 85

"That Was Your Life: A Biographical Approach to Later Life" (1976), 184

theory-building: activity theory, 195, 196, 265; adaptability, 206; disengagement theory, 195, 265; equity theory, 62; grand theory, 194; multidisciplinary research in aging, 193, 195; multidisciplinary theories, 206; small-group cohesion, 2; support convoy, 242; structural functionalism, 196; theory, 194, 200. *See also* ambivalence; intergenerational solidarity; life-course theory; life-span theory

third demographic transition, the, 293

Thompson, E., 107

Thomson, D. W., 297

Thornton, A., 211

Thought Provoking Questions (TPQ), 88

Tinsley, B. J., 107, 108

Tinsley, B. R., 106

Tirrito, T., 202

Tocqueville, A. de, 201, 203

Tolstoy, L., 1

Tomlin, A. M., 111

Toner, B. B., 15

Tornstam, L., 187

Tower, R. B., 318

Townsend, A. L., 318, 319

Townsend, P., 266

transformation of family life, 285–89. *See also* forces accounting for transformation of family life

transitions to adulthood, 104, 109–114, 117, 121

transnational labor migration, 284–88

Treas, J., 299
Troll, L. E., 13
Troutt, D. D., 317
Trozzolo, T. A., 201
Tucker, C. J., 13
Tuljapurkar, S., 271
Turner, B. S., 165, 168, 169
Turner, J. B., 317
Turra, C. M., 317

Uhlenberg, P., 14, 33, 38, 49, 51, 104, 107, 110, 180, 285
Umberson, D., 318
Unemployment Insurance System (UI), 90
Unger, D., 110
United Nations, 160, 274
U.S. Bureau of Labor Statistics, the, 274
U.S. Census Bureau, 109, 110, 214
U.S. census data, 318
University of Michigan's Institute for Social Research, 245, 246
University of Southern California (USC), 197–99
Updegraff, K. A., 12, 13

Valencia Forum of Aging, 272
Van de Kaa, D., 285
Van Tilburg, T. G., 61, 63, 64, 68, 73
Van Volkom, M., 60, 61, 73
Vega, W. A., 317
verticalized family. *See* sibling relationships in verticalized family
Volling, B. L., 12, 13
Voorpostel, M., 59
Vorek, R., 38
Voydanoff, P., 287
Vincent, J., 266, 267, 275, 276
Vincent, J. A., 167, 279
vulnerability, 288, 289

Waite, L. J., 212, 286, 288
Walker, A., 266, 275, 296, 297, 298
Wandersman, A., 108

Wandersman, L. P., 108
Wang, C. P., 251
Ward, R. A., 315, 327
Warner, R. S., 209, 213, 214, 215
Warwick, D. P., 147
Watts, J., 271
Weaver, W., 26
Weinberger, J. L., 140
Weinstein, K. K., 106, 108, 109, 120
welfare state, 293, 295, 296–98. *See also* Nordic social democratic states; Southern European states
Wenk, D., 287
Werner, P., 110
White, H., 141, 142
White, L., 33, 34, 35, 38, 39, 48
White, L. K., 59, 60, 61, 63, 73
Widmer, E., 299
Wiesner, M., 251
Wilhelm, B., 106
Williams, C. L., 15
Wilson, E. B., 196
Wilson, M. N., 110
Windle, M., 251
Wink, P., 211, 220
Winston, P., 86
Wisconsin's Client Assistance for Re-Employment and Economic Support program (CARES), 90
Wise, D., 294
Wittberg, P., 213
Wolff, F. C., 163
women's studies, 200
Wong, R., 37, 317
World Bank, 274
World War II, 71, 179, 202
Worthen, M. F., 15
Wulff, K., 239, 241, 243

Yi, C., 107

Zimmerman, M. K., 288
Zlotnick, C., 239